PATIENT CARE

Basic Skills

FOR THE HEALTH CARE PROVIDER

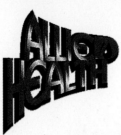

PATIENT CARE

Basic Skills

FOR THE HEALTH CARE PROVIDER

Barbara Acello, MS, RN

To accompany Delmar's
Multiskilling for the Health Care Provider Series

Beverly M. Kovanda, PhD, MS, MT(ASCP), CLP(NCA)
Series Editor

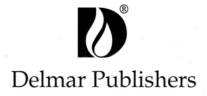

Delmar Publishers

an International Thomson Publishing company I(T)P®

Albany • Bonn • Boston • Cincinnati • Detroit • London • Madrid
Melbourne • Mexico City • New York • Pacific Grove • Paris • San Francisco
Singapore • Tokyo • Toronto • Washington

NOTICE TO THE READER

Cover Design: Scott Keidong's Image Enterprises

Delmar Staff

Publisher: Susan Simpfenderfer
Acquisitions Editor: Dawn Gerrain
Developmental Editor: Marjorie A. Bruce
Project Editor: Brooke D. Graves/Graves Editorial Service
Team Assistant: Sandra Bruce

Art and Design Coordinator: Vincent S. Berger
Production Coordinator: John Mickelbank
Marketing Manager: Katherine Slezak
Marketing Coordinator: Glenna Stanfield
Editorial Assistant: Donna L. Leto

COPYRIGHT © 1998
By Delmar Publishers
a division of International Thomson Publishing Inc.

The ITP logo is a trademark under license.

Printed in the United States of America

For more information, contact:

Delmar Publishers
3 Columbia Circle, Box 15015
Albany, New York 12212-5015

International Thomson Publishing Europe
Berkshire House 168-173
High Holborn
London, WC1V 7AA
England

Thomas Nelson Australia
102 Dodds Street
South Melbourne, 3205
Victoria, Australia

Nelson Canada
1120 Birchmount Road
Scarborough, Ontario
Canada, M1K 5G4

International Thomson Editores
Campos Eliseos 385, Piso 7
Col Polanco
11560 Mexico D F Mexico

International Thomson Publishing GmbH
Konigswinterer Strasse 418
53227 Bonn
Germany

International Thomson Publishing Asia
221 Henderson Road
#05-10 Henderson Building
Singapore 0315

International Thomson Publishing—Japan
Hirakawacho Kyowa Building, 3F
2-2-1 Hirakawacho
Chiyoda-ku, Tokyo 102
Japan

1 2 3 4 5 6 7 8 9 10 XXX 03 02 01 00 99 98 97

Library of Congress Cataloging-in-Publication Data

Acello, Barbara.
    Patient care : basic skills for the health care provider / Barbara
Acello.
        p.   cm.
    Includes index.
    ISBN 0–8273–8423–8
    1. Nursing. 2. Allied health personnel. 3. Clinical competence.
I. Title.
    [DNLM: 1. Nursing Care. 2. Allied Health Personnel. WY 100 A173
1998]
RT42.A25   1998
610.73—dc21
DNLM/DLC
for Library of Congress   97–26953
                                                              CIP

MESSAGE FROM THE SERIES EDITOR

The Multiskilling for Health Care Providers series consists of the *Patient Care: Basic Skills for the Health Care Provider* core text and many separate modular texts. The Multiskilling series offers a comprehensive vision of the diversity and many implications of multiskilling, whether in an acute care setting, home care, hospice, ambulatory setting, long-term care facility, or physician's office. The core text and module subjects have been identified through research as key topics in multiskilling and patient care training across the nation.

The framework for this series is found in the historic evolution of multiskilling, the National Health Care Skill Standards, and 13 years of personal experience in developing academic material and successfully training thousands of multiskilled health care providers in a multitude of nursing and allied health skill areas. The concept referred to as *multiskilling, crosstraining,* and (more recently) *patient care skills* began to gain national awareness in the mid-1980s, as pressures for cost containment in health care intensified. Institutions began to focus on more efficient use of personnel for economic survival. The implications of managed care are far-reaching.

In 1994, the National Health Care Skill Standards were developed through a national collaborative effort of health care organizations, professional organizations, schools, and colleges of higher education. By implementing these standards, we can more effectively serve the needs of a diverse client population and maintain quality care, while increasing the efficiency of staff utilization. Health care costs can be contained; the new technology, which is changing how and where health care is delivered, can be prudently applied. We believe that the skill standards are important and so their intent has been incorporated into the entire series.

The core text, *Patient Care: Basic Skills for the Health Care Provider,* meets the OBRA requirements for basic patient care skills. These skills are required of every health care provider who undertakes client care, regardless of the institutional setting or professional affiliation.

We believe that the core-text-plus-modules concept is the only rational approach to meeting the vastly different academic and training needs in multiskilling, as we re-engineer careers in all health care settings. The modules are flexible, well written, and academically sound. The modular approach is cost-effective. A health care worker's skills can be developed based upon individual goals, institutional needs for retraining, or specific career development. Colleges, hospitals, other health care agencies, technical and career schools, and "tech prep" programs need only purchase the modules that address their unique, customized academic and training needs. Because multiskilling is market-driven, other modules continue to be developed as health care needs are identified and evolve.

The modules are written by credentialed experts in each content area and multiskilling education. They have identified essential and appropriate nursing and allied health skills that can be accurately and safely performed by nonprofessionals to enhance the quality of patient care.

The depth of theory and skills in each module goes beyond other texts, which are usually written from the perspective of one profession rather than by specialists in each identifiable allied health and nursing area. We believe that this principle provides a stronger basis for instruction and facilitates a higher level of quality patient care.

The material in each module is organized in a clear, concise, straightforward manner to make learning easier, because health care institutions are demanding shorter—but intensified—training periods. The pedagogical features enhance retention and simplify learning.

We believe that the Multiskilling series combines the knowledge, experience, successes, and expertise of all of the authors. It provides the tools and flexibility to custom-design a curriculum that truly meets worker/student professional goals, augments valuable skills, and strengthens employability, not only now but as we prepare for the 21st century.

Beverly M. Kovanda, Ph.D., M.S., M.T. (ASCP), CLP (NCA)
Coordinator/Professor
Multicompetency Health Technology

Table of CONTENTS

INTRODUCTION TO THIS BOOK

This book is designed to prepare individuals to provide basic personal care for people in many different health care settings. Economic pressures in health care are forcing health care organizations to improve quality, while at the same time reduce costs. Today's patient care technician is expected to fill many roles in health care. This program provides the student with a turnkey package to which supplemental modules can be added to provide the core curriculum for a multi-skilling program. The complete supplement package was prepared to enable students to function efficiently as patient care technicians, and to provide instructors with comprehensive, cost-effective resources.

The text is also designed to meet the OBRA requirements for a basic nursing assistant training program, and may be used independent of the modules for this purpose. It meets the requirements for training in other settings, where employees are being prepared to deliver basic personal care to patients under the supervision of a licensed professional health care provider. Your instructor will act as your "tour guide" and will help you apply the principles in the book to the health care setting in which you will be working.

The text uses a practical, reality-oriented approach based on "need to know" information. Current issues in health care are emphasized. Patient and caregiver safety and infection control are stressed throughout the book. Where appropriate, real-world solutions to problems and examples are used. The text is designed to assist the student to become a strong clinician. Theory is included when it is necessary to understand the reason for a procedure or to apply the information to other similar clinical situations. In addition to traditional nursing procedures, the text provides lists of general guidelines that describe how to manage many common patient care situations.

Today's health care provider must be sensitive to the needs of a wide variety of individuals. The text explains how to communicate and interact with persons with common disabilities, as well as individuals of different cultural and ethnic backgrounds.

The name used for the person receiving care varies with the health care setting. For purposes of this text, we have opted to use the title "patient" when referring to this individual. Likewise, the name of the caregiver varies with the agency. The text uses the new title "patient care technician" to refer to the person providing care.

ACKNOWLEDGMENTS

The author wishes to thank Kim Davies and Dawn Gerrain of Delmar Publishers for their confidence and support. Marge Bruce, developmental editor at Delmar Publishers, provided creative ideas and invaluable assistance, encouragement, and guidance throughout the development of this manuscript.

Special thanks to Cathy Johnson, LVN, for her ideas and contributions to the basic patient caregiver training program. Laura Fowler, CNA, and Dennis Clarkson, CNA, Jon Acello, and Fran Acello were most helpful and patient during the photo shoots. The staff and residents of Collinsville Care Center, in Collinsville, Texas, and Kern Manor in Pilot Point, Texas, were more than cooperative during the photo shoots. Mrs. Billie Hoyle is the beautiful patient pictured in the section opener. John Foppe provided tremendous inspiration to me and many of my students by setting a positive example and overcoming the obstacles of physical disability to reach, touch, and provide hope and love to others.

The following individuals provided invaluable assistance with the art manuscript:

Daniel J. Barbaro, MD, Fort Worth Infectious Disease Consultants, P.A., Fort Worth, Texas

Kathleen Moore, RN, Parkland Hospital, Dallas, Texas

Arnie Silverman, President, Skil-Care Corporation

Brian S. Loiacono, REACH Resource Center on Independent Living, Dallas, Texas

Will Hipwell, Briggs Corporation

Ginger Butcher, Ross Laboratories

Linda Menditto, Administrative Director, National Pediculosis Association

Pat Cassidy, *Journal of Nurse Assistants*

Roberto Taloria, CNA President, CNA Association of Georgia

Jackie Rak, Hollister, Inc.

Tanya Dartez, Medline Industries

Melenda Newtson, Sammons-Preston Corp.

The following patient care technician instructors, consultants, and facility educational supervisors dedicated many hours to reviews and provided helpful comments during text manuscript development. To each of these individuals, the author and staff of Delmar Publishers extend sincere thanks for a job well done.

Nancy Gobbato, Phoenix College, AZ

Ann Robicheau Kaisen, Yale New Haven Hospital, New Haven, CT

Beverly M. Kovanda, PhD, Columbus State Community College, Columbus, OH

Clara E. McElroy, Florida Health Academy, Bonita Springs, FL

Barbara Matthay, College of DuPage, Glen Ellyn, IL

Joan F. Needham, Consultant, DeKalb, IL

Dolores J. Pederson, Albuquerque Technical Vocational Institute, Albuquerque, NM

INTRODUCTION TO HEALTH CARE

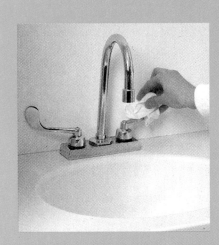

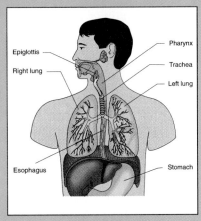

Epiglottis
Right lung
Esophagus
Pharynx
Trachea
Left lung
Stomach

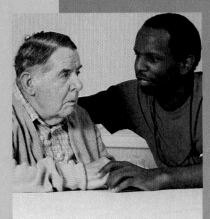

Introduction to Health Care

After reading this chapter, you will be able to:

Spell and define key terms.

List five settings in which health care is delivered and describe the function of each.

Differentiate the role and responsibilities of the patient care technician in each health care setting.

Differentiate care given in an acute care hospital, subacute unit, health maintenance organization, private home, and long-term care facility.

Describe the purpose and function of the interdisciplinary team.

Explain what the chain of command is and describe why using it is important.

Describe some ways to establish meaningful relationships with patients.

Describe at least five desirable qualities of the patient care technician.

Describe responsible behavior and list nine examples of ways to show that you are responsible.

■■■■■ INTRODUCTION TO HEALTH CARE

Welcome to the field of health care! You are on the way to becoming a respected health care worker who provides direct care to ill or injured persons in a variety of health care settings. In most settings, you will provide services under the supervision of a licensed nurse. In some settings, such as physician offices or specialty departments in a hospital, you may be supervised by another licensed health care professional.

Many titles are used to describe the person who gives basic personal care to patients. These include patient care technician, patient care attendant or assistant, nursing assistant, nurse aide, primary caregiver, and health care technician. A newer term is unlicensed assistive personnel (UAP). However he or she is titled, this caregiver is very important to patient comfort and well-being. A multiskilled worker has completed the basic patient care training and has received additional training to perform advanced patient care skills.

Health Care Delivery Sites

Health care is provided in many settings. Many **professional** and nonprofessional workers provide patient care at these sites. The type of care given is determined by the types of services each site delivers, but the basic patient care skills you will learn in this course are used to some degree in all health care settings.

Hospitals. Hospitals give care to **patients** with **acute illnesses**. These patients usually stay in the hospital for a short period of time. When the patient is medically stable, he or she is transferred to a lesser care setting or returns home.

Long-Term Care Facilities. Long-term care facilities care for **residents**. These facilities may be called by many different names: nursing homes, nursing facil-

■ **professional:** *a skilled practitioner who is capable, competent, and efficient*
■ **hospitals:** *institutions that care for people with acute illnesses*
■ **patients:** *persons who are cared for in a hospital*
■ **acute illness:** *illness that develops suddenly and lasts for a short time*
■ **long-term care facilities:** *health care institutions that care for residents with chronic diseases and personal care needs*
■ **residents:** *persons who are cared for in a long-term care facility*

■ **chronic illness:** an illness or disease that lasts for a long time
■ **rehabilitation:** program(s) designed by a therapist to help patients regain lost skills or teach new skills
■ **restorative care:** nursing care designed to assist the patient to attain and maintain the highest level of function possible

■ **subacute care:** a level of care in which the patient has complex care needs but is not critically ill
■ **chemotherapy:** a cancer treatment that uses specific chemical agents or drugs to destroy cancer cells
■ **postoperative care:** care given to patients after surgical procedures
■ **ventilator:** a device used to assist or control breathing

■ **registered nurse (RN):** a nurse who has two to four years of nursing school and has passed a state licensing examination

■ **licensed practical nurse (LPN):** a nurse who has completed one to two years of nursing school and passed a state licensing examination
■ **licensed vocational nurse (LVN):** same as a licensed practical nurse

■ **client:** a person being cared for in his or her own home

ities, convalescent homes, rehabilitation centers, care centers, care facilities, assisting living facilities, and skilled nursing facilities. Long-term care facilities provide care for people who have **chronic illnesses** and others who need personal care. An example of a chronic illness is diabetes. Long-term care facilities also provide **rehabilitation** programs and **restorative care** to help residents overcome the disabling effects of illness and injury and restore them to their maximum potential.

Skilled Nursing Facilities. Often the name of the agency describes the type of care that the facility provides. Some hospitals have units called "skilled units." These units are licensed as long-term care facilities. Many nursing homes are also licensed to provide skilled care. Residents who require skilled care have illnesses or injuries requiring daily services that only a licensed health care professional can provide. These services can involve one or more disciplines within the health care facility. For example, nurses must administer injections and are responsible for complex treatments. The services of a licensed nurse are also required to physically assess the resident's medical condition and take appropriate action if problems are noted. If the resident has many complex needs, planning and monitoring daily care are considered skilled services. Licensed therapy personnel provide skilled therapy on a daily basis to rehabilitate the resident. Skilled nursing facilities provide care for residents with highly specialized medical needs, but who are not unstable or critically ill.

Subacute Units. Care may also be given in **subacute care** centers or units. These units can be part of a hospital or a long-term care facility. Patients in these units have complex medical needs. The subacute unit is a transitional step between the hospital and the skilled nursing facility. The patient is not ill enough to require the services of the acute care hospital, but still requires frequent care by licensed health care personnel. Patients in the subacute unit are less stable than those in the long-term care facility and require close monitoring. They usually require many services from the patient care technician. Subacute care units may provide intensive rehabilitation services, **chemotherapy** for cancer patients, and **postoperative care** for surgical patients. Many patients in subacute units require feeding through intravenous tubes. Some require **ventilator** support.

There are four types of subacute units:
1. Transitional subacute units are a less expensive setting than the acute care hospital and provide 24-hour-a-day coverage by a **registered nurse (RN)**. Rehabilitation therapies are available 7 days a week. Respiratory therapy is available 24 hours a day. A nutritional consultant is available.
2. General medical surgical subacute units provide care for patients who require medical care and monitoring, rehabilitation therapy, and nursing services. RN coverage is provided 24 hours a day. Rehabilitation therapies are available 6 days a week. Respiratory therapy and nutritional consultants are available.
3. Chronic subacute care units provide care for patients with little hope of recovery or return to functional independence. These units usually provide an RN at least 8 hours a day. If an RN is not on duty, a **licensed practical nurse (LPN)** or **licensed vocational nurse (LVN)** is in charge. Restorative nursing care is provided and physical, occupational, and speech therapies are available.
4. Long-term transitional subacute units provide care for medically complex patients or acute ventilator patients. Many different types of physician specialists must be available to care for patients in this type of unit. The unit is directed by an RN with acute care experience. The patients require a high degree of RN intervention because of their acute medical problems. Respiratory therapists and nutritional consultants are available.

Home Care. Care is sometimes given to a **client** in the home by qualified caregivers. Caregivers who work in home health care may be called home health aides, home care aides, or home health assistants.

■ *hospice care:* physical, psychological, and spiritual care provided to patients who have a limited life expectancy and their families

■ *interdisciplinary team:* a group of caregivers who work together for the good of the patient, resident, or client

Hospice Care. Hospice care may be provided in the home or a long-term care facility. Some hospitals have special hospice units. The emphasis is on preventing pain and suffering and making the patient as comfortable as possible. In hospice care, the patient and family are considered a unit. An **interdisciplinary team** works to ensure that the needs of the entire family are met. Team members work to provide the patient the opportunity to die with dignity, in comfortable, familiar surroundings. Support is provided so the patient and family members are not left alone in times of crisis.

Other Types of Health Care Facilities. Health care may also be delivered in many other settings. These include:

- Freestanding clinics and emergency care centers
- Mental health facilities
- Adult group living centers
- Residential care centers and assisted living facilities
- Board and care homes

Financing Health Care

■ *reimburse:* to repay an institution for the cost of services provided

■ *Medicaid:* a program funded by the state and federal governments that pays for health care for individuals with a low income

■ *Medicare:* a program administered by the federal government that helps the elderly and disabled pay for care in the hospital, long-term care facility, and home health care settings

■ *health maintenance organizations (HMOs):* groups of health care providers and hospitals paid by insurance companies to care for patients for a monthly fee

Health care is paid for in many different ways. Some individuals pay for care out of their personal bank accounts. Others pay a premium to insurance companies. When these individuals get sick, the insurance company **reimburses** the facility for the medical care. **Medicaid** is a health care program funded by both the state and federal governments. **Medicare** pays for certain services in the hospital, long-term care facility, and home health care setting. Although most hospitals accept payment from the Medicare and Medicaid programs, some home health agencies, **health maintenance organizations (HMOs)**, and long-term care facilities do not.

Occasionally, other sources pay for health care. The Veterans Administration (VA) has special hospitals to care for veterans with service-related illnesses and injuries. Sometimes the VA also pays long-term care facilities for care provided to veterans. Private agencies in the community may also help pay the cost of care for certain individuals.

The health maintenance organization may be funded by Medicare, Medicaid, or the patient's private money. HMO members are given a list of physicians, clinics, offices, and hospitals where they may go to receive care. The patient must see only certain doctors and go to only designated hospitals, except in certain situations and emergencies. The HMO pays the doctor (or group of doctors) a fee for each member every month. The doctor is paid the fee even if the member does not visit. The doctor or clinic is expected to deliver all care, whenever needed, for this monthly fee. There are no additional payments. Some HMOs have special outpatient clinics in which outpatient surgery, diagnostic testing, patient teaching, and preventive health care are delivered. Medical care may be provided for individuals with acute illnesses. Usually the patient returns home after treatment in the clinic.

■ *preferred provider organization (PPO):* listed physicians and health care agencies that contract with insurance companies to provide health care to insurance company subscribers

■ *OBRA (Omnibus Budget Reconciliation Act):* legislation that made sweeping reforms of the long-term care industry and describes requirements for nursing assistant training

Another common method of paying for health care is through a **preferred provider organization**, or **PPO**. Various insurance companies contract with physicians and health care agencies. When patients become sick, they can choose a physician or agency on the preferred provider list to care for them. The patient's out-of-pocket expenses are reduced as long as the patient uses the physicians and agencies on the list. The patient may go to any other service provider of his or her choosing. However, going to providers who are not on the PPO list will cost the patient more.

■ THE OBRA LEGISLATION

OBRA is an abbreviation for the *Omnibus Budget Reconciliation Act*. The OBRA legislation of 1987 was designed to improve the quality of life, quality of care,

■ *decline:* worsening or deterioration in the resident's physical or mental condition

■ *risk factors:* conditions that have the potential to cause the patient, resident, or client's health to worsen

health, and safety of residents in long-term care facilities. Residents' rights are emphasized. Residents in long-term care facilities have the same legal rights as all other citizens. The facility must maintain a homelike environment that maintains or improves the quality of life.

OBRA also requires facilities to maintain or improve the resident's condition. **Declines** in condition are not allowed unless they are medically unavoidable. The resident's condition is assessed at admission by licensed facility staff and a record is made of this assessment. The facility is expected to maintain or improve the resident's condition compared with how the resident was at the time of admission. For example, if the skin was free from injury on admission, the facility is expected to keep the skin free from injury. If the skin was injured at the time of admission, the facility is expected to take steps to heal the injured area.

The long-term care facility must help the resident function at the highest level possible for the resident's individual situation. To do this, facilities use a written tool developed by the government to assess residents. This tool is called the Minimum Data Set or MDS. It assists facility personnel to identify **risk factors** in advance, so they can address them to prevent the resident's condition from worsening. For example, a resident who is in bed all the time is at risk for skin breakdown and other problems. If the resident does not have bowel and bladder control, the risk of skin problems increases. The MDS identifies the resident's risk and the facility is expected to take steps to prevent it. Declines are addressed in other chapters of this book, but understanding this concept from the beginning of your study is important. Preventing declines is a good practice in all health care settings.

The OBRA laws require caregivers to see the resident in a long-term care facility as a whole person with many strengths and needs. We are not to look at medical problems alone. Needs in one area of life can affect the resident's entire life and well-being. For example, a resident may need help to overcome problems with sadness and depression. If this need is not met, the resident may stop eating, refuse therapy, and eventually give up on living entirely. Many people can be taught to use their own strengths to meet their needs. Again, this is good to remember in all settings where health care is delivered.

The OBRA legislation sets minimum standards that all states must follow to ensure that nursing assistants are trained and qualified to give personal care. The legislation specifies that a nursing assistant must have a minimum of 75 hours of training in certain subject matter to work in health care. Many states require more than 75 hours of training. The skills learned in the nursing assistant program are the basic skills required for entry-level positions in most health care settings.

Before the OBRA legislation, each state decided whether nursing assistants had to receive training to work in health care. The programs varied widely from state to state. Some states had no training requirement. OBRA recognizes that the person receiving care, the health care facility, and the patient care technician all benefit from the training program. The information learned is useful in many different health care settings. The care required by the OBRA legislation translates into good patient care regardless of the setting. However, the OBRA legislation was specifically designed to improve the quality of care in long-term care facilities and skilled units of hospitals.

Benefits of Training the Patient Care Technician

Many people benefit when the patient care technician has been trained and understands the responsibilities of the position. Training assures that all care providers understand basic procedures for patient care.

Benefits to the Person Receiving Care. It is comforting to the patient in a health care agency to know that the staff is properly prepared to deliver care. When a person is sick, he has many worries. Knowing that training is mandatory relieves the patient of worry about the qualifications of the staff caring for him. Additional benefits to the patient are:

- The care given is safe, effective, and of high quality, because the staff is properly trained.
- Changes in condition are rapidly recognized, reported, and treated.
- Patients are satisfied with the care received.
- Quality of life is improved because the staff has a better understanding of patient needs.
- There are fewer incidences of abuse and neglect because of staff understanding of what constitutes abuse and neglect, what causes it, and how to prevent it.

Benefits to the Health Care Agency. The health care agency has a great responsibility for the health, safety, and welfare of its patients. A large amount of trust is placed in employees to deliver the highest possible quality of care. Employees who are trained understand their duties and responsibilities and deliver safe care. Patient care technicians can perform many different skills that cross over into other areas of health care. This enhances the worker's value to the organization and allows more cost-effective delivery of health care to the patient. Other benefits of training to the employer are:

- Decreased staff turnover.
- Improved quality of care, because staff members are better trained to perform procedures.
- Improved safety, so patients and workers have fewer accidents and incidents.
- Better observation and reporting of important changes in condition, which enable timely medical care.
- Lower infection rates, because the staff understands how to prevent infection.
- Enhanced image of the health care facility, because of the qualified caregivers on its staff.
- Enhanced image of the health care industry, because all caregivers are trained and qualified to do their jobs.

Benefits to the Licensed Supervisor. The licensed supervisor is responsible for what happens on the unit each shift. This is a great responsibility. The manager must be able to trust the other workers to take proper care of the patients and report changes in a timely manner. Some benefits of patient care technician training to the supervisor are:

- Observations and reporting of changes in patient condition are improved, because of better understanding of patient needs and training to recognize problems.
- Improved understanding of the role and responsibilities of the patient care technician.
- Consistency by all care providers in performing procedures and delivering care. This uniformity benefits the patient, and the supervisor does not have to worry about variations from standard procedures.
- Improved skill level of caregivers.

Benefits to the Care Provider. The patient care technician benefits greatly from completing a basic skills training program. Benefits to the care provider include the following:

- Information gained in the training program is useful in many areas of your life. In addition to teaching you how to care for patients, you will gain information that will help you care for yourself and family members.

■ The program gives you an improved understanding of your role and responsibilities.

■ Your knowledge and skill level are improved so that you can give safe, high-quality personal care to patients, residents, and clients.

■ Job satisfaction increases because you understand the reasons for what you are doing.

■ You become aware of the factors that cause patient and employee accidents and illnesses so that you can prevent them.

■ You develop a sense of accomplishment, pride in what you are doing, and an improved self-image. Completing the basic skills training program is something to be proud of!

Nursing Assistant Certification

If you are trying to complete a nursing assistant training program, you must understand how to get and keep your certification.

Some states require the employing health care facility to complete a criminal background check on applicants. This background check will show if the applicant has ever been arrested. In these states, if an individual has been convicted of a felony crime, he or she cannot work in a health care facility.

After completing the state-approved course, the nursing assistant must take written and manual competency skills examinations given or sponsored by the state. After passing these examinations, the nursing assistant is entered into the state nursing assistant registry. To keep nursing assistant certification active, you must work in a health care agency for pay every two years. The number of hours you must work during the two-year period varies by state. If you do not work for 24 months or longer, you must complete another nursing assistant training program or refresher course and successfully complete another competency evaluation test to work as a nursing assistant again. Some states will allow you to take the test over without repeating the class. The OBRA legislation requires the nursing assistant to attend a minimum of 12 hours of continuing education each year to remain active. Some states require more than the 12-hour minimum. The facility that you work for will offer these classes. It is your responsibility to attend them to maintain your certification. Your facility is required to evaluate your skills every year to be sure that you can do them in the way you were taught.

Supervision of the Patient Care Technician

In most health care facilities, you will provide personal care to patients under the supervision of a licensed nurse. The nurse who supervises you may be a registered nurse. Some nurses are licensed practical nurses or licensed vocational nurses. The nurse manager will give you your assignment at the beginning of your shift. You will report your concerns and observations to this nurse.

In some health care settings, your supervisor will be another licensed health care professional. This individual may be licensed as a physician, radiologic technologist, or other professional who is educated and licensed to practice in the area in which you are working.

■■■■ INTRODUCTION TO HEALTH CARE SERVICE SETTINGS

Health care is delivered to patients in a variety of settings. Each setting has a specific purpose. Health care agencies are highly specialized and are designed to meet the specific needs of the patients and populations they serve.

The Acute Care Hospital

Hospitals employ many individuals to provide basic patient care. Some hospitals hire or train certified nursing assistants. Some hospitals send their employees to community colleges and technical schools for training. Some agencies require prospective employees to complete these classes before they are hired.

Many additional classes that expand the basic caregiver's scope of practice are available. This is usually called cross-training or multiskilling. The hospital provides continuing education classes and periodic competency evaluation of skills. A multiskilled worker is very valuable to the hospital and can work in many different departments.

A hospital provides care to people with acute illnesses of all types. Some patients have medical problems. Others have surgical problems. Hospitals have special care units for patients who are critically ill. Some patients go to the hospital for outpatient tests, treatment, and surgery. These patients return home the same day, unless complications develop. Patients in the hospital can be any age, from newborn to very old.

Most hospitals are inspected and accredited by the Joint Commission on Accreditation of Healthcare Organizations (JCAHO). This organization sets standards for quality patient care and inspects periodically to ensure that hospitals are meeting the standards. In most states, other regulatory agencies also have authority over hospitals.

Skilled nursing units within the hospital must follow the same laws as long-term care facilities. They follow the training and caregiving requirements in the OBRA legislation. Inspections of hospital skilled units are done by state or federal surveyors who use the same survey tool that is used for long-term care facilities.

The Long-Term Care Facility

Long-term care facilities employ many patient care technicians. Some long-term care facilities provide general care to all types of residents with chronic diseases and personal care needs. Some facilities offer care to residents with special needs, such as those with Alzheimer's disease or those who depend on ventilators and other special equipment.

Long-term care facilities are regulated and inspected by government agencies. Agency representatives visit the facility unannounced to inspect resident care and facility cleanliness. Facilities that are not in compliance with the law must pay penalties and fines according to the nature and severity of the problems surveyors find. The patient care technician has a very important responsibility to follow all laws, rules, and facility policies. If you follow facility policies and do your job in the way that you were trained, you will stay in compliance with the law.

Types of Residents in Long-Term Care Facilities. Long-term care facilities are home to many types of residents. Some will spend the rest of their lives in the facility. Others come to the facility for a short time for rehabilitation and restoration, to regain strength after an acute illness or injury. These residents may then return to their own homes. Regardless of discharge plans, remember that the quality of the resident's life is as important as, or more important than, the length of the resident's stay. As a care provider, you should try to give all residents the highest quality of life possible.

Many residents in the long-term care facility are **geriatric**. Other residents have a physical or mental **disability** that prevents them from taking care of themselves in the community. Some residents may be **mentally retarded**. These residents have low intelligence that prevents them from caring for themselves or living independently. Most can learn new things, but learning may take a long time. Some residents have a **developmental disability**. These individuals may have a physical impairment, a mental impairment, or a combination of both. Individuals with mental retardation or developmental disabilities may not be admitted to skilled nursing facilities unless their medical needs require skilled nursing care. If these residents do not require skilled nursing care, they are usually admitted to special facilities that provide services to meet their highly individual needs and give training in skills to make them as independent as possible, despite their disabilities.

■ **geriatrics:** *care of the elderly*
■ **disability:** *inability to function normally because of a physical or mental problem*
■ **mentally retarded:** *a person with lower than average intellectual development ranging from mild to severe*
■ **developmental disability:** *a severe physical and/or mental impairment that is apparent before the age of 22 and is likely to continue indefinitely*

Not all residents in the long-term care facility are elderly. Some are young and middle-aged adults who have chronic diseases. Still others have infectious diseases. Some specialized long-term care facilities take care of infants and young children.

Subacute Care Units

Rules and regulations for subacute units vary depending on whether the unit is located within a hospital or a long-term care facility. The requirements also vary according to the type of services the subacute unit offers. The patient care technician is very important because the patients in a subacute unit require a great deal of care, monitoring, and observation. These patients have had an acute illness or an acute episode related to a chronic problem. Their condition can change very quickly. They have complex care needs related to medical and surgical problems. They may be connected to several electronic monitoring or caregiving devices and may have tubes in different areas of the body. Patients in a subacute unit are usually dependent on the patient care technician to help them with many activities of daily living. A patient's stay in a subacute unit is usually temporary. If the patient recovers sufficiently, she will be discharged and go home. If her condition becomes chronic and more stable, she will go to a long-term care facility to complete her recovery. If the patient becomes unstable or acutely ill, she will be transferred to a hospital.

Home Health Care

Sometimes care is provided in the home setting. This care may be provided by an independent worker who is hired by the client or family. Most home care is performed by home health agencies. These agencies have many workers who are repsonsible for care and supervision of clients in their homes. Commonly, the patient care technician or nursing assistant is the primary caregiver. In the home care setting, this person may be called a home health aide or home health assistant. This assistant is usually an experienced caregiver who visits the client's home and provides personal care to the client.

Some clients receiving home care are acutely ill and need 24-hour care. Many clients require only short visits daily or several times a week. A visit is usually from 45 minutes to 2 hours in length. Other workers, such as physical, occupational, speech, or respiratory therapists, may also visit the home to perform services for the client.

The caregiver who works in the home does so without direct supervision. A registered nurse is responsible for supervising the care given in the home, but the RN may not be present when the care is actually given. Although the personal care is the same as care provided in other settings, the location is different. Caring for the client in the home may also involve preparing meals, shopping for groceries, and doing light housekeeping and laundry. The patient care technician must follow a plan of care developed by the nurse supervisor. Sometimes you must improvise by using common items in the home so that you can care for the client. A caregiver may not be in the home at all times, so your accurate observations and reports to your supervisor (by telephone and in writing) are very important.

Health Care Clinics and Physicians' Offices

Health care clinics and physicians' offices serve clients of all ages, ranging from newborn to elderly. Many clinics employ patient care technicians to do diagnostic testing and assist with a variety of procedures. Some clinics are part of a hospital and some are freestanding. They are well staffed and equipped to deliver emergency care if the need arises. Some clinics deliver only highly specialized services, such as care of expectant mothers, cancer treatment, or outpatient care of persons with AIDS. Some clinics perform outpatient surgery. In this setting the patient care technician assists with patient flow, movement between examination rooms, and testing. In some clinics, the patient care technician draws blood and performs other diagnostic tests, such as EKGs. The technician may also assist with surgery and monitoring of vital signs in patients recovering from anesthesia. Patient care technicians may help the licensed supervisor with teaching clients the skills needed to manage their problems at home. Some clerical functions are also performed.

THE ELDERLY

Many patients in the hospital, long-term care facility, subacute unit, health maintenance organization, and home care setting are elderly. The elderly are like you in many ways. They have, or have had, families, jobs, homes, and status in the community. Their physical and emotional needs are similar to yours. They may be anxious or frustrated. They often fear the unknown, their illnesses, and dependence on others. A basic understanding of the needs of the elderly is essential to the success of the patient care technician.

Common Myths and Beliefs about the Elderly

■ **myths:** *common beliefs that are not true*

People may believe things about the elderly that are not always true. Myths have no basis in fact. Here are some common myths about the elderly:

■ *Myth:* All elderly people become senile and confused. *Fact:* The truth is that mental confusion does occur in some people, but not all. (The causes of mental confusion are discussed later in this book.) All elderly people *do not* become confused, and mental confusion is not a normal part of the aging process. Many live to be quite old with their mental abilities intact.

■ *Myth:* Old people do not like to be touched. *Fact:* All human beings need to be touched. The elderly are like us in this respect. Touch shows love and respect, and provides comfort to someone who is in physical or mental pain.

■ *Myth:* All old people are irritable and crabby. *Fact:* Everyone gets upset and gets in a bad mood from time to time. The elderly get upset, too. Nevertheless, old people are not more irritable than younger people. Irritability is not determined by age.

■ *Myth:* Old people are unable to do anything for themselves. *Fact:* We all are dependent on other people for certain things. The elderly are like we are. They may depend on others for some things, but can do other things for themselves. A person's worth should not be decided or judged by how independent he is.

■ *Myth:* Old people cannot contribute anything to society. *Fact:* Many elderly people have contributed a great deal to society already, and they continue to make contributions. For example, many presidents of the United States were considered elderly when they were elected to office. Some societies value and respect the elderly because they have a lifetime of experience to share with others. The elderly can teach us many things if we take the time to listen.

RESPONSIBILITIES OF THE PATIENT CARE TECHNICIAN

The person who delivers basic patient care is a very important member of the health care team. You will spend more time with patients than any other caregiver. The patient care technician performs many valuable services to assist the patient and other members of the health care team.

Responsibilities for Providing Personal Care

You will help patients with bathing, personal hygiene, and grooming. You may need to help patients with dressing and undressing. Some patients may need assistance turning and positioning in bed or moving from one place to the other. Some require help with toileting and elimination needs.

Providing Food Service and Mealtime Assistance

A very important responsibility of the patient care technician is seeing that patients receive food and fluids. You are responsible for delivering food trays, special supplements, and snacks. There may be times when you will help patients eat or even feed them. You are also responsible for providing fresh water and encouraging patients to drink enough liquid.

Caring for the Patient's Unit and Belongings

■ **unit:** *the patient's personal space, which includes a bed, chair, overbed table, nightstand, dresser, wastebasket, and closet*

The patient's room is called the **unit**. You are responsible for keeping the unit tidy and safe. You will make beds and handle the patient's clothing and belongings. Treating personal items with care is important. This shows respect for the patient. Many patients bring only their most important possessions with them to the health care facility. This is particularly true in long-term care. It is your responsibility to see that both the patient and her belongings are kept safe.

Observation and Reporting

A very important responsibility of the patient care technician is making observations of patient conditions and reporting changes to the licensed supervisor. The care provider often spends more time with the patient than any other caregiver. Because of this close contact, you may be the first person to recognize a variation from the patient's normal condition. All changes, even if they seem minor, may be important and should be reported to your manager.

Caring for Equipment and Supplies

Many different pieces of equipment are used in the health care facility. Some are used once and thrown away. Others are used for one patient only. Some pieces of equipment are used for many patients, and are cleaned and disinfected between each use. You will learn how to safely care for and use the equipment found in the health care facility. Take your responsibility for using and caring for equipment very seriously!

Recordkeeping, Communication, and Messenger Duties

We communicate in many different ways in the health care facility. These methods are discussed in more detail in Chapter 5. You will be responsible for keeping accurate records in writing and for communicating information to others verbally. For example, you will report changes in patient condition to your supervisor. At times you will be asked to give other departments and staff members pertinent information.

▰▰▰▰ THE INTERDISCIPLINARY TEAM

The health care team is also called the interdisciplinary team. You will work with other members of this team to contribute to the care, health, and well-being of the patient. All team members are important. We need each other and the patient needs us. To be successful, we must work together and cooperate with each other.

Members of the Interdisciplinary Team

■ **care plan:** *a plan developed by the interdisciplinary health care team that describes the goals and approaches that all team members should use when caring for the patient*

Many individuals, both within and outside the health care agency, are members of the interdisciplinary team. We must use whatever resources are necessary to meet our patients' physical, mental, and emotional needs. The goal of the interdisciplinary team is to assist patients to maintain the highest level of physical, mental, emotional, and psychosocial well-being possible. Team members meet shortly after a patient's admission, and periodically after that, to develop a **care plan** for each patient. All team members must know and follow the information on the care plan (Figure 1-1). By doing this, all staff members will use the same approaches and work on the same goals for the benefit of the patient. The patient and family members that the patient wants to be included are also

Mercy Medical	CARE PLAN	02/06/19XX
		FORM # 280L

PROBLEM	SHORT TERM GOAL	APPROACH

(1) Potential for impaired skin integrity
  a) Related to altered circulation in legs
  b) Related to flexion contracture of neck
 	
     ONSET   TARGET   RESOLVE
     02/06/XX   05/07/XX   / /
	(1) Will remain ulcer free (legs) through 5/7/XX
	
	   BEGIN TARGET RESOLVE
	   02/06/XX 05/07/XX / /
	
	(2) Skin intact lower neck through 5/7/XX
	
	   BEGIN TARGET RESOLVE
	   02/06/XX 05/07/XX / /
		(1) R.N. check legs q a.m.
		    DISC: NSG
		
		(2) Elevate legs when up in w/c.
		    DISC: NA
		
		(3) Wash and dry area b.i.d.
		    DISC: NA
		
		(4) Apply 4 x 4 to separate skin surfaces.
		    DISC: NSG NA
		
		(5) Use Mycalog cream for increased redness prn.
		    DISC: NSG

(2) Alteration in comfort
  a) Related to impaired circulation
  b) Related to joint pain
 	
     ONSET   TARGET   RESOLVE
     02/06/XX   05/07/XX   / /
	(1) 2 nocs/week without leg cramps by 5/7/XX
	
	   BEGIN TARGET RESOLVE
	   02/06/XX 05/07/XX / /
	
	(2) States relief of pain with heat packs through 5/7/XX.
	
	   BEGIN TARGET RESOLVE
	   02/06/XX 05/07/XX / /
		(1) Administer Procardia as ordered and assess effectiveness.
		    DISC: NSG
		
		(1) Heat packs to neck, shoulder, knees 5x/wk.
		    DISC: RA

PHYSICIAN / ALT. PHYSICIAN	PHONE NO.	ALLERGIES / NOTES
WASHINGTON, JAMES M.D. KEELEY, JANICE M.D.	(555) 555-8888	PENICILLIN, ASPIRIN

NAME	STATION / ROOM / BED	ADMISSION NUMBER / DATE	SEX	DATE OF BIRTH	CARE PLAN DATE	PAGE #
JAMES, FIONA	NORTH-122-B	33652 10/18/19XX	F	(73) 02/28/19XX	02/06/19XX	1

Figure 1-1 Everyone involved in the patient's care follows the care plan.

members of the interdisciplinary team. The following team members provide most of the direct care services to patients.

Licensed Nurses. Licensed nurses may be either RNs or LPN/LVNs. Nurses direct the care of patients and give medications and treatments.

Patient Care Technician. This team member delivers most of the personal care to the patient under the supervision of the licensed nurse. This caregiver spends more time with the patient than others.

Dietary Staff. Staff members in the dietary department prepare meals and are responsible for ordering groceries, washing dishes, and other kitchen duties.

Licensed Dietitian. This team member writes the menus that the dietary department prepares. The dietitian is responsible for seeing that patients on special diets receive the right food in the proper amount.

Activities. Activity personnel serve the very important function of providing activities for patient enjoyment. Some activities are done to provide exercise for patients. Other types of activities are designed to improve patient self-esteem by making patients feel good about themselves. Activities also provide opportunities for patients to socialize with others.

Social Service. Social workers help meet patients' mental and emotional needs. They also coordinate many functions with personnel and agencies inside and outside the facility to see that patient needs are met. When the patient is discharged to home or to another health care agency, the social worker coordinates the resources the patient will need and makes the transition as smooth as possible.

Physical Therapist. The physical therapist helps patients regain strength and physical function lost because of illness or injury. The goal of the therapist is to help the patient achieve the highest level of function possible.

Occupational Therapist. The occupational therapist also helps patients regain strength and physical function lost because of illness or injury. This therapist often helps patients to relearn self-care skills such as feeding, bathing, grooming, and dressing. The goal of care is for the patient to be as independent as possible. Patients who have lost physical function may be able to use adaptive or self-help devices to be independent. The occupational therapist helps patients obtain these devices and teaches how to use them. The occupational therapist may also fabricate or order splints and other equipment to prevent deformities.

Respiratory Therapist. A respiratory therapist works with patients who have breathing problems and those who need oxygen and other special treatments for the lungs. The goal of respiratory treatment is to have patients receive enough oxygen.

Speech Therapist. The speech therapist works with patients who have diseases or injuries that have affected their ability to speak properly. This therapist also helps patients with swallowing problems to eat and drink without choking.

Physician. The physician is the team member who orders the patient's medical plan of care. Medications, diagnostic tests, and treatments must be ordered by the physician.

Other Team Members. Other members of the interdisciplinary team also provide important services to patients, but are not as involved in delivering basic patient care. Some of these team members are:

- Emergency medical service workers are trained to provide emergency care at the scene of illness or injury.
- Pharmacy workers prepare and dispense medications.
- Medical assistants are trained to provide care and perform procedures in physicians' offices, clinics, and outpatient care centers.
- Medical laboratory workers obtain specimens and conduct laboratory tests, some of which are highly technical. The physician depends on the information provided by the laboratory to properly diagnose and treat the patient.
- Radiology workers operate x-ray and other specialized equipment to view the inside of the body. As with laboratory tests, the physician depends on this information to make a diagnosis and provide treatment.
- Central processing workers provide equipment and materials to many different departments. They are responsible for seeing that equipment and supplies are available and in good working condition. These workers are also responsible for cleaning, packaging, and sterilizing medical equipment.
- Food service workers are responsible for food preparation, tray preparation and delivery, and dishwashing duties.

clergy: a minister of the gospel, a pastor, priest, or rabbi or other religious worker

- Members of the **clergy** are pastors of churches or other religious workers who help patients meet their spiritual needs.
- Medical records workers keep permanent records of the patient's care and treatment.

■ Bookkeeping and office workers are responsible for answering the telephone, recordkeeping, and taking care of business and financial functions.

■ Maintenance workers are responsible for seeing that the building and equipment are safe and in good repair at all times.

■ Laundry workers wash all of the facility linen and keep the nursing units supplied with enough sheets, towels, and other items needed to care for patients. The laundry in most long-term care facilities also washes residents' personal clothing.

■ Housekeeping personnel keep the facility clean and sanitary.

■ Volunteers serve many important purposes in the facility. Some volunteers help with patient activity programs. Others visit patients, read to them, and pass library and hospitality carts.

CHAIN OF COMMAND

■ **chain of command:** *the line of authority in each department*

The **chain of command** is very important to the proper operation of all health care facilities. The chain of command is the line of authority that each department follows in reporting information. You will report your observations, problems, and concerns to your immediate supervisor. If you have a problem with another department, you should report this to your manager. The manager will contact the appropriate person in that department to solve the problem. It is your responsibility to know and follow your facility's chain of command.

RELATIONSHIPS WITH PATIENTS

■ **tactful:** *considerate, polite, and thoughtful*
■ **empathetic:** *being able to understand how someone else feels*

Learning how to establish meaningful relationships with patients is important. Always be kind, **tactful**, **empathetic**, and professional with patients. Find ways to control your emotions if you are angry or upset. Allow patients to express their thoughts, feelings, and emotions without judging them. Try to understand the patients' concerns, even if you do not agree with them. Do not criticize patients to other staff members and avoid criticizing your coworkers to patients. Leave your personal problems at home, and do not discuss them with patients.

DESIRABLE QUALITIES IN THE PATIENT CARE TECHNICIAN

The patient care technician is a special person. The successful caregiver usually likes people, takes responsibility seriously, and believes in the importance of the position.

Personal Qualities

A pleasant demeanor is an important quality for health care workers. You will learn how to communicate and interact with different people. Being pleasant and polite to everyone is important, even if they have not treated you this way. Treat others with respect and dignity. Show a genuine concern for your patients and coworkers. Be available to help others and accept help if you need it. Do not judge other people's feelings. You will become more aware of how to assist patients with their feelings as you learn more about emotional needs. Remember, behavior is influenced by things such as culture, personality, illness, and emotional health. Understanding why others respond as they do will help you accept and deal with people's behavior.

■ **attitude:** *the outer reflection of your feelings*

A positive **attitude** is an important characteristic to bring to your job. Others can see your attitude by your behavior. The tone of your voice and your body language can change the message you are trying to send. Your attitude will be reflected in your work. Be positive about your job and your contribution to patient care.

You must also learn to work as a team player. This means that you depend on other people to help care for the patient. It also means that other people can de-

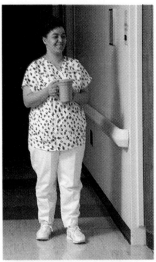

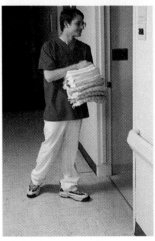

Figure 1-2 A professional appearance sends a message that you feel good about yourself and the job you are doing.

pend on you. Good patient care cannot be accomplished by one person or department. It takes many people and departments working together to meet the patient's needs.

Practice tact. Tact involves the ability to say and do things at the right time. Be sensitive to the problems and needs of others. Do not judge others or give advice. Treat patients and coworkers with courtesy, respect, and consideration. Do not argue, gossip, criticize your employer or others, or use abusive language.

Be proud of what you do and feel good about yourself! It takes a special person to provide basic care to other people. The patient care technician is very important to the operation of many different health care agencies. Work to do the best job that you can. Others will follow your example.

Professional Appearance. Your appearance should be clean, neat, and well groomed at all times (Figure 1-2). A professional appearance gives others confidence in you and sends a message that you feel good about yourself and the job you do. Your facility will have a dress code or uniform that you must wear. Be sure to wear the clothing that your facility requires. Your uniform must be clean and wrinkle-free each day. The color and design of your undergarments should not be visible beneath your uniform.

A name pin is a very important part of your uniform. The name pin identifies you by name and title. Many facilities issue name badges that are also electronically scanned in the time clock. If your facility does not issue a badge, it is your responsibility to obtain one.

Because you will be standing and walking for much of the day, having comfortable, well-fitting shoes is important. Some facilities require athletic shoes or shoes with closed toes that provide good foot support. Your shoes are an important part of your uniform. Keep them clean and in good repair.

Personal Hygiene, Grooming, and Health. Staying clean is one way to maintain your personal health. Take a bath or shower every day. Use a deodorant or antiperspirant. Keep your hair clean and neat. If your hair is long, wear it up or pulled back. Your fingernails should be short and clean; long fingernails can cause injury to patients. Also, potentially harmful germs can grow under nails. Jewelry is kept to a minimum. Many facilities allow only a watch and wedding band. Cologne and after-shaves should not be worn when on duty. Some patients have allergies to fragrances. Patients who are nauseated or have other medical problems may become ill from the scent of perfume or cologne. Others with respiratory problems may have difficulty breathing with a heavy fragrance in the room.

Personal Health and Safety

If you are to do your job well, you must be in good physical and emotional health. You will learn many health and safety principles and practices throughout your study that you can apply to your personal life.

Preventing Physical Illness. Practice the principles of proper nutrition, good health, and personal hygiene taught in this class. Eat three well-balanced meals each day. Avoid fad diets and junk foods. Avoid using alcohol, tobacco, and drugs. These substances endanger you and others.

Get adequate rest. Most people need eight hours of sleep each night. Exercise for at least 30 minutes 3 times a week. This is a good way of keeping your body healthy and helps relieve stress.

See your doctor regularly for checkups and preventive health care. Treat your medical problems early. Do not wait for them to become worse.

Men should practice testicular self-examination monthly. Women should practice breast self-examination each month and have mammograms as recommended by the treating physician.

Preventing physical illness is very important. You will learn principles of infection prevention in Chapter 2. These principles will help you prevent infection and communicable disease.

Preventing Injuries. Safety practices taught in this book will protect both you and your patients. The most common causes of employee injuries in health care facilities are slips, falls, and back injuries caused by improper lifting and moving. Wear a back support for lifting and moving, if this is your preference or the policy of your employer. Lifting and moving are discussed in detail in Chapter 7.

Know and follow your facility policies for reporting injuries of patients or employees, and follow them if an accident or injury occurs.

Emotional Health

Your feelings and behavior are your responsibility and you must work to control them. A sign of maturity is your ability to control your emotions. Ask yourself how your behavior will affect others. If you are upset, leave the area and take time out, if necessary. If you feel angry, upset, or impatient, try to understand why you feel this way. Find acceptable ways to cope with these feelings. Do not take negative comments from patients personally. Often the patient is reacting to a situation, not to you. Try to understand why the patient is acting this way. You must respond with respect and courtesy even if the patient is not kind to you.

■ **stress:** *physical or emotional strain and tension*

Stress in the Workplace. Stress can be harmful to your health. Working in a health care facility can be stressful at times. Your job may be physically or emotionally demanding. Stress is sometimes unavoidable when you are helping other people with their problems. If stress goes unchecked, you may feel overwhelmed and out of control. Personal or family problems may also contribute to the stress you feel. If your physical health is not good, stress may worsen. Burnout is the result of a buildup of stress. Feel good about yourself and the job you are doing. Having good self-esteem helps you cope with stressful situations. Use stress-reducing techniques to help cope with stress or sadness. The goal of stress management is to prevent burnout. Try to think through a problem before you worry about it. Understand that health care is constantly changing and that, to be successful, you must change with it. If stress is caused by change, resolve to accept it. If you know of a stress-relieving technique that works for you, use it.

■ **burnout:** *complete physical, mental, or emotional fatigue or exhaustion*
■ **self-esteem:** *how a person feels about himself or herself*

Ways of Managing Stress. Everyone has certain ways of managing stress. Learn which ways work for you and practice them regularly. Controlling stress is good for you! Some suggestions for controlling stress are:

■ Be nice to yourself. Be aware of your own needs.

■ Replay the good things that you have done in your mind. Dwell on these things and not on mistakes you have made.

■ Do something that you enjoy and have fun.

■ Exercise.

■ Take a break and relax in a pleasant atmosphere (Figure 1-3).

■ Sit with your feet up and your eyes closed and relax for a few minutes. Take a few deep breaths. Try to think of a pleasant scene or event. Imagine that you are there.

■ Use specific relaxation techniques, audiotapes, or videotapes.

■ Soak in a warm bath.

■ Listen to quiet music.

■ Find a hobby you enjoy.

■ Talk with a friend.

■ Get in touch with nature. Contact with plants and animals has been proven to reduce stress.

■ Watch a funny movie or do something to make you laugh. Laughing is a good stress reliever.

■ Sing. Singing relieves stress.

■ Have someone give you a massage.

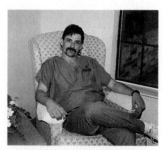

Figure 1-3 Relaxing in a pleasant, comfortable atmosphere is a good way to relieve stress.

Proper Equipment

Health care facilities and agencies have different requirements for equipment that you will be expected to provide. By law, the health care facility is required to supply you with well-fitting gloves and other protective equipment. Gloves and personal protective equipment are used when some care is given, to prevent the spread of infection, as is explained in detail in Chapter 2. In most cases you will be expected to furnish your own uniform and name pin. Some facilities expect their employees to provide a **gait belt**, back support belt, blood pressure cuff and stethoscope, watch with a second hand, pen, and pocket-size note pad. Know and follow your facility policies.

■ *gait belt: a heavy canvas belt used to assist the patient with ambulation; may also be called a transfer belt*

Responsible Behavior

Responsible behavior is very important for workers in health care professions. If a member of the health care team is not responsible, patients and coworkers suffer. Because you care for the health and welfare of human beings, you must take your job duties very seriously. Think how you would feel if a family member was a patient of a health care facility. You would want the best care possible for your loved one. To deliver the best care, all team members must demonstrate responsible behavior.

■ *responsible behavior: behavior that is dependable and trustworthy*

Health care facility rules must be followed even if you do not agree with them. Learn and profit from constructive criticism. Responsible behavior includes:

■ Reporting to work on time on the days that you are scheduled.

■ Keeping absences to a minimum. If you must be absent, follow your facility policy for reporting your absence. Notify the facility as early as possible so that they can call in a replacement. If the facility does not know you will be absent, care will suffer and your coworkers will have to work much harder than usual.

■ Keeping your promises to patients and staff members.

■ Doing tasks that you are assigned to do quickly and accurately.

■ Demonstrating initiative. This means doing things that you see need to be done without waiting to be told to do them.

■ Cooperating with other staff members in all departments.

■ Being **dependable**, so that patients and coworkers will trust you to do your job to the best of your ability.

■ *dependable: trustworthy; able to be relied on*

■ Reporting mistakes if you make them.

■ Giving proper notice of resignation if resigning from your position is necessary. Most facilities require a minimum of two weeks notification.

Organizing Your Work

Practice organizing your work. Organization is not something that can be taught in the classroom. The *principles* of organization can be taught, but it is up to you to learn, practice, and master them. Organizing your work means learning how to set **priorities**. It also means that you anticipate your own supply needs and patients' personal needs. Bring needed items to the room before you begin your care. This will save time and steps. If you can plan and prepare to meet these needs in advance, the quality of care you give will be better and the job will be much easier for you.

■ *priorities: things that are very important that must be taken care of first*

Manage Your Time Well. Report for duty at your assigned time. Listen to the report and get your assignment from your supervisor. Set your priorities to make the most of your day. Setting priorities makes the job easier. Good organization also reduces stress.

When organizing your work, rate each assignment in order of importance. Do not become frustrated if your priorities change or must be adjusted partway through the shift. Priorities are constantly changing in health care because of patient illness and other emergencies.

After you have established your priorities, plan your work for the most efficient use of your time. Identify tasks that you can group together. For example, a well-organized worker can make the bed while the patient is sitting in a chair or washing at the bathroom sink. Plan your schedule around patient meal times. Plan for tasks that will require special equipment or someone else to help you.

Check on all of your patients before beginning your assignment. Take care of immediate needs. List special procedures that must be done and the time, such as positioning and turning patients according to an assigned schedule. Check to see if patients are scheduled for tests, apppointments, or other activities during your shift.

Remember that while you are at work, you are on duty. You are being paid to work the whole time. Report to your supervisor when you go on break. Return from lunch and breaks on time. If you run out of things to do, help your coworkers or perform tasks that need to be done on your unit. Do these things without being told.

Other Qualities of the Successful Patient Care Technician

The successful employee delivers quality care to the patients in the health care facility. Always do things in the manner in which you were trained. Taking shortcuts can be dangerous. Do not do things that you were not taught to do. For example, giving medication is not taught in a PCT class, so this is something that you cannot do without additional training. If you are not sure how to do a procedure, consult your supervisor or check the procedure manual.

■ *compassion:* kindness
and mercy

Inform your supervisor if you will be unable to get a job done. Conduct yourself as a professional at all times. Being compassionate and empathetic with patients and families shows you care and sets a good example for others.

Continue to Learn and Grow

This class is just the beginning of your career. Health care changes daily and it is your responsibility to keep up. You can learn much from your coworkers and by reading books and journals. Attend continuing education classes offered by your employer.

Professional organizations, support groups, and publications are available for nursing assistants and other patient care technicians. Participating in a professional organization or support group will help you learn and grow. Different resource organizations use many names for the patient care technician in their titles, but most meet the needs of all patient care technicians.

Protect Yourself Legally

Follow your facility policies and procedures even if you do not agree with them. This protects you as an employee and ensures that you will do your job in accordance with the law. Anticipate patients' needs and meet them in a timely manner. Protect the rights of patients and residents in your health care facility. These rights and your legal responsibilities are discussed in detail in Chapter 4.

KEY POINTS IN CHAPTER

- *Hospitals provide care to patients with acute illnesses.*
- *Long-term care facilities provide care to residents with chronic illnesses and those who need personal care.*
- *Subacute care is given to patients who have complex medical or rehabilitation needs.*
- *Skilled nursing facilities provide care to patients who are medically stable, but require daily skilled services and intervention by licensed health care professionals.*
- *Health care clinics provide care, procedures, and diagnostic testing to clients in outpatient settings.*

KEY POINTS IN CHAPTER

Home care is provided to clients in their own residences by qualified caregivers.

The OBRA legislation was designed to improve the quality of life for residents of long-term care facilities. OBRA also specifies requirements for nursing assistant training.

A decline is a worsening of a resident's condition. Declines are not allowed under OBRA unless they are directly related to medical problems.

The health care agency, person receiving care, supervisor, and patient care technician all benefit from basic care skills and nursing assistant training and certification.

The patient care technician is supervised by a licensed nurse or other licensed health care professional. The supervisor varies with the setting in which the technician works.

Basic patient care skills include providing personal care, providing food service and mealtime assistance, making observations and reporting, caring for the patient's unit and belongings, caring for equipment and supplies, keeping records, and performing messenger duties.

The interdisciplinary team is a group of caregivers who contribute to the care, health, and well-being of the patient.

The chain of command describes the lines of authority used in the health care facility for reporting information.

Developing good relationships with patients is important.

Desirable qualities are professional appearance, good personal hygiene and grooming, good personal health, responsible behavior, dependability, and good organizational skills.

REVIEW QUIZ

Multiple Choice Questions

1. People with acute illnesses are usually cared for in:
   a. home care.
   b. hospitals.
   c. long-term care facilities.
   d. physicians' offices.

2. The person who receives care in the long-term care facility is the:
   a. client.
   b. patient.
   c. resident.
   d. charge nurse.

3. The OBRA legislation:
   a. is concerned with improving the quality of life for residents in long-term care facilities.
   b. describes requirements for nursing assistant training.
   c. requires the facility to maintain or improve residents' condition.
   d. all of the above.

4. Benefits of patient care technician and nursing assistant training to the health care facility include all of the following *except:*
   a. the patient care technician can give medicine to patients.
   b. quality of care to patients is improved.
   c. infection rates are lower because the caregiver understands how to prevent infection.
   d. the image of the health care facility is improved.

5. What is the minimum number of hours of continuing education that the nursing assistant must have every year?
   a. Two.
   b. Four.
   c. Eight.
   d. Twelve.

6. Personal care is provided to patients under the supervision of the:
   a. administrator.
   b. clergy.
   c. licensed health care professional.
   d. social worker.

7. The term *geriatrics* means:
   a. care of patients in the hospital.
   b. care of the elderly.
   c. care of the client in the home.
   d. none of the above.

8. Your uniform should:
   a. be neat and clean.
   b. include a name pin.
   c. include well-fitting, comfortable shoes.
   d. all of the above.

9. Responsible behavior includes:
   a. working at least three of every five days that you are scheduled.
   b. calling your facility in advance if you are unable to come to work.
   c. doing only those tasks that you want to do.
   d. all of the above.

10. The interdisciplinary team includes the:
    a. patient.
    b. licensed nurse.
    c. patient care technician.
    d. all of the above.

True/False Questions

11. ___ All old people become senile and confused.

12. ___ Old people are always very crabby.

13. ___ It is important to understand what the OBRA laws require regarding patient declines.

14. ___ Everyone involved with the patient's care should follow the care plan.

15. ___ The patient is a member of the interdisciplinary team.

Short Answer/Fill in the Blanks

16. The OBRA laws require long-term care facilities to maintain or _____ residents.

17. A _____ illness is one that lasts for a long time.

18. Health care workers must expect risk factors and act to prevent _____.

19. It is important to handle the patient's belongings with _____.

20. A _____ employee is one whom patients and coworkers trust.

21–25. List five members of the interdisciplinary team.

21. _____   24._____

22. _____   25._____

23. _____

26. To maintain nursing assistant certification, you must work in a health care facility for pay for a specified period of time every _____ years.

CHAPTER 2

Infection Control

- **medical asepsis:** practices used in health care facilities to prevent the spread of infection
- **infection control:** same as medical asepsis.
- **infection:** a state of sickness or disease caused by pathogens in the body
- **nosocomial infection:** an infection acquired by a patient while in a health care facility
- **localized:** confined to a specific area of the body
- **generalized:** spread throughout the entire body
- **susceptibility:** the ability of the body to resist disease
- **immune system:** part of the circulatory system that recognizes invading microorganisms and works to eliminate them from the body
- **microorganisms (microbes):** living germs that cannot be seen with the eye

MEDICAL ASEPSIS

Medical asepsis is also called infection control. Preventing the spread of infection is a very important responsibility. By practicing infection control, health care workers prevent the spread of infection to many people. These practices protect both you and your family members, patients and their family members, other staff members, and visitors to the health care facility.

Nosocomial infection is a serious risk for health care facility workers and patients. Some infections are localized. Signs of a localized infection are redness, swelling, and drainage. An infection can also be generalized. Signs of a generalized infection are fever, chills, pain, disorientation, fatigue, and nausea. Report any signs or symptoms of infection to your supervisor.

Susceptibility is the ability of the body to resist disease. If the immune system recognizes a harmful microbe, the body's natural defenses are stimulated. The body then works to eliminate the germ and prevent infection. Some diseases weaken and destroy the immune system. The ability of the body to resist infection is determined by age, presence of an underlying disease, health, nutritional state, and certain medications. When the immune system is weakened, the patient's body is unable to defend itself and infection results. Patients with certain diseases, the elderly, and patients receiving cancer treatments often have weakened immune systems.

Microorganisms, also called microbes, are present everywhere in the environment. Some are harmless and do not cause disease. Normal flora are healthy and helpful to the function of the body. For example, the normal flora in the

■ *normal flora:*
microorganisms that are
healthful and necessary for
the body to function correctly;
they are not harmful in the
area in which they reside, but
can cause infection if spread to
other parts of the body
■ *pathogen: a*
microorganism that
causes disease
■ *bacteria: one-celled*
microorganisms that can
cause disease
■ *antibiotics: medications*
used to eliminate pathogens
from the body
■ *viruses: tiny pathogens*
that cause disease
■ *disinfection: a cleaning*
process that destroys most
microorganisms; a chemical is
usually used to disinfect
reusable items
■ *sterilization: processes*
used to kill all microorganisms
■ *antiseptic: chemical agent*
designed to cleanse the skin
■ *direct contact: the spread*
of infection by touching
■ *indirect contact:*
touching objects, equipment,
or dishes contaminated with
harmful microorganisms

digestive tract help break down food and turn it into waste products. However, when these organisms gain access to an area of the body where they do not belong, they may cause disease.

Pathogens cause disease. Bacteria are microorganisms that can be eliminated with antibiotics. Viruses cause many diseases but cannot be eliminated by antibiotics. We can destroy many pathogens in the environment by a process known as disinfection. This commonly involves scrubbing or soaking an item with a special chemical or cleaning agent. The item is rinsed well to remove all traces of the chemical. Sterilization can be done by using heat, gas, or chemicals. An antiseptic is used to cleanse the skin and as a scrub to remove microorganisms before certain invasive procedures. Antiseptics should not be used on equipment or for cleansing environmental surfaces.

SPREAD OF INFECTION

Infection is spread by many methods. Table 2-1 lists common ways microbes are spread. The most common methods are by contact and in the air. The spread of infection by contact occurs in two different ways. Infections spread by direct contact are caused by touching a patient or host directly. A handshake is an example of direct contact. Your hands pick up the pathogen from the patient's hands. If the pathogen can enter your body through broken skin or the mucous membranes of your eyes, nose, mouth, or genital area, an infection will result. Pathogens may also be spread by indirect contact. This involves touching environmental surfaces, linen, supplies, or equipment that have pathogens on them (Figure 2-1). You pick up the pathogen on your hands and spread it to the inside of your body through nonintact skin or by touching your mucous membranes.

Infection may also be spread by the airborne route. Pathogens spread by this method are very tiny and lightweight, and enter the air in respiratory secretions. They travel long distances in the ventilation system, in dust, or in moisture par-

Table 2-1 Common Ways Microbes Are Spread

Airborne
■ Microbes carried by moisture or dust particles in air are inhaled

Droplet
■ Droplet spread within approximately 3 feet (no personal contact); droplet nuclei are inhaled
  - Coughing   Laughing
  - Sneezing   Singing
  - Talking

Contact
■ *Direct contact* of health care provider with patient:
  - Touching
  - Toileting (urine and feces)
  - Bathing
  - Secretions or excretions from patient
  - Rubbing
  - Blood, body fluid, mucous membranes, or nonintact skin

■ *Indirect contact* of health care provider with objects used by patients:
  - Clothing
  - Bed linens
  - Personal belongings
  - Personal care equipment
  - Instruments and supplies used in treatments
  - Dressings
  - Diagnostic equipment
  - Permanent or disposable health care equipment

Common Vehicle
■ Spread to many people through contact with items such as:
  - Food   Medication
  - Water   Contaminated blood products

Vector-Borne
■ Intermediate hosts such as:
  - Flies   Rats
  - Fleas   Mice
  - Ticks   Roaches

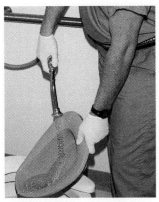

Figure 2-1 This bedpan has been disinfected and rinsed after use.

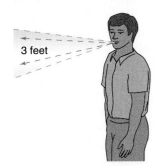

Figure 2-2 The droplets from a sneeze usually do not spread more than three feet from the patient.

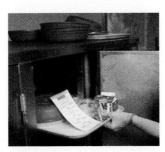

Figure 2-3 Food is one method of common vehicle transmission of infection.

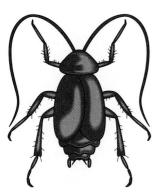

Figure 2-4 Vectors can carry microbes from one place to another.

ticles in the air. Because of their weight, these pathogens do not drop to the ground quickly and are easily inhaled.

Pathogens may also enter the air and spread infection by the droplet method. Pathogens spread by droplets are larger and heavier than those spread by air. Because of their size and weight, they usually do not spread beyond three feet from the host (Figure 2-2). Understanding the difference between the **airborne** and **droplet methods of transmission** is important so you can follow proper procedures to prevent infection from spreading.

Infections can also be spread by a common **vehicle.** Examples of common vehicles are food, water, or medication containing pathogens (Figure 2-3). The pathogens are taken into the body by eating and drinking.

Vectors (Figure 2-4) are insects and small animals that can carry disease-causing microorganisms.

Chain of Infection

The **chain of infection** describes six factors necessary for an infection to develop. The **source** represents the germ that causes disease. The **host** or **reservoir** is the place where the germ can grow. A **carrier** is a person who is infected with a disease that can be spread to others. The carrier may not know of the infection. **Transmission** is the method by which the disease is spread. The **portal of entry** is the place in the body where the germ enters. Pathogens can enter the body through any opening, such as a tiny cut or crack in the skin. They can also enter through the mucous membranes of the eyes, nose, mouth, or genital area. If any part of the chain of infection is broken, the disease will not spread. Figure 2-5

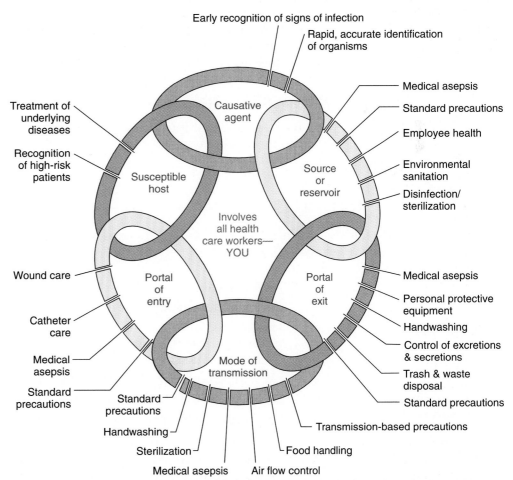

Figure 2-5 The chain of infection. If one link of the chain is broken, the infection cannot spread to others. The picture shows ways that health care workers can break each link in the chain.

Table 2-2 Elements in the Chain of Infection

Causative Agent	Source or Reservoir	Portal of Exit	Mode of Transmission	Portal of Entry	Susceptible Host
Bacteria	People	Blood	Direct contact	Mucous membranes	Chronic diseases
Fungi	Medicine	Moist body fluid	Indirect contact	Nonintact skin	Immunosuppression
Viruses	Food	Droplets	Airborne	Urinary tract	Surgery
Parasites	Water	Secretions	Droplet	GI tract	Diabetes
	Equipment	Excretions	Contaminated equipment and environmental surfaces	Respiratory tract	Elderly patients
		Skin	Common vehicle		Burns
			Vectors		Cardiopulmonary disease

airborne method of transmission: when very small microorganisms suspended in dust and moisture in the air are inhaled by a susceptible host

droplet method of transmission: when microorganisms are spread by secretions produced when laughing, talking, singing, sneezing, or coughing; these microorganisms are large and usually do not spread more than three feet in the air

vehicle: food, water, or other items in or on which pathogens can live and multiply

vector: an insect, rodent, or small animal that spreads disease

chain of infection: description of the factors necessary for an infection to spread

source: a pathogen that causes disease

host (reservoir): the place where a disease-causing germ can grow

carrier: a person who can give a disease to others; the person may not know of or show symptoms of the infection

transmission: the way in which a germ is spread

shows breaks in each link of the chain of infection. Using one of the methods listed next to any link will break the chain and prevent an infection from developing. Table 2-2 lists some common elements in each link of the chain.

PREVENTING THE SPREAD OF INFECTION

You have learned that infective organisms are everywhere in the environment. You can meet your very important responsibility to prevent the spread of infection in many ways.

General Guidelines for Reducing the Spread of Infection

- Wash your hands often.
- Keep the patient's unit neat, tidy, and sanitary.
- Clean equipment after each use. This includes small items used in the patient's room and larger permanent items such as the bathtub and shower chair.
- Handle and dispose of soiled material properly.
- Assist patients to bathe and maintain personal cleanliness.
- Practice good personal hygiene.
- Handle food properly.
- Handle clean and soiled linen correctly.
- Keep clean and soiled items separate.
- Perform procedures in the way that you were taught to do them, without taking shortcuts.

■ **portal of entry:** *the place where a pathogen enters the body*

Separation of Clean and Soiled Items and Equipment

To prevent infection, clean and soiled items must be kept separate. Clean items are either new, wrapped articles or reusable articles that have been washed or cleaned by staff. Soiled items are things used by a patient or brought into a patient's room. The items are considered soiled even if they were not used to care for the patient. They must be cleaned or disinfected when they are removed from the room. For example, if linen is brought into a patient's room, but is not needed, it cannot just be removed from the room and used in the care of another patient. It must be placed in the soiled linen hamper and washed before it is used again.

General Guidelines for Separating Clean and Soiled

- Keep the food cart, housekeeping cart, and clean linen cart separated from the soiled linen hamper by at least one room's width (Figure 2-6).
- Remove housekeeping carts from the hallway when food trays are being served. Some facilities also require that soiled linen hampers be removed from the hallway when food is being served.
- Many long-term care and psychiatric facilities have pets. They should not enter areas where food is being prepared or served.
- Wash soiled items in the soiled utility room. After they are clean, move them to the clean utility room for storage. Be sure that items are dry before storing them.
- Bring only needed linen and supplies into the patient's room.
- Avoid carrying trash, linen, or other contaminated items next to your uniform (Figure 2-7).
- Dispose of trash contaminated with blood or body fluid according to facility policy. It is usually placed in covered biohazard containers.
- Keep the patient's toothbrush covered when not in use. The toothbrush should be labeled with the patient's name.

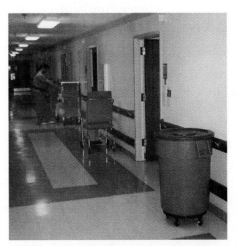

Figure 2-6 The clean linen cart and soiled linen hamper should be separated by a distance equal to the width of one room.

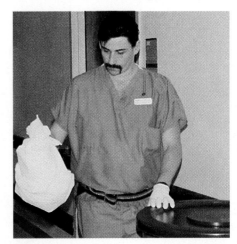

Figure 2-7 Soiled linen is carried away from your uniform.

continues

General Guidelines for Separating Clean and Soiled, *continued*

■ Wear gloves if needed when caring for patients. Wash your hands before applying gloves. Use gloves for the care of one patient only. After each patient, remove the gloves and wash your hands again.

■ After you have used gloves for patient contact, they are contaminated. Take care not to contaminated clean supplies, linen, equipment, or environmental surfaces with them. The best way to do this may be to remove one glove and use your ungloved hand for touching these things.

■ Dispose of used gloves according to facility policy. Generally they are not discarded in the open wastebasket in the patient's room. Some facilities place extra plastic bags in the bottom of the wastebasket. If throwing soiled gloves and other items into the wastebasket is necessary, remove the bag, tie it, and take it with you when you leave the room. Replace it with a new bag from the bottom of the wastebasket.

■ Follow facility policy for carrying soiled items in the hallway. If use of gloves is necessary, remove one glove. Carry the soiled item in the gloved hand. Use the ungloved hand to turn on faucets, open doors, and touch items considered clean. Follow the same procedure when emptying bedpans and urinals in patient bathrooms. Use the ungloved hand to open the door, turn on faucets, and flush the toilet (Figure 2-8).

■ Cover bedpans and urinals when you are carrying them.

■ Do not store lab specimens in a refrigerator with food or beverages. A separate refrigerator or cooler, marked with the biohazard emblem, should be used for lab specimens.

■ Follow your assignment and facility cleaning schedule for washing and disinfecting patient care items. You will use a special cleaner to disinfect reusable items. The friction created by wiping is important to remove microorganisms. You may be asked to date and initial items after they are cleaned.

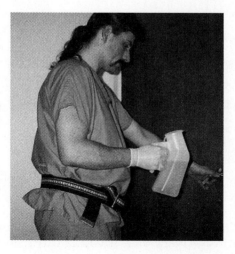

Figure 2-8 One-glove technique for handling contaminated equipment. The glove is removed from one hand, allowing the caregiver to open doors and turn on faucets without causing contamination.

continues

General Guidelines for **Separating Clean and Soiled,** *continued*

■ When working in two-bed rooms, clearly mark each patient's drinking glass and water pitcher, bedpan, urinal, emesis basin, and personal care items so that they do not accidentally get mixed up.

■ Use liquid soap whenever possible. If patients have individual bars of soap, keep them from getting mixed up. Soap should be stored in a container that allows extra water to drain from the bottom of the bar.

■ Cover food and beverages when you carry them in the hallway.

■ Monitor patient rooms for snacks and other food items. They should be stored in a covered or closed container.

■ Additional guidelines for handling of clean and soiled linen are listed in Chapter 8.

■ Additional guidelines for handling food and beverages are listed in Chapter 10.

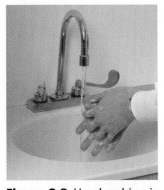

Figure 2-9 Handwashing is the most important method of preventing infection.

■■■ HANDWASHING

Handwashing is the most important method used to prevent the spread of infection (Figure 2-9). You can pick up microbes on your hands and introduce them to your own body. You can also transfer the microbes on your hands to patients. If your hands touch a clean object, the microbes on your hands may be transferred there. This is a potential source of indirect contact transmission. The purpose of handwashing is to clean the hands and prevent microorganisms from spreading. Handwashing should take a minimum of 10 to 15 seconds. If your hands are visibly soiled, you will need to take longer. The longer the handwashing, the more microorganisms are eliminated. The most important part of the handwashing procedure is the friction caused by rubbing your hands together. The friction removes the microbes from your hands.

General Guidelines for Times When Handwashing Should Be Done

■ When coming on duty

■ After picking up anything from the floor

■ Before and after caring for each patient

■ Before applying and after removing gloves

■ After personal use of the toilet or using a tissue to blow your nose

■ After you cough or sneeze

■ Before and after applying lip balm

■ Before and after manipulating contact lenses

■ Before and after eating, drinking, or smoking

■ Before handling a patient's food and drink

■ After contact with anything considered soiled or contaminated

continues

General Guidelines for Times When Handwashing Should Be Done, *continued*

- Before handling any item considered clean
- Immediately before touching nonintact skin (if you are already wearing gloves, change them)
- Immediately before touching mucous membranes (if you are already wearing gloves, change them)
- After touching nonintact skin, mucous membranes, blood, or any moist body fluid, secretions, or excretions, even if gloves were worn during the contact
- Whenever your hands are visibly soiled
- After touching equipment or environmental surfaces that could be contaminated
- Any time your gloves become torn
- Before you go on break and at the end of your shift before you leave the facility

PROCEDURE

OBRA

1 HANDWASHING

1. Turn on warm water. Use a paper towel to turn the faucet on if this is your facility's policy.

2. Wet your hands. Keep your fingertips pointed down.

3. Apply soap from the dispenser.

4. Rub your hands together vigorously to create lather. Rub the hands together in a circular motion for 10 to 15 seconds. Rub all surfaces of the hands. Keep your fingertips pointed down (Figure 2-10).

5. Rub the fingernails against the palm of the opposite hand. Clean the nails with a brush or an orange stick if they are soiled.

6. Rinse your hands from the wrist to the fingertips. Keep the fingers pointed down.

7. Dry your hands with a paper towel.

8. Use a clean, dry paper towel to turn off the faucet (Figure 2-11). Do not touch the faucet handle with your hand.

9. Discard the paper towel.

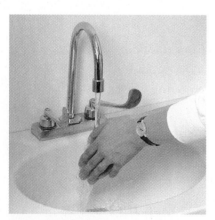

Figure 2-10 Keep your fingers down when washing your hands.

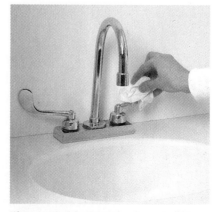

Figure 2-11 Turn the faucet off by using a paper towel.

■ ***bloodborne pathogens:*** *microbe-caused diseases that are spread through contact with blood or body fluid*
■ ***nonintact skin:*** *skin that is broken, chapped, or cracked*
■ ***mucous membranes:*** *tissues of the body that secrete mucus; these areas open to the outside of the body*
■ ***secretions:*** *drainage, discharge, or seeping from the body*
■ ***excretions:*** *human waste products eliminated from the body*
■ ***hepatitis B:*** *an infection of the liver caused by a virus; can cause liver cancer and death*
■ ***hepatitis C:*** *an infection of the liver caused by a virus; can be spread through contact with blood or body fluids and by eating raw seafood*
■ ***HIV disease:*** *disease caused by the human immunodeficiency virus, which may progress to AIDS; spread by direct or indirect contact with blood and body fluid*
■ ***AIDS (acquired immune deficiency syndrome):*** *a progressive fatal disease caused by the HIV virus and spread by contact with blood or moist body fluids*
■ ***jaundice:*** *a yellow color of the skin caused by hepatitis and other liver diseases*

Rules for Handwashing

Never wash your gloved hands. Handwashing damages the gloves so they will not protect you. Remove gloves, wash your hands, then reapply a clean pair of gloves.

■ Avoid leaning against the sink during the handwashing procedure. The inside of the sink and the faucet handles are considered contaminated.

■ Avoid splashing your uniform when washing your hands.

■ Keep your fingertips pointed down during the handwashing procedure.

■ Bar soap can hold microorganisms on its surface. Use liquid soap whenever possible.

■ Turn the faucets on with a paper towel if this is your facility's policy.

■ Always turn the faucets off with a clean, dry paper towel.

■■■ BLOODBORNE PATHOGENS

Bloodborne pathogens are microbes that cause disease and are spread through contact with blood, **nonintact skin**, **mucous membranes**, **secretions**, **excretions**, or any moist body fluid except sweat. Many diseases can be transmitted by contact with these substances. **Hepatitis B**, **hepatitis C**, **HIV disease**, and **AIDS** are commonly spread through contact with blood and body fluids.

Hepatitis B is a virus that causes an infection of the liver. This disease infects approximately 300,000 people a year. Of these, roughly 12,000 are health care workers. The virus causes about 7,000 deaths each year. Individuals with hepatitis B may have no symptoms at all, but may still be infectious. These people are carriers of the disease. The presence of hepatitis B can be diagnosed only by a blood test. You probably cannot tell that the carrier is sick by appearance. Some people have only mild symptoms that mimic the flu. Some common symptoms of hepatitis B disease are fever, aches and pains, nausea, and fatigue. The urine may turn dark in color. The skin, mucous membranes, and white area of the eyes may appear **jaundiced** or yellow in color. A person is sometimes able to transmit the disease even after he has recovered from the symptoms. Many people who have had hepatitis B have permanent liver damage and are disabled for life.

Human immunodeficiency virus is the virus that causes HIV disease and AIDS. When a person first becomes infected, she is called "HIV Positive, or HIV+." A newer term for this is to say that the individual has HIV disease. Most, but not all, people with HIV disease develop AIDS over time. After exposure to HIV, a person may have no symptoms at all. Sometime between one week and six months later, the exposed person may develop fever and flu-like symptoms. When this occurs, the blood converts from HIV-negative to HIV-positive. This can be very confusing because some individuals can go for longer periods before the blood converts from negative to positive. Some people convert from negative to positive but do not experience the flu-like symptoms. These people do not know that they are HIV positive. The only way to know for sure is to do a blood test. Once a person converts to HIV positive, it may take 6 to 10 years or more for AIDS to develop. Even if AIDS does not develop, the HIV-positive person becomes a lifelong carrier and can spread the virus to others.

As the disease progresses, the immune system is destroyed. When the blood count reaches a certain level, the patient develops AIDS, and becomes prone to many illnesses and infections because of the immune system destruction. Normally the immune system would prevent these infections from causing illness. A person with AIDS may have a chronic fever and swelling of the lymph nodes, particularly in the neck, armpits, and groin. Weight loss, diarrhea, and night sweats are common. The patient feels very tired. He may develop white patches called *thrush* (Figure 2-12) inside the mouth and throat. Occasionally, Kaposi's sarcoma develops (Figures 2-13A and 2-13B). This is a form of cancer in which

Figure 2-12 Oral thrush in an AIDS patient. (Courtesy Daniel J. Barbaro, M.D., Fort Worth, Texas)

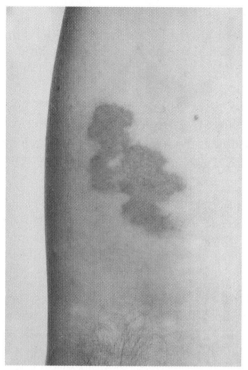

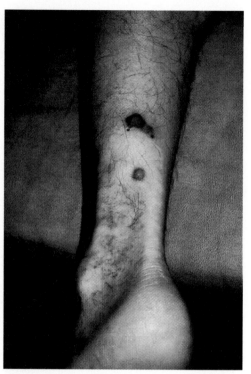

Figure 2-13A Typical purple lesions caused by Kaposi's sarcoma.

Figure 2-13B Raised Kaposi's sarcoma lesions. (Courtesy Daniel J. Barbaro, M.D., Fort Worth, Texas)

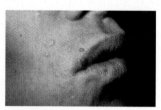

Figure 2-14A Oral herpes simplex molluscum. (Courtesy Daniel J. Barbaro, M.D., Fort Worth, Texas)

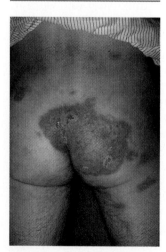

Figure 2-14B Chronic herpes in an AIDS patient. (Courtesy Daniel J. Barbaro, M.D., Fort Worth, Texas)

raised, purple spots appear on the skin. Many individuals develop chronic herpes (Figures 2-14A and 2-14B). People with advanced AIDS may develop mental confusion, emotional problems, and loss of motor control. When these individuals enter the health care facility for care, they are often in the end stage of the disease. Caring for them may be emotionally trying because many are young adults. AIDS is the primary cause of death in males aged 25 to 44. The staff may feel that these individuals are too young to die and have not had a chance at life. Many have young families and children. When caring for patients with AIDS, the staff must support each other, and may need outside resources to help them deal with their feelings about the disease.

AIDS is seen in all races and socioeconomic groups. State and federal laws prohibit discrimination against persons with AIDS. Some health care workers have contracted the HIV virus at work, but the total number of work-related cases is small. Estimating the number of new AIDS cases each year is very difficult. It is projected that there will be 1.5 million AIDS cases in the United States by the year 2000, and that 80% of all people with AIDS die within 3 years. However, new drug treatments appear to be extending lives, and this statistic may soon change. Remember that AIDS is *not the same* as HIV disease. People with HIV disease do not usually die within three years. The best way to prevent AIDS is to know how it is transmitted. Take measures to protect yourself both at work and in your personal life.

Over the past few years, great strides have been made in treating HIV disease and AIDS. A laboratory test called the *viral load* is used as an indicator of when and how to medicate. By monitoring the viral load, the physician knows when to change the patient's medications. Several different types of drugs are used in combination to treat the HIV virus in the body. These drugs do not eliminate the disease; treatment is geared to controlling symptoms. The combination drug therapy is effective in many patients because each drug works on a different part of the HIV virus in the body. The drugs control the new viruses that are produced in the body each day, but they do not reverse damage that was done before the patient began drug therapy. Taking the drugs exactly as ordered is important, because the HIV virus can become drug-resistant in a very short time. Taking the drugs as ordered increases the time during which the patient will benefit from the drugs before resistance develops. Because of the progress in treating the HIV virus, HIV disease and AIDS are now viewed as chronic, manageable diseases rather than fatal illnesses.

Because hepatitis B and HIV are spread by blood and body fluid contact, the diseases are seen in heterosexual, homosexual, and bisexual individuals. People who use intravenous drugs and share needles with others are at particularly high risk. Children born to mothers who are HIV positive may also be infected. People who received blood from 1978 to 1984 may have contracted HIV from the blood transfusion. Since 1984, donor blood has been routinely tested for HIV. You cannot contract HIV from donating blood at a blood bank or hospital.

You can contract HIV and HBV by contacting the virus through your nonintact skin (when cut or chapped skin touches blood or a body fluid containing the virus). The virus can also be passed by contact with the mucous membranes of the eyes, nose, mouth, and genital area. You cannot contract the virus through casual contact or airborne transmission.

The hepatitis B virus is much more contagious than the HIV virus. Imagine that one-quarter teaspoon of hepatitis B virus is mixed into a 24,000-gallon swimming pool of water. Someone draws a quarter teaspoon of that water into a syringe and injects you with it. Although the virus is diluted well, you will become HBV positive. Now imagine that 10 people are in the room. Someone takes one-quarter teaspoon of HIV and mixes it into a quart of water. A quarter teaspoon of this solution is injected into each person. Only one person in the room will become HIV positive. Hepatitis B is thus a much greater threat to health care workers than HIV. We now know that some people do not contract HIV because of certain elements within their cells. A vaccine is available to prevent hepatitis B. If your job involves handling blood or body fluids routinely, your employer is required to provide you with the vaccination free of charge. The vaccine is given in a series of three injections over several months. Presently, there is no vaccine to prevent HIV or AIDS. Employers are also required to have an **exposure control plan** that describes what to do if you contact blood or body fluid. Always report accidental contact with blood or body fluid to your supervisor immediately. The employer will treat you according to the established plan, draw blood samples, and may begin a combination of drugs to prevent HIV and HBV from developing. This medical care will continue over a long period of time.

■ *exposure control plan:* *a written program the employer is required to have; describes what to do if an employee contacts blood or body fluids*

■ PROTECTION FROM EXPOSURE TO PATHOGENS BY USING STANDARD PRECAUTIONS

Health care workers can take measures to prevent the spread of infection to themselves and others. These measures are called **standard precautions** (Figure 2-15). We cannot tell whether someone has a disease or infection by appearance. Therefore, we must use standard precautions in the care of all patients regardless of their disease or diagnosis. Standard precautions protect workers against many diseases besides AIDS and hepatitis B. Standard precautions involve the use of **personal protective equipment (PPE)** when performing certain tasks. Personal protective equipment protects the health care worker from contracting a disease from a patient. It also protects the patient from contracting a disease from a microbe passed from the worker's hands.

■ *standard precautions:* *measures that health care workers use to prevent the spread of infection to themselves and others*
■ *personal protective equipment (PPE):* *equipment worn to protect the health care worker and the patient from contact with disease-causing pathogens; also called barrier equipment*

Guidelines for Selection and Use of Personal Protective Equipment

Standard precautions are used whenever the health care worker anticipates contact with blood or any moist body fluid (except sweat), secretions, and excretions. They are also used anytime there may be mucous membrane contact. If either you or the patient has nonintact skin, personal protective equipment

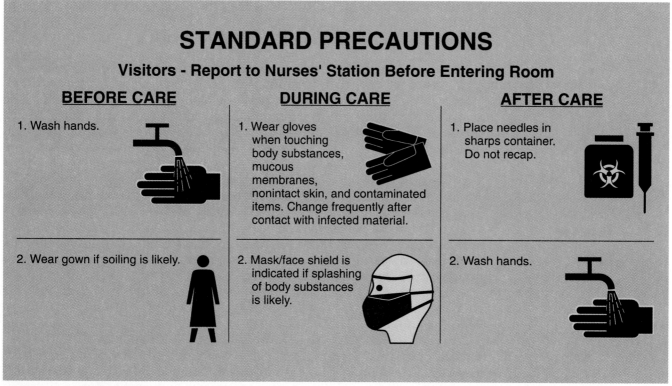

Figure 2-15 Standard precautions are used by all caregivers for all patient care. It is your responsibility to learn the principles of standard precautions and apply them. (Compliments of Briggs Corporation)

should be used. Equipment is worn during some direct patient care tasks. Personal protective equipment is also worn during cleaning procedures when contact with blood or body fluids is likely. It is your responsibility to select the personal protective equipment according to the task being done. Table 2-3 will guide you in choosing personal protective equipment for common tasks.

Personal protective equipment will protect you only if it fits properly, is free from defects, and is used regularly in the way that you were taught. You must study and learn the principles of standard precautions so you can use good judgment and apply them correctly. The purpose of using standard precautions is to prevent the spread of infection. Always follow the standard precautions and transmission-based precaution policies and procedures for your facility.

Rules for Standard Precautions

Certain common procedures apply to using standard precautions in all patient care. It is up to the patient care technician to anticipate and select the correct type of personal protective equipment and use handwashing before and after every procedure.

Handwashing. Handwashing is done before doing any patient care or procedure. It is also done before applying and after removing gloves. Even when gloves are worn, picking up a microbe on your hands is possible. Handwashing is also done immediately if your hands contact blood or any moist body fluid except sweat. Handwashing is also performed at the end of each procedure, after gloves are removed.

Barrier Precautions. Personal protective equipment is also called barrier equipment. Using barrier precautions involves wearing gloves for handling or touching blood, any moist body fluid (except sweat), secretions, excretions, mucous membranes, and nonintact skin. If your gloves become visibly soiled, you should remove them, wash your hands, and apply a clean pair of gloves. When

Table 2-3 Examples of Personal Protective Equipment in Basic Patient Care

Note: There are exceptions to every rule. Use this chart as a guideline only. Add personal protective equipment if special situations, such as splashing, exist. Follow your facility policies for use of protective equipment in routine tasks.

Patient Care Task	Gloves	Gown	Goggles/ Face Shield	Surgical Mask
Controlling bleeding with squirting blood	Yes	Yes	Yes	Yes
Wiping a wheelchair, shower chair, or bathtub with disinfectant solution	Yes	No	No	No
Emptying a catheter bag	Yes	Yes, if facility policy	Yes, if facility policy	Yes, if facility policy
Serving a meal tray	No	No	No	No
Giving a back rub to a patient who has intact skin	No	No	No	No
Brushing a patient's teeth	Yes	No	No	No
Helping the dentist with a procedure	Yes	Yes, if facility policy	Yes	Yes
Cleaning a patient and changing the bed after an episode of diarrhea	Yes	Yes	No	No
Taking an oral temperature with a glass thermometer (gloves are not necessary with an electronic thermometer)	Yes	No	No	No
Taking a rectal temperature	Yes	No	No	No
Taking a blood pressure	No	No	No	No
Cleaning soiled patient care utensils, such as bedpans	Yes	Yes, if splashing is likely	Yes, if splashing is likely	Yes, if splashing is likely
Shaving a patient with a disposable razor	Yes, because of the high risk of this procedure for contact with blood	No	No	No
Giving eye care	Yes	No	No	No
Giving special mouth care to an unconscious patient	Yes	No, unless coughing is likely	No, unless coughing is likely	No, unless coughing is likely
Washing the patient's genital area	Yes	No	No	No
Washing the patient's arms and legs when the skin is not broken	No	No	No	No

Table 2-4 Changing Gloves

Always wash your hands before applying and after removing gloves. Never touch equipment or surfaces in the environment with a contaminated glove.

Change Your Gloves:
- Before each patient contact
- After each patient contact
- Immediately before touching mucous membranes
- Immediately before touching nonintact skin
- After you touch a patient's secretions or excretions, before moving to care for another part of the body

- After touching blood or body fluids, before moving to care for another part of the body
- After touching contaminated environmental surfaces or equipment
- Any time your gloves become visibly soiled
- If your gloves become torn

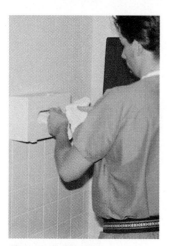

Figure 2-16 Gloves should fit properly and be conveniently located.

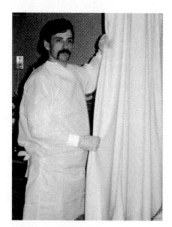

Figure 2-17 The gown may be paper, plastic, or cloth. It is chemically treated so it is water-resistant.

using barrier precautions, you should remove your gloves, wash your hands, and reapply clean gloves *immediately* before contact with mucous membranes and nonintact skin. Gloves (Figure 2-16) are also worn for touching dressings, tissues, infective items, and contaminated surfaces or equipment. You may have to change your gloves and wash your hands several times during the care of one patient. Use Table 2-4 to guide you as to when to change your gloves.

Your facility is required to have barrier equipment available in a variety of sizes in locations where use can reasonably be anticipated. Do not carry glove use to the extreme. Use gloves when necessary, but do not use them for all patient contact. Using gloves at all times sends a negative message. It says that the patient is untouchable. Touching is very important to all human beings. Gloves should be used only when contact with blood, body fluids, secretions, excretions, mucous membranes, or nonintact skin is likely. Be careful not to contaminate clean equipment, supplies, or environmental surfaces with used gloves.

A gown (Figure 2-17) is worn anytime your clothing may contact blood or other body fluids. The gown must be fluid-resistant. Many cloth gowns are specially treated to resist fluid.

A face shield (Figure 2-18A) or goggles (Figure 2-18B) and a mask are worn during procedures when body fluids or secretions may splash into your face. A good rule is that you can wear a mask without eye protection, but you should never wear eye protection without a mask. An alternate type of mask with a plastic eye shield attached may also be used (Figure 2-18C). The facial barriers protect the mucous membranes in your eyes, nose, and mouth from contacting pathogens. It is your responsibility to anticipate what you will need and put it on before you begin a procedure. Check the equipment before you use it. If it is cut or torn, it will not protect you and should be replaced. If you tear your gloves during a procedure, remove them as soon as possible. Wash your hands and put

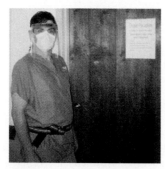

Figure 2-18A A full face shield is always worn with a mask.

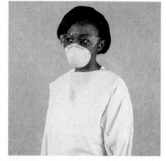

Figure 2-18B Goggles are always worn with a mask.

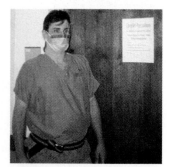

Figure 2-18C An alternate type of face mask with an eye shield attached.

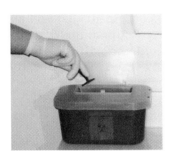

Figure 2-19 Razors and blades are disposed of in a sharps container.

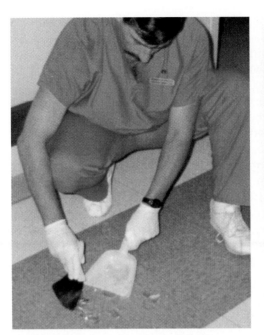

Figure 2-20 Use a broom and dustpan when cleaning up broken glass to avoid injury.

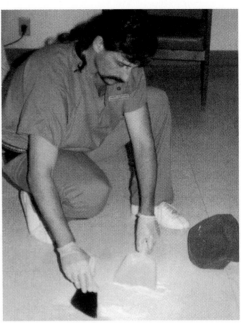

Figure 2-21 This absorbent powder has turned a body fluid spill into a solid material that can be swept up. The floor is disinfected after the powder is removed.

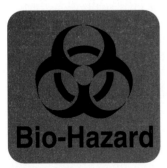

Figure 2-22 The biohazard emblem has an orange or red background with a contrasting color symbol.

■ *biohazardous waste: disposable items that are contaminated with blood or body fluids*

on a new pair of gloves before continuing. If your skin accidentally contacts blood or body fluid, wash the area immediately. Report the contact to your supervisor.

Personal protective equipment is discarded, laundered, or decontaminated according to facility policy after use. Be sure to replace what you have used so it is available the next time it is needed.

Needle and sharp precautions are also used. Handle needles, razors, and other sharp objects with care. Needles are never cut, bent, broken, or recapped by hand. After using a sharp object, dispose of it in a puncture-resistant "sharps" container (Figure 2-19). The sharps container should not be overfilled. The cap is placed on the container when it is three-quarters full. The cap is designed so that it cannot be snapped back off after it is closed. The sealed sharps container is stored until it can be picked up with the other biohazardous waste.

If you must clean up broken glass, always wear gloves. Avoid picking up glass with your hands. Use a broom and dustpan (Figure 2-20), forceps, or other mechanical method. Protect your hands from being cut. Dispose of the broken glass in a puncture-resistant container.

Follow your facility policy for cleaning up spills of blood or body fluid. Many facilities use an absorbent powder to soak up the fluid. After the fluid has been absorbed, sweep it up (Figure 2-21). Wipe the area with a facility-approved disinfectant. If your facility uses bleach as a disinfectant, it should be mixed in a container using 1 part bleach to 10 parts of water. Some facilities are now using a different concentration of bleach solution for cleaning blood spills, because research has shown that a much lower concentration can eliminate bloodborne pathogens. Know and follow your facility policies. The container should be labeled with the contents and the date it was mixed.

Items that have contacted blood or body fluids are biohazardous waste. Dispose of linen and trash contaminated with blood or body fluids according to your facility policy. Contaminated trash is discarded in containers marked with the biohazardous waste emblem (red or orange background with a black biohazard symbol; see Figure 2-22). Biohazardous waste requires special handling when it is removed from the facility. Having biohazardous waste removed is very expensive, so do not place non-biohazardous materials into this trash container.

Biohazardous trash is stored in a special holding area until it can be safely removed.

Body fluids such as urine can safely be disposed of in a drain connected to a sanitary sewer. Your instructor will teach you facility policies for handling and disposing of biohazardous waste.

Laboratory specimens are always considered potentially infectious. They are collected in covered containers. The containers are placed in sealed plastic transport bags with a biohazard emblem on them before they are transported to the lab. If a specimen must be refrigerated, it should not be stored in a refrigerator with food or beverages. A separate refrigerator or cooler, marked with a biohazard emblem, is used to hold laboratory specimens.

Each facility has policies and procedures for cleaning equipment that will be reused for patient care. If the equipment may have been contaminated with blood or body fluid, always use personal protective equipment. Utility gloves may be better for cleaning duties than the disposable gloves used in patient care. The chemicals used for cleaning make the pores of the disposable gloves too large. Although you probably cannot see this defect, the large pores may allow microbes to pass through the gloves to your hands. Follow your facility policy for use of gloves.

ISOLATION MEASURES

■ **isolation:** *measures used when a patient has an infectious disease to prevent the spread of pathogens*

■ **reverse isolation (protective isolation):** *used in some health care facilities to protect patients with weakened immune systems from contacting pathogens in the environment*

Isolation measures are used when a pathogen is present in a patient. Isolation is used to prevent others from contracting the disease. Some facilities place patients with diseases of the immune system in **reverse** or **protective isolation**. These patients do not have a contagious disease. Because of their immune system disorder, they can catch diseases easily. They are isolated to prevent them from contracting pathogens from others and from the environment. Patients with other conditions, such as burns, and those receiving cancer treatment may also be placed in protective isolation.

When caring for a patient in isolation, remember that you are isolating the pathogen and not the patient. Isolation can be very difficult for a patient emotionally. The patient may feel unclean, unwanted, and untouchable. Staff and visitors must wear personal protective equipment when they are in the room. Sometimes this is upsetting to the patient. A confused patient may be very frightened of staff wearing isolation garments. Because of the difficulty of putting on personal protective equipment, staff may not visit patients as often. This too can be difficult for the patient. Do everything you can to teach the patient about the purpose of the isolation. Check on her frequently, and avoid making her feel unclean, unwanted, and unloved. Use the least amount of isolation possible to contain the pathogen. Extra precautions beyond those that are required to prevent the spread of disease are unnecessary.

Transmission-Based Precautions

■ **Centers for Disease Control and Prevention (CDC):** *a federal agency that studies diseases and makes recommendations on protective measures*

The **Centers for Disease Control and Prevention** (CDC), recommend three types of transmission-based precautions. Standard precautions are always used in addition to transmission-based precautions. The type of precautions used is selected by the nurse manager and physician according to how the disease is spread. Transmission-based precautions are used because ordinary cleanliness and standard precautions may not protect you or others from the spread of certain pathogens. Patients with the same disease or germ may share a room. Otherwise, a private room is used to confine the pathogen to the patient's unit.

■ **airborne precautions:** *practices that health care workers use to protect themselves from airborne pathogens*

Airborne Precautions. **Airborne precautions** (Figure 2-23) are used for patients whose disease is spread by the airborne method of transmission. The type of pathogen involved is very tiny and lightweight. It can be suspended on dust and moisture in the air and travel for long distances in the ventilation system. Because of the mode of transmission, special precautions are taken to contain the microbe. A private room is necessary. This room must have a special ventilation

AIRBORNE PRECAUTIONS
In Addition to Standard Precautions

Visitors - Report to Nurses' Station Before Entering Room

BEFORE CARE	DURING CARE	AFTER CARE

BEFORE CARE

1. Private room and closed door with monitored negative air pressure, frequent air exchanges, and high-efficiency filtration.

2. Wash hands.

3. Wear respiratory protection appropriate for disease.

DURING CARE

1. Limit transport of patient/resident to essential purposes only. Patient resident must wear mask appropriate for disease.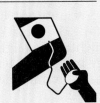

2. Limit use of noncritical care equipment to a single patient/resident.

AFTER CARE

1. Bag linen to prevent contamination of self, environment, or outside of bag.

2. Discard infectious trash to prevent contamination of self, environment, or outside of bag.

3. Wash hands.

Figure 2-23 Airborne precautions. (Compliments of Briggs Corporation)

■ **negative-pressure environment:** *a description of the ventilation system used in an airborne precautions room; the room air is drawn upward into the ventilation system and is either specially filtered or exhausted directly to the outside of the building*

■ **high-efficiency particulate air (HEPA) filter mask:** *respirator used to protect employees working in rooms of patients who have diseases spread by air*

system that prevents the pathogen from escaping into the rest of the facility. In a normal hospital room, the air is forced downward from the ventilation system. In an airborne precautions room, the ventilation is reversed so that room air is drawn upward into the vents. This creates a **negative-pressure environment.** The ventilation is either specially filtered or exhausted directly to the outside of the building. This room has 6 to 12 complete changes of air per hour. The door to the room is always kept closed.

Staff entering the room must wear a special mask, called a **high efficiency particulate air (HEPA) filter respirator** or **mask** (Figure 2-24). This mask has very small pores that prevent the pathogen from entering. The mask must be fit tested by a professional to be sure it fits the employee and does not leak. Each time you apply the mask, you must check the fit. After the HEPA mask is professionally fit tested, the employee must also have a medical exam to be sure

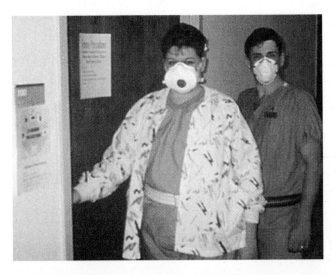

Figure 2-24 Disposable and reusable HEPA masks.

that use of the HEPA mask is not dangerous to her health. Men with facial hair cannot wear HEPA masks because the facial hair prevents a tight seal. If a man with facial hair must enter the room, he must wear a special hood. Because of the fit testing and health examination requirements, facilities may select only certain employees to work in isolation rooms where airborne precautions are used. When working in an airborne precautions room, no other personal protective equipment is necessary unless it is needed to apply the principles of standard precautions.

In hospitals and long-term care facilities, special rooms are designated as airborne precautions rooms. These rooms are ready at all times so that a patient can be moved into them immediately if a disease that is spread by air is diagnosed. Hospitals, HMOs, and other outpatient clinics may also have rooms with negative air pressure set up for certain procedures and diagnostic testing. Procedures that may involve splashing or spraying of respiratory secretions into the air are performed in these rooms. Staff assisting with such procedures wear HEPA masks and other personal protective equipment appropriate to the procedure.

A **PFR95 respirator** (Figure 2-25) or **N95 respirator** (Figure 2-26) may be worn instead of the HEPA mask. Some health care workers prefer these masks because they are lighter in weight and are more comfortable to wear. Like the HEPA mask, they must be fit tested by a qualified professional. The worker must also have a health examination. These masks are also fit tested each time they are worn (Figure 2-27).

■ **PFR95 respirator:** *a mask with very small pores that may be worn when caring for patients in airborne precautions*

■ **N95 respirator:** *a mask with very small pores that may be worn when caring for patients in airborne precautions*

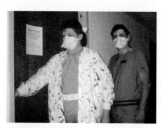

Figure 2-25 The PFR95 mask is preferred by some caregivers because it is light in weight but still offers good protection against airborne pathogens. It is used once, then discarded.

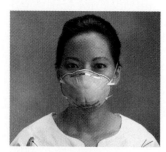

Figure 2-26 The N95 mask is used once, then discarded. (Courtesy of 3M Health Care)

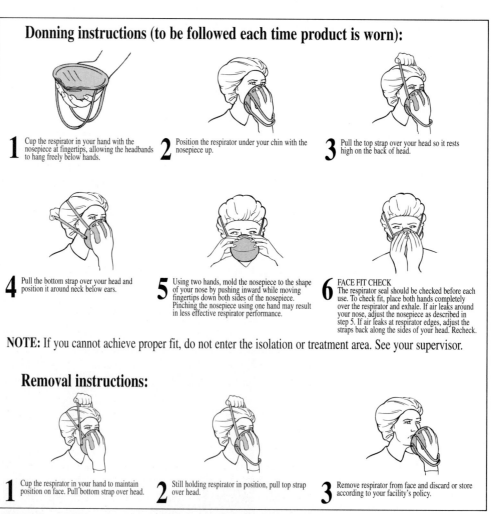

Figure 2-27 All masks worn in airborne precautions are fit tested each time they are put on. (Courtesy of 3M Health Care)

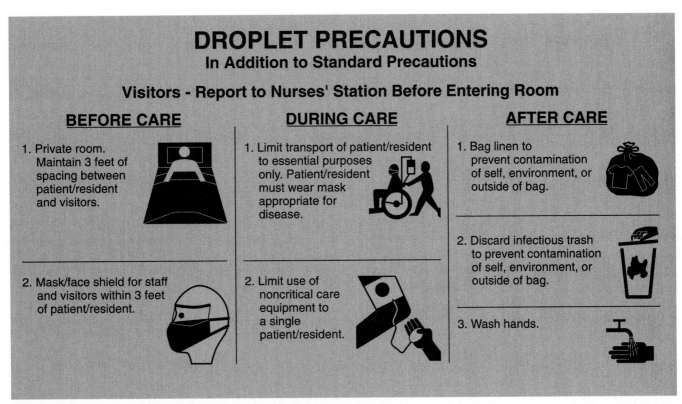

DROPLET PRECAUTIONS
In Addition to Standard Precautions

Visitors - Report to Nurses' Station Before Entering Room

BEFORE CARE	DURING CARE	AFTER CARE
1. Private room. Maintain 3 feet of spacing between patient/resident and visitors.	1. Limit transport of patient/resident to essential purposes only. Patient/resident must wear mask appropriate for disease.	1. Bag linen to prevent contamination of self, environment, or outside of bag.
2. Mask/face shield for staff and visitors within 3 feet of patient/resident.	2. Limit use of noncritical care equipment to a single patient/resident.	2. Discard infectious trash to prevent contamination of self, environment, or outside of bag. 3. Wash hands.

Figure 2-28 Droplet precautions. (Compliments of Briggs Corporation)

Droplet Precautions. Droplet precautions (Figure 2-28) are used for some patients whose infection is spread in the air. An example of a disease for which droplet precautions are used is influenza. The pathogen is spread by the droplets in mucus from oral, nasal, and respiratory secretions. The droplets usually remain within three feet of the patient. The secretions containing the pathogen are too large and heavy to be carried in the air currents. A private room is necessary, but special ventilation is not used. Regular surgical masks are worn. The pathogen is too large to fit between the pores of the surgical mask. The door to the room does not have to be kept closed unless direct care is being performed because the organism stays within three feet of the patient. No other personal protective equipment is necessary unless it is needed to practice standard precautions.

Contact Precautions. Contact precautions (Figure 2-29) are used when personnel may pick up the pathogen by direct or indirect contact. The microbes that spread disease by contact are usually found in infections of the skin and urine. Standard precautions are used in addition to contact precautions. Gloves are worn whenever you enter the room. No other personal protective equipment is necessary until you anticipate having direct contact with the patient or with environmental surfaces. When contact is expected, you must wear a gown to cover your uniform. Additional personal protective equipment is used only if you think that splashing of secretions is likely. If you think this may happen, you will need a face shield or goggles and a surgical mask to protect the mucous membranes in your eyes, nose, and mouth.

Special Circumstances. Patients may have infections that are transmitted by more than one method. A patient may have an infection, such as a cold, that is spread by the droplet method. The patient may also have a separate infection of the skin. Some diseases, such as chickenpox, are spread by more than one method. In this case, two types of isolation are used in addition to standard precautions. Table 2-5 lists common diseases and the type of transmission-based precautions used for each.

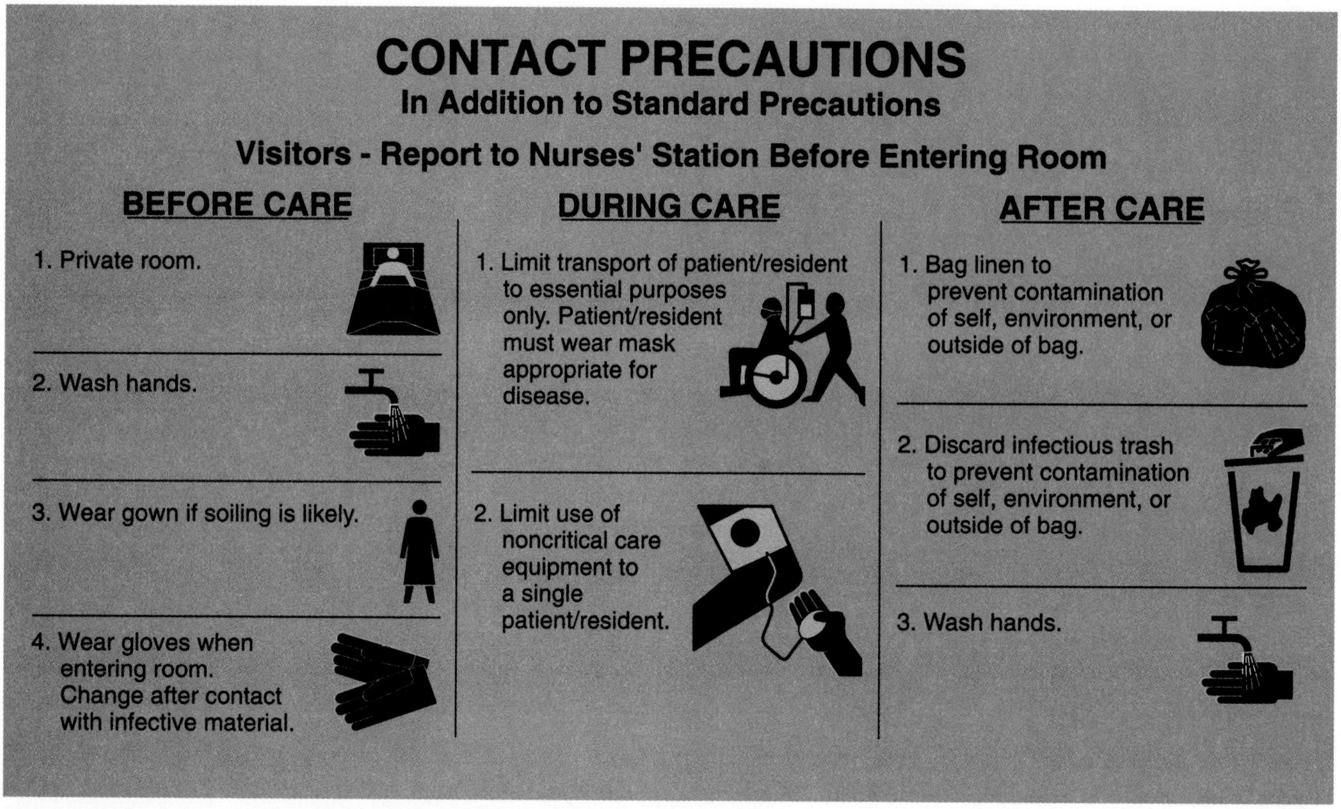

CONTACT PRECAUTIONS
In Addition to Standard Precautions
Visitors - Report to Nurses' Station Before Entering Room

BEFORE CARE	DURING CARE	AFTER CARE
1. Private room.	1. Limit transport of patient/resident to essential purposes only. Patient/resident must wear mask appropriate for disease.	1. Bag linen to prevent contamination of self, environment, or outside of bag.
2. Wash hands.		2. Discard infectious trash to prevent contamination of self, environment, or outside of bag.
3. Wear gown if soiling is likely.	2. Limit use of noncritical care equipment to a single patient/resident.	
4. Wear gloves when entering room. Change after contact with infective material.		3. Wash hands.

Figure 2-29 Contact precautions. (Compliments of Briggs Corporation)

Table 2-5 Diseases Requiring Transmission-Based Isolation Precautions

Use standard precautions in addition to other types of precautions listed.

Disease or Condition	Type of Precautions	Disease or Condition	Type of Precautions
AIDS	Standard	Infected pressure sore with no drainage	Standard
Chickenpox	Airborne and Contact	Infected pressure sore with heavy drainage	Contact
Diarrhea	Standard	Infectious diarrhea caused by a known pathogen	Contact
Drug-resistant skin infections	Contact		
German measles	Droplet	Measles	Airborne
Head or body lice	Contact	Mumps	Droplet
Hepatitis, type A	Standard. Use contact if diarrhea or incontinent patient.	Oral or genital herpes	Standard
		Scabies	Contact
Hepatitis, other types	Standard	Syphilis	Standard
HIV disease	Standard	Tuberculosis of the lungs	Airborne
Impetigo	Contact		

General Guidelines for Isolation Handwashing

- Roll your sleeves up to your elbows.
- Wash your hands and forearms following the procedural guidelines for handwashing.
- Wash your hands:
  - Before entering an isolation room
  - After removing the isolation gown and gloves
  - Before and after removing an isolation mask
  - Immediately before leaving the isolation room; use a paper towel to turn the doorknob when leaving the room
  - Any other time handwashing is required to practice standard precautions
  - Anytime your hands touch a contaminated or potentially contaminated surface

PROCEDURE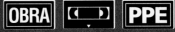

2 APPLYING AND REMOVING PERSONAL PROTECTIVE EQUIPMENT: DISPOSABLE GLOVES, GOWN, MASK, PROTECTIVE EYEWEAR

Applying Disposable Gloves

1. Wash your hands.
2. Remove clean gloves from the box.
3. Put hands into the gloves, adjusting the fingers for comfort and fit.
4. Pull cuffs of gloves over the sleeves of the gown, if worn.

Removing Disposable Gloves

1. Grasp the outside of the glove on the nondominant hand at the cuff. Pull the glove off so that the inside of the glove faces outward. Do not touch the skin of your wrist with the fingers of the glove.
2. Place this glove into the palm of the hand that is still gloved.
3. Put the fingers of the ungloved hand *inside* the cuff of the gloved hand. Pull the glove off inside out. The first glove removed should be inside the second glove.
4. Discard gloves into a covered container or isolation trash, according to facility policy.
5. Wash your hands.

Putting on Gown

1. Wash your hands.
2. Hold the clean gown by the neck in front of you, letting it unfold. Do not let the gown touch the floor.
3. Place your arms in the sleeves and slide the gown up to your shoulders.
4. Slip your hands inside the neck band and grasp the ties. Tie them at the neck.
5. Cover your uniform at the back with the gown and tie the ties at the waist. The gown must completely cover your clothing.

Removing Gown

1. Remove gloves, if worn.
2. Wash your hands.
3. If a mask is worn, untie the bottom ties of the mask, then the top ties.
4. Discard the mask.
5. Untie the waist ties of the gown.
6. Untie the neck ties of the gown and loosen it at the shoulders by touching only the inside of the gown.

continues

PROCEDURE **2** *continued*

7. Grasp the neck ties and pull the gown off inside out.

8. Roll the gown away from your body. Discard according to facility policy.

9. Wash your hands.

Applying Surgical Mask

1. Wash your hands. Remove a mask from the box by holding the ties.

2. Cover your nose and mouth with the mask.

3. Pinch the metal nose piece over the bridge of your nose until it fits comfortably.

4. Tie the top tie (or stretch elastic over the top of your head or ears, depending on the type of mask used).

5. Tie the bottom tie.

6. Wash your hands.

Removing Surgical Mask

1. Remove gloves, if worn.

2. Wash your hands.

3. Untie the neck tie of the mask.

4. Untie the upper tie.

5. Remove the mask by touching only the ties.

6. Discard according to facility policy.

7. Wash your hands.

Applying Protective Eyewear

1. Wash your hands and apply the surgical or HEPA mask.

2. Apply the goggles and secure the elastic strap around the back of your head, or apply the face shield.

3. Wash your hands.

Removing Protective Eyewear

1. Remove your gloves and wash your hands.

2. Lift the protective goggles or face shield.

3. Remove the surgical or HEPA mask.

4. Wash your hands.

Identifying Patients in Isolation. Most facilities post signs on the door to the patient's room when a patient is in isolation. The sign provides directions on personal protective equipment to wear and describes precautions to take. Some facilities feel that posting signs on the door of the patient's room is an invasion of the patient's privacy. These facilities usually post a stop sign on the door that advises you to check with the supervisor before entering the room. Before caring for these patients, you must get verbal directions from the supervisor or look for an isolation sign on the cover of the patient's chart or other designated location.

Sequence for Applying and Removing Personal Protective Equipment

There are times when you must wear full isolation garments in a patient's room. If you will be using your watch in the room, you should remove it first and place

General Guidelines for Putting on Personal Protective Equipment

- Wash your hands.
- Put on the isolation mask.
- Put on the isolation gown.
- Put on the isolation gloves.
- Apply goggles or face shield, if needed.

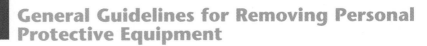

General Guidelines for Removing Personal Protective Equipment

- Untie the front waist tie (only) of the isolation gown.
- Remove gloves.
- Wash your hands.
- Untie the neck tie of the gown and remove it.
- Wash your hands.
- Remove protective eyewear, if worn.
- Remove your mask.
- Wash your hands.

it on a clean paper towel. You will carry the watch on the towel. The sequence in which you apply and remove your personal protective equipment is important.

Exiting the Isolation Room

If you used your watch in the isolation room, pick it up after removing your personal protective equipment and put it on your wrist. Holding the clean upper side of the paper towel, pick up the towel and discard it in the trash. Obtain a clean paper towel from the dispenser and use it to open the door of the room. After the door is open, discard the towel before you leave the room. The door may be left open in contact and droplet precautions if this is the patient's preference. Wash your hands again after leaving the room if this is your facility policy.

▄▄▄ DRUG-RESISTANT ORGANISMS

Drug-resistant organisms are pathogens that cannot be eliminated by the usual antibiotics. Additional pathogens, including HIV, are developing drug-resistant strains daily. These microbes have become a problem because eliminating them may be difficult or impossible. If antibiotics are available to kill the pathogen, they are often very expensive. These antibiotics may also have severe side effects, such as kidney, liver, and hearing damage. The elderly are particularly vulnerable to these side effects. Pathogens become drug-resistant for several reasons:

1. People went to the doctor and received antibiotics for minor conditions for which antibiotics were not necessary. Over the years, many unnecessary antibiotics have been prescribed.
2. People who were taking antibiotics stopped taking them when they felt better, but before finishing the whole prescription. The pathogens that were still in the body built up resistance to the antibiotic. The next time the pathogen was exposed to the antibiotic, the drug had no effect.

Methicillin-Resistant *Staphylococcus Aureus*

■ *methicillin-resistant staphylococcus aureus (MRSA): a common pathogen in health care facilities that causes illness or infection; resists treatment with most antibiotics*

Methicillin-resistant *staphylococcus aureus* (MRSA) is a common drug-resistant organism found in health care facilities. MRSA is very difficult to control and treat. It causes many different types of infections, including respiratory, skin, and urinary infections. As with the other pathogens discussed earlier, you cannot always tell that the person has an infection. MRSA is spread primarily by direct and indirect contact. Occasionally it is spread through the respiratory and urinary tracts. Use of standard precautions will prevent the spread of MRSA, particularly in urine and in skin infections. Contact precautions are used if the patient has known MRSA in a wound or urine. Droplet precautions are used when a patient is known to have MRSA in the respiratory tract.

Vancomycin-Resistant *Enterococcus*

Vancomycin-resistant *enterococcus* (VRE), is a newer drug-resistant organism. It originates in the colon, but can cause severe infections in other parts of the body. This organism is spread by contact. Standard precautions will also prevent the spread of this pathogen.

■■■■ TUBERCULOSIS

Tuberculosis (TB) is a disease that has been with us for many years. The incidence of tuberculosis was steadily declining until the 1980s, when it began increasing. Many cases of tuberculosis that we see today are drug-resistant. Tuberculosis is spread only through the airborne method, but the organism is very small and can travel long distances in the air. Tuberculosis can occur in many different sites in the body, but it is always spread by air and not through contact.

Signs and Symptoms of Tuberculosis

Signs and symptoms of tuberculosis are feeling tired and sleepy all the time, fever, night sweats, weight loss, cough, coughing up blood-tinged mucus, chest pain, and shortness of breath. When a patient has tuberculosis, airborne precautions are used. A HEPA mask is worn and the room must have negative-pressure ventilation. A patient can usually be removed from isolation after two to three weeks of antibiotics, but treatment will continue for six months to a year.

Testing for Tuberculosis

Health care facilities are required to test patients and employees periodically for the presence of the organism that causes TB. Skin testing is done. Health care facilities are currently using a two-step test for initial testing and a one-step test thereafter. Employees are tested upon employment, then every 3 to 12 months. The frequency of testing is determined by how high the risk of infection is in your health care agency and community. If the skin test is positive, the employee is referred to a physician or public health agency for follow-up. A chest x-ray and other lab tests are done. If the tests are negative, another x-ray will be required if the employee later develops symptoms suggesting tuberculosis. A positive skin test does not mean that an individual has TB. It means that she has been exposed to the pathogen that causes tuberculosis and that further testing and treatment may be indicated. Individuals over the age of 35 are not always treated because the drugs used to treat TB can cause complications in persons of this age. The decision on whether to treat is left to the individual, the personal physician, and the local health authority.

Treating Tuberculosis

Tuberculosis is treated with a combination of antibiotics. It is very important to take the antibiotics exactly as ordered and for as long as directed, to prevent drug-resistant tuberculosis from developing. If the individual is not treated, the TB germ can remain in the body for many years. It may become active sometime in the future. In some people it never becomes active.

Tuberculosis in the Long-Term Care Facility

Tuberculosis should be taken very seriously in long-term care facilities. Many elderly residents were exposed to TB years ago when the disease was common. Their skin tests are positive, indicating that the microbe is in the body and that they were not treated. As residents age, their immune systems weaken and the tuberculosis microbe may become active. Fatigue is often the only sign of TB in the elderly, so a number of people can be infected before the disease is detected.

■ *head lice: human
parasites that feed off blood;
cannot be contracted from
contact with pets or other
animals*
■ *parasites: tiny animals
that survive by feeding off
humans or other animals*
■ *nits: the eggs left by lice;
if untreated, the eggs will
hatch into more lice*

HEAD LICE

Head lice are **parasites**. Fleas and ticks are common examples of parasites.

Head lice are spread primarily by direct contact with an infected person. You cannot contract head lice from pets and animals. They may also be spread by sharing personal belongings such as brushes, combs, ribbons, caps, clothing, and bedding with others. Head lice do not hop, jump, or fly, but they can crawl very quickly. When performing hair care, check patients for **nits** (Figure 2-30B). These are tiny, oval eggs that are yellow-white in color. They are firmly attached to the hair and may be very difficult to remove. Empty nit cases are shown in Figure 2-30A. These nits have hatched into live lice—tiny brown insects about

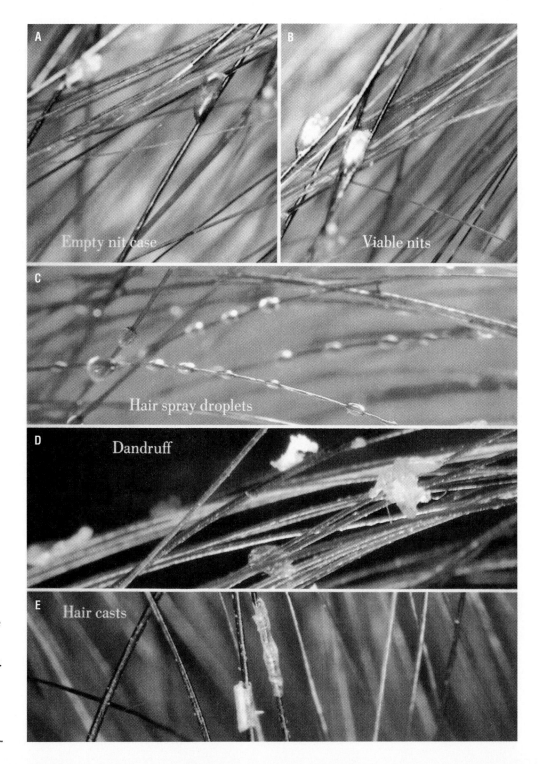

Figure 2-30 A-E Nits are eggs that attach firmly to the shaft of the hair and are difficult to remove. It may be difficult to differentiate one condition from another. Notify the nurse manager if the hair appears unusual. (Courtesy of Hogil Pharmaceutical Corporation)

the size of a sesame seed which move away from light quickly. Figure 2-30C shows how hair spray drops appear on the hair. Figure 2-30D is a magnified picture of dandruff. Figure 2-30E shows hair casts and plugs, which occur when oil glands in the scalp are overactive. They are easily removed. It may be difficult to differentiate nits from other conditions of the scalp. Notify the supervisor for further assessment if you find any abnormalities.

Treatment for Head Lice

■ *lice: parasites that feed on animals and humans*

If you suspect nits or lice are present, notify the supervisor immediately. You will be directed to wear gloves for further patient contact. You must also wear gloves and a gown when handling the patient's clothing or linen. The supervisor will contact the physician and obtain an order for a special medicated shampoo to kill the parasite. The patient's hair must be washed with this shampoo. Shampoos containing the chemical lindane are toxic to some people, and so are not recommended. Contact isolation is used for 24 hours after the patient is treated. A special comb is used to remove nits from the hair. If the nits cannot be removed by combing, it may be necessary to snip the hair with eggs attached with a pair of safety scissors. The supervisor will inspect the patient's scalp the day after the medicated shampoo to look for additional lice and nits. You may be directed to check other patients for the presence of head lice, because this parasite is highly contagious.

As with other diseases, some head lice have become resistant to the medicated shampoos used to eliminate them. If the lice cannot be killed with a shampoo, the only way to remove them is by checking the head and eliminating them manually. It may be necessary for two people to check the head simultaneously, because the lice can run very fast.

All clothing and linen must be bagged and sent to the laundry for washing. Furniture and personal items in the room must be vacuumed to eliminate lice in the environment. Vacuuming is safer and more effective than using pesticide sprays. After vacuuming, wipe environmental surfaces with a facility-approved disinfectant to eliminate microorganisms left from the outside of the vacuum cleaner. Previously, toxic sprays were used to eliminate lice from environmental surfaces and personal belongings, but this is no longer recommended.

▆▆▆▆ SCABIES

■ *scabies: a skin condition caused by a mite; causes a rash and severe itching and is highly contagious*
■ *mite: a tiny parasite that cannot be seen with the eye*

Scabies is a disease of the skin caused by a parasite called a mite (Figure 2-31). Scabies is highly contagious and is spread by direct and indirect contact. It causes a rash (Figure 2-32A) and severe itching of the skin. The rash may be seen in the webs of the fingers, inside the wrists, outside the elbows, and/or in the underarm, waist, and nipple area. It is also sometimes seen in the genital area in men and around the knees (Figure 2-32B) and lower buttocks. One type of scabies causes scaling of the skin on the palms of the hands and soles of the feet. If you notice a rash in these areas, notify the supervisor immediately. As with head lice, you will be directed to wear a gown and gloves for further patient contact.

Treatment for Scabies

Special medicated creams and lotions are used to kill the mite. Treatments containing the chemical lindane are toxic to some people, and so are not recommended. Some strains of scabies have become resistant to common treatments.

The patient's nails should be clipped before beginning the procedure. The medicated treatment is worked into and around the fingernail area with a cotton swab. The patient must not be bathed before or after the lotion is applied. You may be directed to apply the lotion to the patient's entire body, not just the rash area. It is not applied to the eyelids or lips. Wear a gown and gloves when applying this treatment. The lotion remains on the patient's skin for 12 to 24 hours, then is washed off in the tub or shower. If the patient washes her hands during this period, the lotion should be reapplied. Depending on the so-

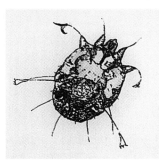

Figure 2-31 The scabies mite cannot be seen without a microscope. (Courtesy of L. E. Morris and Donna J. Lewis, "Management of Chronic, Resistive Scabies: A Case Study," *Geriatric Nursing* 16 (Sept./Oct. 1995): 230–37)

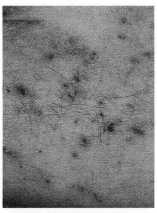

Figure 2-32A Typical rash of scabies on the back. (Courtesy of L. E. Morris and Donna J. Lewis, "Management of Chronic, Resistive Scabies: A Case Study," *Geriatric Nursing* 16 (Sept./Oct. 1995): 230–37)

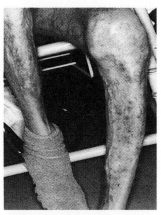

Figure 2-32B Typical rash of scabies on the legs and knees. (Courtesy of L. E. Morris and Donna J. Lewis, "Management of Chronic, Resistive Scabies: A Case Study," *Geriatric Nursing* 16 (Sept./Oct. 1995): 230–37)

lution used, the patient may require another treatment several days to several weeks later. It takes about a month from the first treatment for the rash to disappear. The patient may experience itching even after the scabies are eliminated. You may be directed to check other patients for the appearance of a rash. Facility personnel who have had direct contact with the host patient may also be treated to prevent the spread of the mite.

The patient's room, clothing, and linen must also be cleaned. The room and furnishing should be vacuumed well to capture mites in the environment. If items cannot be vacuumed, they are bagged in a sealed plastic bag for 14 days. The mite cannot live beyond this time without food. Some facilities expose the bags to extreme heat or cold to kill the mite more quickly. The mattress is turned and vacuumed, then wiped with a facility-approved disinfectant to remove microorganisms left from the outside of the vacuum cleaner. Contact isolation is usually used for 24 hours after the patient is treated. If the patient requires a second treatment, the cleaning procedure is repeated for clothing, linen, and furnishings.

Drug Resistance. As with other microorganisms, lice and scabies have become resistant to some of the pesticides commonly used in shampoos and body lotions. When treating for head lice or scabies, it is important to use the products exactly as directed. When treating head lice, removal of nits is important; otherwise the nits will hatch into live head lice. If live parasites are noted after a patient has been treated, it is recommended that the treatment product be discontinued. Products for treating lice and scabies are pesticides and repeated use can cause toxicity and other serious complications. Manual removal of lice and nits, using a comb, tweezers, or double-sided tape, is recommended.

KEY POINTS IN CHAPTER

Medical asepsis *refers to practices used in health care facilities to prevent the spread of infection.*

Microorganisms are everywhere. Pathogens are microorganisms that cause disease.

The most common methods of spread of infection are airborne, droplet, direct contact, and indirect contact.

KEY POINTS IN CHAPTER

— *The patient care technician plays an important role in preventing the spread of infection.*

— *The care provider must know which items are considered clean and soiled. These items must be separated to prevent the spread of infection.*

— *Handwashing is the most important method used to prevent the spread of infection.*

— *Bloodborne pathogens are microbes that cause disease through contact with blood, any moist body fluid except sweat, secretions, excretions, nonintact skin, and mucous membranes. HIV disease and hepatitis B are two diseases that are spread by contact with bloodborne pathogens.*

— *Hepatitis B is a greater threat to health care workers than HIV.*

— *Standard precautions are measures used in the care of all patients to prevent the spread of disease.*

— *The care provider is responsible for selecting and using the correct personal protective equipment for the procedure being performed.*

— *Needles, razors, and other sharps are disposed of in puncture-resistant biohazardous waste containers.*

— *Trash or linens that have contacted blood or body fluids are biohazardous waste.*

— *Isolation can be difficult for the patient emotionally.*

— *A HEPA mask is used when a patient is in airborne precautions. A PFR95 or N95 respirator may also be worn.*

— *A surgical mask is used when a patient is in droplet precautions.*

— *A gown and gloves are used when a patient is in contact precautions.*

— *Standard precautions are used in addition to other isolation measures.*

— *Drug-resistant organisms are a problem in health care facilities. Their spread can be prevented by medical asepsis and use of standard precautions.*

— *Tuberculosis is a growing public health problem that is detected by a skin test and treated with antibiotics.*

— *Head lice and scabies are highly contagious and require the use of contact precautions for 24 hours after the patient is treated.*

REVIEW QUIZ

Multiple Choice Questions

1. Medical asepsis is:
   a. a surgical technique.
   b. practices used to prevent the spread of infection.
   c. of concern only to licensed personnel.
   d. part of the chain of infection.

2. An infection that develops when a person is a patient in a health care facility is called a/an:
   a. facility infection.   c. nosocomial infection.
   b. acquired infection.   d. delayed infection.

3. Some factors that affect the body's natural ability to resist disease are:
   a. age and overall health.
   b. nutritional status and presence of other diseases.
   c. some medications.
   d. all of the above.

4. The system that detects pathogens in the body and stimulates the body's defenses to prevent disease is the:
   a. immune system.
   b. nervous system.
   c. genitourinary system
   d. respiratory system.

5. Infections can be spread by:
   a. direct contact.   c. vectors.
   b. inhaling a microbe.   d. all of the above.

6. An example of common vehicle method of transmission is:
   a. touching a contaminated object.
   b. eating contaminated food.
   c. inhaling droplets in the air.
   d. all of the above.

7. Droplets usually are confined to a space within:
   a. 3 feet of the patient.   c. 12 feet of the patient.
   b. 6 feet of the patient.   d. 24 feet of the patient.

8. Pathogens spread by the airborne method:
   a. are confined to a space within three feet of the patient.
   b. pose no threat to others.
   c. travel long distances in the ventilation system.
   d. none of the above.

9. The six factors necessary for an infection to spread are called the:
   a. mode of transmission.   c. portal of exit.
   b. reservoir of infection.   d. chain of infection.

10. Care providers should practice _____ _____ in the care of all patients.
    a. standard precautions   c. skin precautions
    b. substance isolation   d. isolation precautions

11. The most important measure health care workers use to prevent the spread of infection is:
    a. wearing a mask.
    b. handwashing.
    c. surgical asepsis.
    d. wearing a gown when close contact with the patient is anticipated.

12. Handwashing should be performed
    a. when coming on duty and when leaving at the end of the day.
    b. after personal use of the toilet.
    c. before applying and after removing gloves.
    d. all of the above.

13. Handwashing should be done for a minimum of:
    a. 3 seconds.   c. 10 seconds.
    b. 5 seconds.   d. 60 seconds.

14. A vaccination is available to protect health care workers from:
    a. AIDS.   c. herpes.
    b. hepatitis B.   d. all of the above.

10. Hepatitis B and AIDS are spread by:
    a. blood and body fluid contact.
    b. the inhalation method.

c. casual contact.
d. all of the above.

16. Gloves should be worn when:
    a. serving meal trays.   c. taking a blood pressure.
    b. passing ice.   d. brushing a patient's teeth.

17. The transmission-based precautions category in which a gown is routinely worn during close patient care is:
    a. airborne precautions.   c. droplet precautions.
    b. contact precautions.   d. universal precautions.

18. When working in an airborne precautions room, you should wear a:
    a. HEPA mask (or equivalent).
    b. surgical mask (or equivalent).
    c. gown.
    d. face shield.

19. Trash that is contaminated with blood or body fluid is identified by:
    a. using a black bag.   c. the biohazard emblem.
    b. a circle with a slash through it.   d. none of the above.

20. Apply personal protective equipment in this order:
    a. gloves, gown, mask.   c. gown, mask, gloves.
    b. mask, gown, gloves.   d. gloves, mask, gown.

21. Drug-resistant organisms:
    a. are of no concern to the patient care technician.
    b. can be eliminated easily with most antibiotics.
    c. are a threat to patients and health care workers.
    d. are very uncommon.

22. Tuberculosis is:
    a. a growing public health concern.
    b. a disease that was eliminated in the 1960s.
    c. easily treated.
    d. none of the above.

23. Head lice and scabies are:
    a. the same as nits.   c. parasites.
    b. fomites.   d. all of the above.

24. When a patient has scabies, he will be placed in:
    a. airborne precautions.   c. droplet precautions.
    b. contact precautions.   d. secretion precautions.

True/False Questions

25. ____ The term *infection control* refers to practices that reduce the spread of infection in the health care facility.

26. ____ Susceptibility is the ability of the body to resist disease.

27. ____ Hepatitis B destroys the immune system.

28. ____ A handshake is an example of indirect contact spread of infection.

29. ____ A microbe that is capable of causing disease is a pathogen.

30. ____ The objective of using medical asepsis is to break the chain of infection.

31. ____ Always wear gloves on both hands when carrying contaminated items in the hallway.

32. ____ It is not necessary to wash your hands after gloves are removed.

33. ____ Standard precautions are used in the care of all patients.

34. ____ Gloves should be changed immediately before contact with mucous membranes.

Short Answer/Fill in the Blanks

35.–40. List six times when you should wash your hands.

35. _____

36. _____

37. _____

38. _____

39. _____

40. _____

3

Safety and Emergencies

OBJECTIVES:

After reading this chapter, you will be able to:

Spell and define key terms.

Describe measures to keep the environment safe.

List three measures to prevent burns in the health care facility.

Describe safety factors to consider when using heat and cold applications.

Describe safety factors to use when caring for a patient who is using oxygen.

List the three elements necessary to start a fire.

Describe your responsibilities in a fire, tornado, hurricane, earthquake, and bomb threat.

Describe what to do if you find a patient in an emergency situation.

List seven guidelines to follow in an emergency.

THE IMPORTANCE OF SAFETY IN THE HEALTH CARE FACILITY

■ **accident:** *an unexpected, undesirable event*
■ **incident:** *an occurrence or event that interrupts normal procedures or causes a crisis*
■ **incident report:** *a special form that is completed for each accident or unusual occurrence in a health care facility; describes what happened and contains other important information*
■ **factual:** *known to be true*
■ **resolved:** *through, over, completed*

Safety is everyone's concern. Special safety measures are noted throughout this text. Every employee of the health care facility is responsible for keeping the environment safe and preventing accidents. Accidents often result in injuries, which can range from minor to serious. An incident is an occurrence that disrupts the normal procedures and routine of the facility. It may be the result of an accident. A fall is an accident, but it is also an incident. If a confused patient wanders away but is returned unharmed, an incident has occurred. An incident report (Figure 3-1) is completed by the supervisor on all accidents and incidents. The incident report states what happened, describes injuries, lists witnesses, and notes special notifications of the doctor or patient's family. Information written on the incident report is always factual. If you are asked for information about an incident, state only what you *know* to be true, not what you *think* may have happened. You may be asked to do extra monitoring of the patient until the signs of the incident are resolved.

Most accidents can be prevented. Accidents can happen to patients, visitors, and employees. Everyone benefits from a safe environment. The most common accidents in health care facilities are falls and burns.

Physical and Mental Changes That Increase the Risk of Incidents

Physical and mental changes occur with aging and as a result of certain diseases. Many of these changes affect the patient's awareness of hazards in the environment, increasing the risk of incidents. Factors that influence patient safety include:

■ Changes in vision affect the patient's ability to see unsafe conditions. Other changes in vision may make patients unable to judge distance.

■ Changes in hearing may affect the patient's ability to hear warnings or approaching carts or equipment.

RESIDENT INCIDENT REPORT

IF INJURY SERIOUS, GIVE IMMEDIATE NOTICE TO THE ADMINISTRATOR
AND DIRECTOR OF NURSING SERVICE   **NOTE:** PLEASE COMPLETE IN DETAIL

INSTRUCTIONS: Completed report to D.O.N. for review and filing in Administrator's Office. Make detailed report in Nurses Notes/Resident Records.

DATE OF OCCURRENCE _1/4/97_ PLACE _Room 304_   TIME _4³⁰_ AM (PM)

NAME _Jane Walther_   TEMP _98⁴_ BLOOD PRESSURE _134/88_ PULSE _80_ RESPIRATIONS _16_

ASSISTANCE NEEDED (Partial or Total)	FUNCTIONING (Partial or Total)	MENTAL STATUS*** Yes No	BEHAVIOR PROBLEMS 1-Minimum 2-Moderate 3-Maximum
P T Ambulation	P T Bedfast	(Y) N Lucid	2 Confused
P T Amb. w/Cane, Crutch, Walker	P T Fecal Incontinent	Y (N) Labile	0 Withdrawn
(P) T Transferring	P T Urinary Incontinent	(Y) N Disoriented	0 Hyperactive
(P) T Wheelchair Mobility	(P) T Blindness	Y (N) Comatose	0 Wanders
P T Bedside Chair	P T Deafness	Y (N) Semi-Comatose	0 Suspicious
(P) T Bathing	P T Aphasia	(Y) N Forgetful	0 Combative
(P) T Dressing	P T Speech Problem	Y (N) Controlled with	2 Supervised for Safety
P T Grooming		Medication	0 Causes Mgt. Problems

RESTRAINTS ORDERED: ☐ YES ☒ NO ☐ NOT APPLICABLE   ***Complete this section **ONLY IF** mental status contributed to incident/accident

IF NOT USED, WHY? _____

WAS PRN MEDICATION ADMINISTERED BEFORE INCIDENT? ☐ YES ☒ NO ☐ NOT APPLICABLE

NAME OF DRUG ADMINISTERED & TIME ADMINISTERED _____

DESCRIPTION OF INCIDENT (include circumstances under which incident occurred): _Resident attempted to transfer self from bed to w/c unassisted. No witnesses to incident. Res. was found on floor. Brakes to w/c were not locked. Footrests to w/c were in down position. Res. had socks on feet, but no shoes. States "I slipped"._

INDICATE ON FIGURES PART OF BODY AFFECTED AND DESCRIBE EXTENT OF INJURY:

Bruise (L) temple
Skin tear (R) forearm
Bruise (L) ankle

PHYSICIAN'S NAME _John Dennis, D.O._

PHYSICIAN NOTIFIED: DATE _1/4/97_   TIME _450/_ AM (PM)

PHYSICIAN'S ORDERS, TREATMENT OR STATEMENT: _Cleanse skin tear & apply dry dressing._

HOSPITALIZED: ☐ YES ☒ NO NAME OF HOSPITAL _____

N511 (R 4/92)

Figure 3-1 An incident report is completed for all incidents and accidents even if there are no injuries. The report gives only factual information.

■ **tremor:** *involuntary shaking*

■ **reflexes:** *unconscious or involuntary movements*

■ **Tremors,** or shaking, occur with some diseases. This affects the patient's balance and increases the risk of falls.

■ Changes in the blood vessels may cause patients to become dizzy when they stand up.

■ **Reflexes** are slowed in the elderly and by some diseases. Reflexes are automatic reactions that cause us to pull away from danger. Because some individuals react more slowly, they cannot move away quickly. For example, if you place your hand under water that is very hot, you quickly pull away. If a patient with impaired reflexes placed her hand under hot water, she would remove her hand more slowly and might be burned.

■ Some patients suffer mental changes that cause them to be confused and forgetful. These patients may not use good judgment or not be aware of common dangers.

■ Some patients may be weak because of an illness or injury. This may cause them to fall.

■ Some medications' side effects cause dizziness, visual disturbances, and other problems that increase the risk of injury.

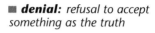

■ **denial:** *refusal to accept something as the truth*

Some patients may not be aware that their activities can be harmful. They may resent the staff's efforts to protect them. They feel that they can protect themselves. Patients may also be in **denial**. They are afraid that if they admit to having a need they will no longer be independent. All caregivers must talk with patients about safety. Explain what you are doing to keep the environment safe. Explain safety to patients in procedures that you do. Always be alert to safety factors when you enter and leave a room.

Providing a Safe Environment

You can do many things to make the health care facility safe. If you notice an unsafe condition that you can correct by yourself, do so immediately. Report unsafe conditions that you cannot correct to your supervisor or the proper person in your facility. Set a good example for others by using safe practices.

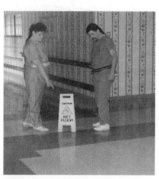

Figure 3-2 A "wet floor" sign is used to call attention to slippery spots.

Safety in the Hallways. Everyone is responsible for keeping the hallways safe. If you notice a spill on the floor, wipe it up immediately and place a "wet floor" sign (Figure 3-2). Keep all equipment and supplies on the same side of the hallway. Your goal is to have one side of the hallway free so that patients can walk safely without having to go around large pieces of equipment or wheelchairs. Follow your facility policy for separating items considered clean and soiled. Pick up anything dropped on the floor.

Never run in the hallways. Teach patients to use the handrails when they walk in the hallway. If you are transporting patients or equipment in the hall, watch where you are going. Approach corners slowly and look before you go around them. Take care when approaching or going through swinging doors. Back wheelchairs and stretchers in and out of elevators and down ramps.

Safety in the Patient's Room. Be sure there is enough light in patients' rooms. Visual changes that result from aging and disease make it difficult to see in dim lighting. However, avoid bright lights that shine directly into the patient's eyes. Remove any items that have fallen on the floor. Arrange the furniture so it is against the walls, not in the middle of the room. Other safety considerations for the patient's room are described in Chapter 8.

Avoid dressing patients in long clothing or gowns that may cause them to trip. Avoid clothing or linen that may get caught in the wheels of a wheelchair. If patients will be walking or transferring from the bed to a wheelchair, they should have nonslip soles on their slippers or shoes.

Follow your facility policy for use of electrical appliances such as televisions, radios, heating pads, and hair dryers in patient rooms. If you observe an electrical hazard, notify the proper person immediately. Follow your facility policy for removing the equipment from service.

Perform procedures in the way you were taught and do not take shortcuts. Shortcuts may injure you and others.

All patients should have a call signal within reach at all times. Even patients who are mentally confused must have a call signal available. Answer all call signals as soon as possible. If patients are unable to get up from the bed or chair, make sure that needed personal items are also within reach. If the patient has to bend or stretch to reach an item he needs, he may lose his balance and fall.

If you notice items in a room that you think are unsafe, follow your facility policy for removing them, or ask your supervisor for advice. Common items such as nail polish remover and denture cleaning tablets can be harmful if swallowed by a confused patient.

Safety in the Bathroom. Many accidents occur in the bathroom. Patients may be in a hurry to get to the bathroom. They may lose their balance, slip, trip, and fall. Sometimes they slip on water on the floor. Always check the bathroom for safety. Leave a night light or the bathroom light on for patients who get up at night to use the bathroom.

Check hot water temperatures with a thermometer before bathing patients. Water temperatures are regulated in health care facilities to keep the water from getting too hot, but sometimes the regulators fail. The hottest temperature allowed by law may be too hot for some patients. Use a thermometer so that you know the exact temperature of the water. Turn hot water on last and off first. Follow your facility policy for using bath oil. Some health care facilities do not allow it because it makes the tub very slippery. Use shower chairs in the shower. Do not leave patients alone in the bathtub or shower.

■ *chemicals: substances that may be harmful if they touch the skin or mucous membranes, and are usually dangerous if swallowed*

Safe Use of Chemicals. Many different chemicals are used in health care facilities. Most cleaning products are chemicals. Some cosmetics contain chemicals. Chemicals can be harmful if swallowed. Some will burn the skin or eyes. Some are harmful if inhaled. Keep all chemicals in their original containers. Never pour them into an unmarked container. The labels on cleaning products will have a warning if the chemical is dangerous. Cosmetic products are not required to have these labels. Use chemicals according to the directions on the package. Cleaning products should be stored in a locked area when not in use. Avoid storing them in the same area as food or beverages. If you are using a cleaning product in a patient care area, you must be able to see it at all times. Never put a bottle down and turn your back on it.

■ *Material Safety Data Sheets (MSDS): information sheets on chemicals used in the workplace that list the health hazards, safe uses, and emergency procedures for chemical exposure*

The Hazardous Communication Right to Know program is designed to make employees aware of the correct use and hazards of chemicals used in the work place. The health care facility is required to keep **Material Safety Data Sheets (MSDS)** (Figure 3-3) for all chemicals used. Know the location of these information sheets in your department. The Material Safety Data Sheets give instructions for safe use, identify health risks, and describe first aid and safety precautions.

Safety with Mentally Confused Patients. Besides the safety practices already discussed, keep sharp objects and plants away from persons who are mentally confused. If you are not sure about the safety of an item, check with your supervisor.

Equipment Safety. Use equipment only according to manufacturers' directions. If you have not been taught to use electrical or mechanical equipment, do not use it. If you feel that a piece of equipment is unsafe, follow your facility policy for notifying the proper person. Many facilities use a "lockout-tagout" system. Under this system, a locking device is placed on the equipment in a way that prevents the equipment from being used. A special tag identifies the equipment as broken and warns the reader not to use it (Figure 3-4). Always follow your facility policy for reporting and removing unsafe or broken equipment from service.

■ *lockout: placing a locking tag on a broken piece of equipment so it cannot be used*
■ *tagout: placing a tag on a piece of broken equipment that warns not to use the equipment until it is repaired*

Answering Call Signals

Your health care facility will have policies for staff to follow in answering call signals. The call signal may be the only way for the patient to get help in an emergency. Remember, all patients should have a call signal available at all times.

Most facilities require all staff to answer patients' call signals, whether they are assigned to care for the patient or not. Facilities usually have two types of call signals. One is the regular signal used in patient rooms (Figure 3-5A). The other is an emergency signal (Figure 3-5B) used in bathrooms, tub, and shower rooms. Become familiar with both types of signals. Regular call signals should be answered as soon as possible, usually within three minutes or less. Emergency call signals should be answered immediately.

When you answer a call signal, knock on the patient's door and wait for a response before entering. Identify yourself and ask how you can help. Turn the call signal off. Do what the patient asks, if possible, or notify the proper person of the patient's request.

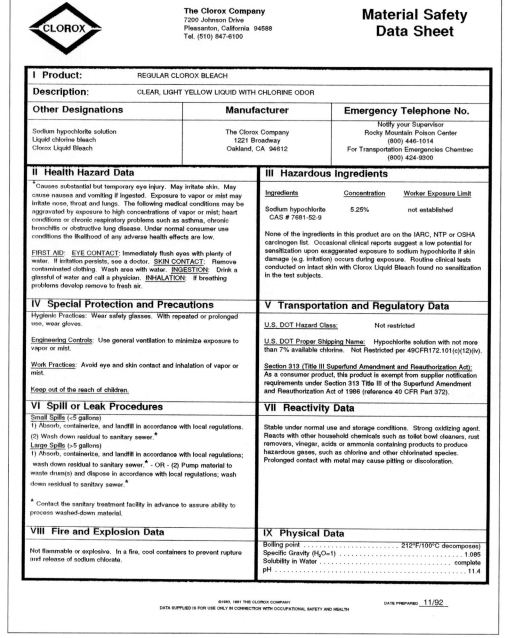

The Clorox Company
7200 Johnson Drive
Pleasanton, California 94588
Tel. (510) 847-6100

Material Safety Data Sheet

I Product: REGULAR CLOROX BLEACH

Description: CLEAR, LIGHT YELLOW LIQUID WITH CHLORINE ODOR

Other Designations	Manufacturer	Emergency Telephone No.
Sodium hypochlorite solution Liquid chlorine bleach Clorox Liquid Bleach	The Clorox Company 1221 Broadway Oakland, CA 94612	Notify your Supervisor Rocky Mountain Poison Center (800) 446-1014 For Transportation Emergencies Chemtrec (800) 424-9300

II Health Hazard Data

*Causes substantial but temporary eye injury. May cause nausea and vomiting if ingested. Exposure to vapor or mist may irritate nose, throat and lungs. The following medical conditions may be aggravated by exposure to high concentrations of vapor or mist; heart conditions or chronic respiratory problems such as asthma, chronic bronchitis or obstructive lung disease. Under normal consumer use conditions the likelihood of any adverse health effects are low.

FIRST AID: EYE CONTACT: Immediately flush eyes with plenty of water. If irritation persists, see a doctor. SKIN CONTACT: Remove contaminated clothing. Wash area with water. INGESTION: Drink a glassful of water and call a physician. INHALATION: If breathing problems develop remove to fresh air.

III Hazardous Ingredients

Ingredients	Concentration	Worker Exposure Limit
Sodium hypochlorite CAS # 7681-52-9	5.25%	not established

None of the ingredients in this product are on the IARC, NTP or OSHA carcinogen list. Occasional clinical reports suggest a low potential for sensitization upon exaggerated exposure to sodium hypochlorite if skin damage (e.g. irritation) occurs during exposure. Routine clinical tests conducted on intact skin with Clorox Liquid Bleach found no sensitization in the test subjects.

IV Special Protection and Precautions

Hygienic Practices: Wear safety glasses. With repeated or prolonged use, wear gloves.

Engineering Controls: Use general ventilation to minimize exposure to vapor or mist.

Work Practices: Avoid eye and skin contact and inhalation of vapor or mist.

Keep out of the reach of children.

V Transportation and Regulatory Data

U.S. DOT Hazard Class: Not restricted

U.S. DOT Proper Shipping Name: Hypochlorite solution with not more than 7% available chlorine.   Not Restricted per 49CFR172.101(c)(12)(iv).

Section 313 (Title III Superfund Amendment and Reauthorization Act): As a consumer product, this product is exempt from supplier notification requirements under Section 313 Title III of the Superfund Amendment and Reauthorization Act of 1986 (reference 40 CFR Part 372).

VI Spill or Leak Procedures

Small Spills (<5 gallons)
1) Absorb, containerize, and landfill in accordance with local regulations.
(2) Wash down residual to sanitary sewer.*
Large Spills (>5 gallons)
1) Absorb, containerize, and landfill in accordance with local regulations; wash down residual to sanitary sewer.* - OR - (2) Pump material to waste drum(s) and dispose in accordance with local regulations; wash down residual to sanitary sewer.*

* Contact the sanitary treatment facility in advance to assure ability to process washed-down material.

VII Reactivity Data

Stable under normal use and storage conditions. Strong oxidizing agent. Reacts with other household chemicals such as toilet bowl cleaners, rust removers, vinegar, acids or ammonia containing products to produce hazardous gases, such as chlorine and other chlorinated species. Prolonged contact with metal may cause pitting or discoloration.

VIII Fire and Explosion Data

Not flammable or explosive. In a fire, cool containers to prevent rupture and release of sodium chlorate.

IX Physical Data

Boiling point . . . . 212°F/100°C decomposes)
Specific Gravity (H$_2$O=1) 1.085
Solubility in Water . . . . complete
pH 11.4

©1983, 1991 THE CLOROX COMPANY
DATA SUPPLIED IS FOR USE ONLY IN CONNECTION WITH OCCUPATIONAL SAFETY AND HEALTH

DATE PREPARED 11/92

Figure 3-3 Material Safety Data Sheets provide important information and instructions on chemical use, health risks, first aid, and safety precautions.

Patient Identification Systems

■ **identification band:** *a plastic bracelet, usually worn on the wrist or ankle, that contains the patient's name and other identifying information*

Many types of identification systems are used by health care facilities. The most common is the identification band system, which used a plastic band placed around the patient's wrist. Some facilities use color-coded identification bands for specific purposes. For example, many facilities use pink or red bands to identify patients with diabetes, or for patients receiving blood transfusions. Some facilities use self-adhesive colored dots on the identification band. These dots have special meanings. For example, a patient on a low-salt diet may have a blue dot on his identification band. Find out the meaning of these markings, if used by your facility.

Many long-term care facilities place the resident's name on the door of the room. Some also place the resident's picture by the door. Sometimes special decorations, such as bows or decorated hats, are placed on the doors to help con-

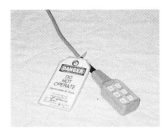

Figure 3-4 A tag is locked to a broken piece of electrical or mechanical equipment to warn others not to use it.

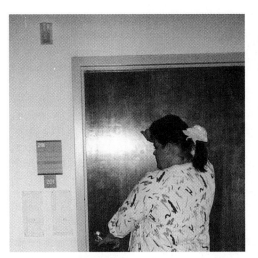

Figure 3-5A The light above the door in this health care facility is white, indicating a regular call signal.

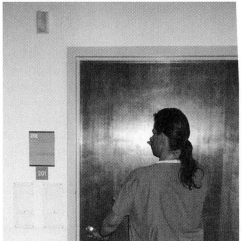

Figure 3-5B The light above this door is red, indicating an emergency signal. Some facilities use a blinking light as an emergency signal.

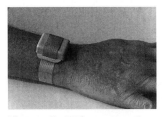

Figure 3-6 The magnetic sensor band is used in addition to the regular identification band. It sets off an alarm if the patient tries to leave through an outside door. (© 1996 RF Technologies. Used by permission.)

fused residents find their rooms. They are directed to find the "blue bow" or the "yellow hat" when they are looking for their rooms.

Some long-term care and psychiatric facilities use special identification systems for confused residents who may be endangered if they wander away. These devices (discussed in detail in Chapter 12) have a distinctive appearance. You can assume that if a patient is wearing one, she is at high risk of leaving the facility and will require close monitoring. Commonly, the devices are bracelets with a magnetic sensor built in (Figure 3-6). The sensors are similar to the devices used in stores to prevent shoplifting. The sensor allows the resident to move freely about the facility. If the resident tries to leave through an outside door, though, an alarm will sound. The bracelets are usually put on the dominant hand to make them difficult to remove.

Always identify patients before giving care. Check the patient's identification band and call the patient by name. Some patients will answer to any name they are called, so make sure that you have the right patient before giving care.

Burn Prevention

Burns are a leading cause of injury, particularly in long-term care. Patients with some diseases do not feel heat as acutely. Hot water may burn them during bathing or treatments. Occasionally, hot liquids spilled on patients result in burns. Unsafe cigarette smoking is also a leading cause of burns.

Cigarette Smoking. Know and follow your facility policy for cigarette smoking. If you smoke, do so only in designated areas. Most facilities do not allow smoking at all. Some facilities allow smoking outside; others do not allow smoking anywhere on the property. Some facilities do not allow patients to keep smoking materials. Many require that patients be supervised when they smoke. Patients are not allowed to smoke in their rooms except in special circumstances, and then only with direct supervision. Provide large, deep ashtrays for patients to use. Empty ashtrays only into metal cans with lids.

Thermal Burns. Thermal burns are caused by flame or hot liquids touching the skin. Be sure that you do not serve very hot food or liquids to patients. Help patients who are confused or who have poor hand control.

HEAT AND COLD APPLICATIONS

Heat and cold applications are used for many different purposes in health care facilities. Moist applications can be hot or cold. In this type of application, water touches the skin. Dry applications are those in which no water touches the skin. Some dry applications have water inside them, such as a hot water bottle. However, the outside of the application stays dry and the skin does not get wet. Sometimes dry applications are used to maintain the temperature of moist applications.

A localized application is used to apply heat or cold to a specific area of the body. An example of this type of application is an ice bag applied to a swollen ankle. A generalized application is used to apply heat or cold to the patient's entire body. An example of this type of application is the cooling or tepid sponge bath to reduce a patient's temperature. Many facilities use cooling blankets for this purpose.

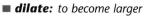 **localized application:** *applied to a specific area of a patient's body*
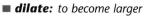 **generalized application:** *applied to the patient's entire body*
 tepid: *lukewarm*

General Principles for Using Heat and Cold Applications

Localized heat and cold applications that touch the patient's skin should have a protective cover. Covers are usually made out of flannel. Pillowcases and towels are also used. Some facilities use a thin layer of protective foam. Check with your supervisor for the type of cover to use. If the device you are using has a metal cap, such as a hot water bottle or ice collar, face the cap away from the patient. The metal in the cap can conduct heat or cold and injure the patient.

Many patients have impaired sensation because of aging or disease. Check the patient's skin under the application every 10 minutes. If the skin under a heat application appears very red, or if a dark area appears, stop the application and notify your supervisor. When using a cold application, stop the application and notify the supervisor immediately if the patient's skin appears blue, pale, white, or bright red. If the patient is shivering and cold, remove the application, cover the patient with a blanket, and notify your supervisor.

Applying Heat and Cold

 dilate: *to become larger*
 edema: *swelling*

Heat applications dilate the blood vessels to bring heat to an area. Heat may be used to relieve pain or edema. Local cold applications are used to relieve pain and prevent or relieve edema. Cold applications can also be used to stop or control bleeding. Cooling reduces the blood flow to the area. Generalized cooling may be used to reduce body temperature—that is, to cool the entire body. The elderly may be very sensitive to heat and cold. Help the patient into a comfortable position that she can maintain for the duration of the treatment. Expose only the part of the body that you will be treating.

Follow all safety rules to prevent spills and falls. If the patient has a dressing covering the area to be treated, ask your supervisor for assistance. Wear gloves if your hands will contact blood, moist body fluids (except sweat), secretions, excretions, nonintact skin, or mucous membranes. Always check the temperature of the solution to be used with a thermometer. You may need to add more liquid to the solution during the treatment to maintain the temperature. When

General Guidelines for Using Heat and Cold Applications

Before using a heat or cold application, you should know the:
- Type of application
- Area of the patient's body to be treated
- Length of time the application is to stay in place
- Proper temperature of the application
- Safety precautions to use
- Side effects to watch for

you are done with the treatment, pat the skin dry. Make the patient comfortable. Clean and put away used equipment. Remove gloves, if worn, and dispose of them according to facility policy. Wash your hands. Report to your supervisor that the procedure was completed and the patient's reaction.

OXYGEN SAFETY

When we breathe, we take in oxygen from the air. Oxygen is necessary for life. Some diseases and conditions cause the patient to be unable to take in enough oxygen. In these cases, the doctor will usually order additional oxygen to be given by an oxygen delivery system. The doctor will order how much oxygen is to be used. She will also specify the method of oxygen delivery and the length of time it is to be applied. As a patient care technician, you should not start, stop, or change the flow rate of oxygen unless you are trained to do this and your facility policy allows you to do so. Even in facilities that allow this, the technician cannot change the flow rate unless directed to do so by the RN. However, you must know how to check the flow rate and general safety measures to use when oxygen is in use. You must also be aware of where oxygen is stored in your facility, as the supervisor may send you for the oxygen supply in an emergency. In many facilities, the patient care technician is also responsible for the maintenance and cleaning of oxygen equipment. Know and follow your facility policy.

Usually, the patient receiving oxygen will need the head of the bed elevated. Elevating the head of the bed makes it easier to breathe. Follow the instructions on your assignment sheet and the patient's care plan.

Oxygen Delivery Systems

Several types of oxygen delivery systems (Figure 3-7A and 3-7B) are used in health care facilities. Oxygen may be piped in through the wall. Most long-term care facilities and home care agencies use oxygen tanks or concentrators. The oxygen concentrator takes in room air, converts it to oxygen, and delivers it to the patient. Oxygen also comes in a liquid canister (Figure 3-7C). This canister delivers a higher concentration of oxygen than a concentrator, but is portable and convenient. It does not require electricity to operate. The canister is quiet compared with a concentrator, which has an electric motor and makes a humming noise.

Oxygen can be very drying and uncomfortable for the patient. Dry oxygen can thicken the patient's respiratory secretions, making breathing more difficult.

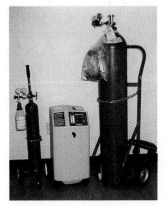

Figure 3-7A Oxygen comes in tank and concentrator form.

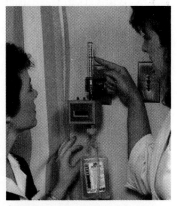

Figure 3-7B This facility has oxygen that is piped in through the wall.

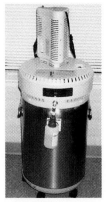

Figure 3-7C This liquid oxygen container has the portability and convenience of an oxygen concentrator, but is able to deliver a higher concentration of oxygen.

■ **humidifier:** *a device that adds moisture to the oxygen supply before the oxygen is delivered to the patient*

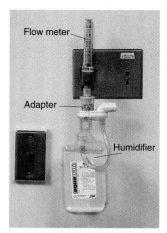

Figure 3-8 Oxygen humidifier

Usually the oxygen passes through water in a **humidifier** to add moisture before it reaches the patient (Figure 3-8). You may be responsible for checking and filling the humidifier with distilled water. The water level in the humidifier should always be at or above the "minimum fill" line on the bottle. Two types of humidifiers are commonly used. *Refillable humidifiers* are usually washed with soap and water every 24 hours. They are rinsed well, then refilled with distilled water. A sticker is attached to the bottle showing the date and time it was changed. Your facility policy may also require you to initial the sticker when you change the bottle. The *prefilled* type of humidifier is usually changed once a week, or according to manufacturers' directions. A sticker is also attached to this bottle showing the date. Cleaning and changing the bottles may be your responsibility.

Oxygen is given through a flow meter that shows how many liters of oxygen are being delivered to the patient each minute. Although you will not be responsible for adjusting this meter, you should check it each time you are in the room to be sure it is set at the proper rate. If you notice a difference from the ordered rate, report this important information to your supervisor. The gauge on tank oxygen also shows how much oxygen is left in the tank. Oxygen in tanks is measured in pounds. Follow your facility policy for checking this gauge and notify your supervisor before the tank is empty. Many facilities consider tanks to be empty when the pressure reaches 500 pounds. The tanks are changed when this pressure is reached.

Oxygen Equipment. The most common devices for oxygen delivery are cannulas and masks (Figure 3-9). The doctor will order the type of equipment to use. You must observe the skin under the device to be sure that it does not become irritated from the elastic that holds the device in place. Report any skin problems to your supervisor. Patients receiving oxygen may need extra liquids to drink. They may also need frequent care of the mouth and nose. Sometimes patients feel warm and will perspire heavily. Extra bathing and linen changes may be necessary. You may need to adjust the temperature in the room and help the patient change into lightweight clothes. The care plan and your assignment sheet will provide information on how and when to do these procedures.

Being unable to breathe is very frightening. Patients who are receiving oxygen may need reassurance and emotional support. Check on the patient frequently and spend as much time in the room as possible. Difficult breathing makes it hard to talk, and the patient may be unable to hold a normal conversation. Just being with the patient without talking is very reassuring.

Use of Oxygen in an Emergency

There are several differences between routine oxygen use and use of oxygen in an emergency. In an emergency, high concentrations of oxygen are necessary. A concentrator will not deliver an adequate amount of oxygen for emergencies. Concentrators cannot deliver liter flows over 5. Most facilities use piped-in oxygen or small, portable tanks for emergency purposes. Oxygen is usually delivered through a mask for emergency purposes. In an emergency, oxygen may be de-

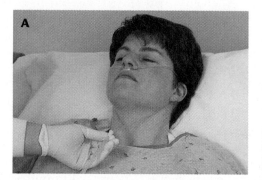
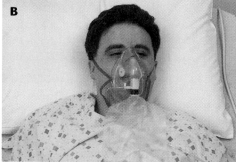

Figure 3-9 Oxygen is commonly delivered through a **A.** cannula or **B.** mask.

General Guidelines for Safe Use of Oxygen

Extra oxygen in the air may cause objects to burn or explode. By itself, oxygen is not explosive. The patient's gown and linen on the bed absorb oxygen from the air. Special precautions should be taken when oxygen is in use.

- Post "Oxygen in Use" signs over the bed and on the door of the room, or according to facility policy.
- Some electrical appliances can cause sparks. Check with your supervisor before using a hair dryer, electric shaver, fan, radio, or television.
- Never use **flammable** liquids such as nail polish remover or adhesive tape remover.
- If tank oxygen is used, it should be secured in a base or chained to a carrier or the wall.
- Smoking is not allowed when oxygen is in use, and smoking materials must be removed from the room.
- Wool and synthetic blankets and clothing should not be used. Use a cotton blanket to cover the patient.
- Some facilities remove the call signal and replace it with a manually operated bell. The call signal may cause a spark.
- Avoid sparks. Static electricity can start a fire.

■ *flammable:* combustible; catches fire or burns readily

livered dry if necessary. If water is used, tap water can be used until distilled water can be obtained. The distilled water has no therapeutic benefit. It is used because the minerals in tap water may crystallize and damage the oxygen delivery system. Use of tap water for a short time will not damage the equipment.

■ FIRE SAFETY

Health care facilities are built with safety features that prevent fires from spreading. These safety features include doors that close automatically when the fire alarm sounds, automatic sprinkler systems, smoke detectors, and fire exits. Fire alarms and fire extinguishers are located on the walls in the hallways. The facility will have an evacuation plan posted (Figure 3-10). Many materials used on the floors, doors, walls, and furnishings are fire rated. This means that they take longer to burn. Nevertheless, fire prevention is a very important responsibility. Despite the built-in safety features, health care facilities catch fire. Many lives can be lost.

Your facility will have periodic fire drills. Take these drills seriously and follow instructions. It is important that your actions in a fire drill become automatic, so that if a real fire starts, you will react properly. Find the evacuation plan on your unit and become familiar with the escape routes. Know the location of fire alarms and fire extinguishers. Your facility may conduct in-services to teach you how to use a fire extinguisher.

Three elements are necessary for a fire to start: oxygen, fuel, and a spark or source of ignition (Figure 3-11). Oxygen is in the air. Wood, paper, linens, and other materials provide fuel. Two of the three elements necessary for fires are everywhere, so the only thing missing is the spark, or source of ignition.

Careless and unsupervised smoking is a major cause of fire in health care facilities. Follow facility smoking policies. Check for and remove smoking materials from patient rooms, if this is your facility policy. Another common cause of fire is electrical problems. Avoid overloading electrical outlets. Report frayed

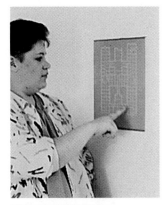

Figure 3-10 Become familiar with the evacuation plan for your unit.

■ **RACE System:** *the steps to be followed in case of fire*

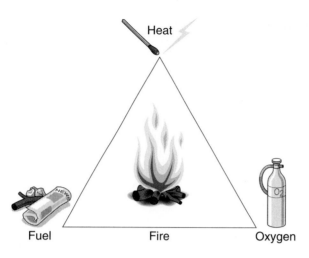

Figure 3-11 Three elements are necessary to start a fire.

Heat

Fuel   Fire   Oxygen

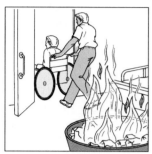

Remove

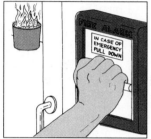

Activate

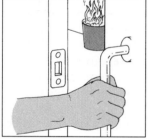

Contain

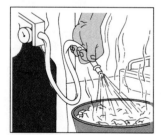

Extinguish or

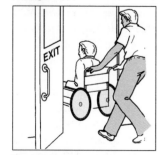

Evacuate

Figure 3-12 The RACE System

wires or other problems with electrical equipment to the proper person. Tag bad equipment out if this is your facility policy. Store flammable materials correctly, and dispose of trash and other wastes in the proper location.

Steps to Take in a Fire Emergency

In a fire emergency, remain calm—do not panic. Most facilities use the **RACE System** (Figure 3-12). The patient is removed from immediate danger. After the alarm is sounded (Figure 3-13), the fire is contained by closing doors and windows. Patients are moved behind the doors to keep them safe. Closing doors and windows slows the spread of fire. The hallways are cleared of patients and pieces of equipment that will burn. If the fire is large and spreading rapidly, patients may be evacuated from the building. If possible, use a fire extinguisher to put out the fire. Fire extinguishers are rated A, B, C, or according to the type of fire they are used on.

- A is used for trash, wood, and paper fires
- B is used for flammable liquids, such as grease and oil
- C is used for electrical fires.
- ABC is used on any type of fire.

Fire extinguishers are used by aiming the spray at the base of the fire. Remembering the word *PASS* will help you remember how to use the fire extinguisher:

- P   Pull the pin out of the upper extinguisher handle.
- A   Aim the extinguisher at the base of the fire.
- S   Squeeze the handle to discharge the contents of the extinguisher.
- S   Sweep the extinguisher from side to side while keeping it aimed at the base of the fire.

In a fire, smoke is very dangerous. If you are in a smoke-filled area, stay as close to the floor as possible. If you can crawl to an exit, cover your mouth and stay on your knees. The floor has the most oxygen available, because smoke rises. Before entering a room, touch the door with the back of your hand (Figure 3-14). *If the door is hot to the touch, do not open it.* If you are trapped in a room and the door is very hot to the touch, stay in the room and place wet blankets or towels under the door to keep smoke out.

■■■■ OTHER TYPES OF EMERGENCIES

When a natural disaster occurs, many people can be injured in a short period of time. Know what natural disasters are possible in your area and find out what evacuation or safety measures are necessary to prevent injury. If evacuation is anticipated, you may be instructed to tell ambulatory patients to stay out of bed and to get bedfast patients up in wheelchairs so that they can be moved quickly. Your health care facility will have a disaster plan describing what actions to take if a disaster strikes. Regardless of the type of emergency, remaining calm is important.

Tornado Safety

■ **tornado watch:** *a state of alert suggesting that conditions are right for a tornado to develop*

■ **tornado warning:** *a state of alert that occurs when a tornado is in the area*

Although rare in some parts of the country, a tornado can occur anywhere. All facilities have specific policies for natural disasters. Know and follow the policy of your facility. Your community will be placed under a **tornado watch** if conditions are favorable for a tornado to develop. A **tornado warning** is given when a tornado is actually in the area. Health care facilities do not evacuate patients during a tornado watch. Someone is designated to monitor the weather in case the situation changes. During a tornado warning, you may be required to help with evacuation of patients. This means that all patients will be moved to the basement, if the facility has one. Frequently patients are moved to a strong area in the center of the building. Patients should not be moved to areas where there are windows, as there is a chance that the glass will break. Evacuation must be done very quickly, as tornadoes strike with little warning. If patients cannot walk, they are moved in a wheelchair or bed. You may be instructed to cover patients with blankets to protect them from flying debris. You may also be required to close the room doors, fire doors, windows, and curtains facing the direction of the oncoming tornado. Next, open the doors, windows, and curtains on the opposite side of the building, if there is enough time. Do not go near the windows during the storm. Follow your supervisor's directions until the tornado has left the area.

Hurricane Emergencies

Some facilities are in coastal areas that are at risk for hurricanes. Hurricanes are not like other emergencies because they can be predicted in advance and there is adequate time to evacuate patients before the hurricane strikes. If a hurricane warning occurs, facility management may give the order to evacuate patients to an area farther inland. Medications and patients' charts are also moved. Follow the directions of facility management during the evacuation procedure.

If patients are not evacuated, you may be instructed to move them into interior rooms or hallways. As with a tornado, patients should be protected from flying glass and other debris. Close the doors to rooms and fire doors. Do not block the emergency exits.

Earthquakes

During an earthquake, the ground shakes. It may cause building destruction and fires. Windows may break and objects may fly around. Earthquakes occur suddenly and without warning. If an earthquake strikes, remain calm. Cover or protect your head from flying debris. Take cover under a large heavy object, if possible.

After the earthquake, check patients for injuries. Do not move injured patients unless they are in danger. Clean up spills on the floor to prevent falls. Do not smoke or use matches or open flames. Earthquakes can rupture gas lines, creating a fire hazard. Be prepared for aftershocks. Use a flashlight to see, if needed. Do not try to use electrical appliances. Listen to a battery-operated radio for emergency information.

Bomb Threat

Occasionally, a health care facility will receive a phone call warning of a bomb. A bomb threat should be taken very seriously. Facility management may order the building to be evacuated quickly. Law enforcement and fire officials will be notified. They will search the facility for a bomb and may help with the evacuation. If you answer the telephone and the caller tells you that a bomb is in the building, stay on the line for as long as possible and obtain as much information as possible. Ask where the bomb is or where it will explode, and at what time. Be very alert to the sound of the caller's voice, and try to determine age,

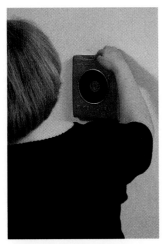

Figure 3-13 After patients are removed from danger, pull the fire alarm.

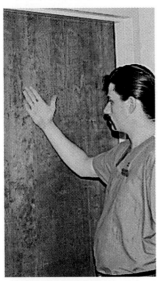

Figure 3-14 When you suspect a fire, touch the door with the back of your hand. If it feels hot, do not open the door.

sex, and other identifying factors (such as an accent). Listen for any background noises, such as music, church bells, or machinery. This information will be useful to the police later when trying to identify the caller. Follow your supervisor's directions in evacuating the facility. Law enforcement authorities will advise facility management when it is safe to return.

▄▄▄ OTHER SAFETY REQUIREMENTS

Many government agencies regulate safety in health care facilities. Some laws pertain to the patient care technician. These agencies routinely inspect health care agencies and respond to complaints about unsafe conditions. Health care facilities receive citations and fines if unsafe conditions exist, or if workers are not following safe practices.

Occupational Safety and Health Administration

■ *Occupational Safety and Health Administration (OSHA):* a government agency responsible for developing and enforcing job safety health standards to protect employees

The Occupational Safety and Health Administration (OSHA) is an agency of the federal government that is responsible for overseeing employee safety in the workplace. OSHA's role is to see that the worker is protected. Other agencies deal with patient safety. For years, OSHA inspected other types of businesses, but not health care facilities. This has changed, however, and in recent years OSHA has become one of the agencies that inspects and has regulatory authority over health care facilities.

OSHA inspects facilities to see if they are following governmental safety requirements. For example, facilities must have an eyewash station within a reasonable distance of where chemicals are used. They are also required to have a total body wash station. This protects employees in case chemicals are splashed into their eyes or spilled on their bodies. Most health care facilities designate the shower or tub rooms for this purpose. OSHA also monitors Material Safety Data Sheets. The inspectors monitor the use of infection control precautions and isolation procedures and check to see that the facility is following guidelines to prevent the spread of infectious diseases.

Safety should be taken very seriously. This will keep your facility in compliance with the various inspecting agencies and protect employees and patients from illness and injury.

The Safe Medical Devices Act

The Safe Medical Devices Act of 1991 requires a health care facility to notify the United States Food and Drug Administration (FDA) of any death or serious injury caused by any medical device or equipment. This federal agency investigates all reports of serious injury and death. Using medical equipment according to manufacturers' directions is important to prevent injury. Do not use electrical or mechanical equipment unless you are trained to do so.

Concealed Handgun Laws

Some states allow citizens to carry concealed weapons. Even in these states, guns *may not* be carried into a health care facility. Law enforcement personnel are exempt from this requirement. If a visitor is carrying a concealed handgun, he must leave it in his car before entering the facility. If you notice any individual carrying a gun, notify your supervisor immediately.

Violence in the Health Care Facility

Violence in the workplace is increasing in our society. Health care facilities are not exempt from incidents of violence. Episodes have occurred in both rural and urban communities. Many health care facilities have violence prevention programs. The goal of this training is to eliminate or reduce worker exposure to conditions that can lead to injury. OSHA has developed guidelines for preventing violence in the health care facility and many employers use these guidelines to implement safety programs and train their employees.

Potential causes of violence in the health care facility include:

- The prevalence of handguns and other weapons
- Acute and chronically mentally ill patients
- The availability of drugs in the health care facility, making it a likely robbery target
- The increasing number of gangs and gang members in many communities
- Unrestricted movement of the public in clinics and health care facilities
- Drug and alcohol abuse
- Distraught family members and other individuals who must wait for long periods in clinics and emergency departments, leading to anger and frustration
- Low staffing levels during meals and at other times when staff is busy caring for patients and unable to observe activity in the hallways
- Health care workers doing community work, often in high-crime areas
- Poorly lit parking lots, garages, and ramps
- Lack of staff awareness and attention to risk prevention, such as locking doors and reporting suspicious individuals to supervisors

Violence Prevention. The patient care technician should follow all facility policies and procedures involving safety and security. Other things you can do to prevent potential incidents are:

- Report suspicious individuals or other potential safety hazards to your supervisor.
- If you are responsible for a secured area, control access to the area and keep it locked.
- Participate in facility continuing education programs to learn how to recognize and manage escalating agitation, assaultive behavior, or criminal intent.
- Attend classes on cultural diversity that offer sensitivity training on racial and ethnic issues and differences.
- Report assaults or threats of assaults to a supervisor or manager immediately.
- Avoid wearing jewelry that could injure you if a patient or other individual attacks you.
- Avoid entering seclusion rooms alone.
- Avoid remote, dark areas when you are alone.
- Exercise caution in elevators, stairwells, and unfamiliar homes and apartments. Immediately leave the area if you believe a hazard exists.
- Use the "buddy system" if personal safety may be threatened.
- If a patient or other person is "acting out," or you believe you may be assaulted, do not let the person come between you and the exit.

EMERGENCY PROCEDURES

When an emergency occurs in a health care facility, the licensed supervisor is usually responsible for treatment of the patient. You should follow your supervisor's instructions and assist as directed. Sometimes, however, you must act immediately to keep the patient from serious harm.

Caring for a Patient Who Has Fainted

- *syncope:* fainting

Fainting, or syncope, occurs when the blood supply to the brain is not adequate. This sometimes occurs as a result of medical problems when patients sit or stand too quickly. The medical condition causes a temporary decrease in the

General Guidelines to Follow in All Emergencies

- ■ If you discover a patient who is ill or injured, stay with the patient and call for help. Your facility will teach you the policy for getting help. Some facilities instruct employees to call out. Others instruct you to pull the call signal or bathroom emergency signal. Nevertheless, do not leave the patient alone while you get help.
- ■ If the patient has fallen and is on the floor, do not move her unless she is in immediate danger. Moving may worsen an injury. The supervisor will check the patient and give permission for the move.
- ■ Stay calm and do not panic.
- ■ Start emergency measures that you are trained to do while you wait for help to arrive.
- ■ Once the supervisor arrives, do as he directs.
- ■ Know facility procedures and phone numbers for reporting emergencies and completing incident reports.
- ■ Know the location of emergency equipment and supplies in your unit so you can get them quickly if instructed to do so.

■ **level of consciousness:** *the degree of awareness or alertness, which ranges from fully awake and alert to confusion and unconsciousness*

PROCEDURE

3 EMERGENCY CARE FOR THE PATIENT WHO HAS FAINTED

1. Stay with the patient and call for help.
2. Lower the patient's head to increase the blood supply to the brain.
   a. If the patient is standing, help him sit or lie down.
   b. If the patient is sitting, have him lean forward and place his head between his knees.
   c. Once the patient is lying down, elevate his legs. Support them on pillows, if possible. This will increase the blood flow to the brain. Keep the patient's head flat.
3. If the patient is nauseated or vomiting, position him on the side. If this is not possible, turn the patient's head to the side.
4. Loosen any tight or restrictive clothing.
5. Apply a cool, wet towel to the forehead.
6. Check the patient's vital signs as directed by your manager. You may be asked to monitor them at 5- to 15-minute intervals until the patient's condition is stable.
7. Keep the patient quiet, with his head lowered, until directed by the supervisor.
8. Help the patient sit up gradually. Be prepared to act if the patient faints again.
9. Leave the patient in a position of comfort and safety. Usually the patient is returned to bed with the side rails up until he has recovered. Leave the call signal and needed personal items within reach.
10. Wash your hands.
11. Report to the supervisor:
    a. The time the patient fainted and how long he was unconscious.
    b. The patient's appearance when the incident occurred.
    c. Any measures that you took to assist the patient and the results.
    d. Visual problems, change in color, excessive perspiration.
    e. Presence of nausea, vomiting, changes in color or temperature of the skin, and changes in the patient's **level of consciousness**.
    f. Vital signs.

blood flow to the brain, and the patient may lose consciousness. The purpose of emergency treatment for this condition is to restore the blood supply to the patient's brain and prevent injury. During this procedure, you will be required to take the patient's vital signs: temperature, pulse, respiration, and blood pressure. You will learn these procedures in Chapter 13.

Caring for a Patient Who Is Having a Seizure

A seizure is caused by a disturbance of the impulses in the brain. Epilepsy, other diseases, injuries, medication, fever, and infection can cause seizures. A seizure is also called a *convulsion*. There are many different types of seizures. Some appear mild, others appear severe. Characteristics are described in Table 3-1. The most common types of seizures are related to epilepsy. Some patients have a sen-

Table 3-1 Seizure Characteristics

Type of Seizure	Signs of Seizure Activity	Comment
Generalized Tonic-Clonic Seizure (Grand Mal Seizure)	May be preceded by an aura. Patient loses consciousness. Convulsive activity, characterized by rigid stiffening of muscles and jerking movement of the arms and legs. Saliva runs from the mouth. Patient's color may change because of lack of oxygen. Incontinence of bowel and bladder.	Usually lasts 3 to 4 minutes. The patient may be very tired after the seizure and may have a headache. The patient may be mentally confused, have slurred speech, and be very weak. The patient will not remember the seizure.
Absence Seizure (Petit Mal Seizure)	Staring, blinking, or stopping what the patient is doing. The patient may stare blankly. One muscle group may twitch or jerk.	Petit mal seizures usually last less than a minute, but may occur many times a day.
Simple-Partial (Jacksonian)	Muscle spasms of the face, hands, or feet. Starts at one extremity, such as an arm or leg, and progressively moves upward on that side of the body.	May spread to other areas in the brain, resulting in a grand mal seizure.
Complex-Partial (Psychomotor)	Abnormal acts, irrational behavior or loss of judgment due to a temporary change in consciousness. Automatic behavior, such as typing or eating, may continue normally. Patient may uncontrollably smack the lips, wander aimlessly, or uncontrollably twitch part of the body.	Usually lasts only a few seconds. The patient usually does not remember the seizure.
Myoclonic	Consists of one or more myoclonic jerks. The patient remains conscious but cannot control the muscle movement.	The patient is aware that an extremity is jerking but is unable to stop it. The patient remains conscious throughout and can remember the seizure activity.
Status Epilepticus	Multiple seizures occurring simultaneously with no break between seizures.	Status epilepticus may be precipitated by sudden withdrawal of antiseizure medications, fever, or infection. This type of seizure is dangerous and can lead to decreased mental function, neurological impairment, and death.

PROCEDURE
PPE

4 EMERGENCY CARE FOR A PATIENT WHO IS HAVING A SEIZURE

1. Stay with the patient and call for help.

2. Use standard precautions if contact with blood or moist body fluids (except sweat) is likely.

3. If the patient is in bed, remove the pillow and raise the side rails.

4. If the patient is not in bed, gently lower the patient to the floor, protecting her head.

5. Turn the patient on her side. If this is not possible, turn the head to the side. This allows secretions to drain from the patient's mouth.

6. Move any hard objects, or pad objects that may injure the patient with pillows, blankets, or other available items such as chair cushions.

7. Loosen tight and restrictive clothing.

8. Provide privacy by asking onlookers to leave, closing the door to the patient's room, and pulling the privacy curtain.

9. Avoid restraining the patient in any way.

10. Do not try to place any object in the patient's mouth. Doing this could break her teeth and cause injury to the patient and you.

11. Check the patient's vital signs as requested by the supervisor. You may be instructed to check vital signs frequently until the patient is stable.

12. Assist the supervisor as directed. The supervisor may need to suction the patient, administer oxygen, or give medication to stop the seizure.

13. When the seizure stops, tell the patient where she is and what happened. Assist her to bed. The patient will be very tired. Allow her to sleep.

14. Leave the patient in a position of comfort and safety. Leave the call signal and needed personal items within reach.

15. Remove gloves, if worn, and dispose of them according to facility policy.

16. Wash your hands.

17. Report to the supervisor:

   a. Any change in the patient before the seizure, such as an aura, confusion, or change in behavior.

   b. Loss of bowel or bladder control, eyes rolling upward, rapid blinking, tongue biting.

   c. Time the seizure started and stopped.

   d. A description of the way the seizure looked, including the body parts involved.

   e. Condition of the patient after the seizure.

   f. Vital signs.

■ **aura:** *a sensation of smell, taste, or bright light that precedes the onset of a seizure*
■ **fractures:** *broken bones*
■ **immobilize:** *to support an area in a way that prevents movement*

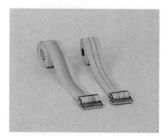

Figure 3-15 Different types of gait belts. (Courtesy of Skil-Care Corp.)

sation called an aura immediately before a seizure. A seizure is a serious medical emergency. The goal of seizure care is to prevent injury.

Caring for a Patient Who Has Fallen and Has a Suspected Fracture

Falls are common emergencies in health care facilities. In the elderly, the bones become more brittle and lose calcium during the aging process. The joints are not as flexible as they were when the patient was younger. Because of these aging changes, fractures, or broken bones, occur more readily in this age group. Sometimes fractures are obvious right away. An area of the body may appear swollen or deformed. If the fracture occurs in a hip, the leg on the affected side may appear shorter than the other and may be rotated outward. There may be bleeding from an injury. The purpose of emergency treatment for falls is to prevent injuries and to assist patients who have suspected fractures.

   If you are walking with a patient who starts to fall:

■ Keep your back straight, your feet about 12 inches apart, and your knees bent.

■ If the patient is wearing a gait belt (Figure 3-15), hold the center back of the belt firmly with an underhand grasp. Ease the patient down your legs

PROCEDURE

5 EMERGENCY CARE FOR FALLS AND SUSPECTED FRACTURES

Assisting the Patient After a Fall

1. Stay with the patient and call for help. Reassure the patient.

2. Use standard precautions if contact with blood or moist body fluids (except sweat) is likely.

3. Do not move the patient until the supervisor has examined her and given approval.

4. Check the patient's vital signs and assist her to bed as instructed by the supervisor.

5. Leave the patient in a position of comfort and safety. Place the call signal and needed personal items within reach.

6. Wash your hands.

7. The supervisor may direct you to monitor the patient's vital signs frequently until she is stable.

Assisting the Patient with a Suspected Fracture

1. Stay with the patient and call for help. Reassure the patient.

2. Use standard precautions if contact with blood or moist body fluids (except sweat) is likely.

3. Do not move the patient until the supervisor has examined him and given approval.

4. Keep the patient as quiet as possible.

5. **Immobilize** the injured area (Figure 3-16) so it cannot be moved. If the area appears out of shape, bent, or deformed, do not attempt to straighten it.

6. Check the patient's vital signs and assist him to bed as instructed by the supervisor.

7. If a fracture is suspected, several staff members must assist the patient to bed. One staff member is assigned to move the injured extremity. Other staff members will move the rest of the patient's body. A sheet or other lifting device may be used to move the patient.

8. Leave the patient in a position of comfort and safety. Leave the call signal and needed personal items within reach.

9. Wash your hands.

10. The supervisor may direct you to monitor the patient's vital signs frequently until he is stable.

11. You may also be directed to apply a cold treatment to the injured area.

12. Observe for and report:

   a. The time of the fall.

   b. The cause of the fall, if known. Do not guess. Report only what you know to be true.

   c. Measures taken to break the fall.

   d. Measures taken to assist the patient.

   e. Known injuries, such as bleeding, deformities, bruises, or changes in the patient's level of consciousness.

   f. Appearance of the injured area and steps taken to immobilize it.

   g. Witnesses to the fall.

   h. Vital signs.

   i. Any additional information needed to fill out the incident report.

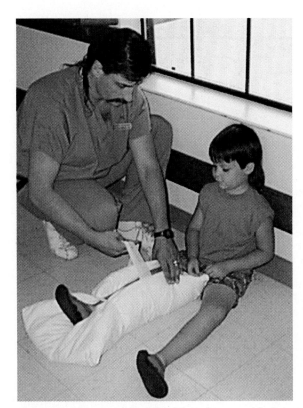

Figure 3-16 Immobilize the joint above and below a suspected fracture.

PROCEDURE

6 APPLICATION OF COLD PACKS TO STRAINS AND BRUISES

1. Notify the supervisor of the injury.

2. If the patient is on the floor, stay with him and call for help.

3. Do not move the patient until the supervisor examines him.

4. Wash your hands.

5. Place the patient in a comfortable position.

6. Use standard precautions if contact with blood or moist body fluids (except sweat) is likely.

7. Prepare the cold pack as directed by the supervisor and according to facility policy:

    a. Place a cloth or flannel cover over the cold pack.

    b. Apply the cold pack next to or on top of the injured area, as directed. If the patient complains that the cold pack increases the pain, remove it and consult your manager.

    c. Secure the cold pack in place, if necessary. You may need to prop it or tie it in place with a gauze bandage.

    d. Check the area under the cold pack every 10 minutes, and remove it if numbness or discoloration of the skin occurs.

    e. Remove the cold pack after 30 minutes.

    f. Reapply the cold pack as directed.

8. Wash your hands.

9. Leave the patient in a position of comfort and safety. Leave the call signal and needed personal items within reach.

10. Observe for and report:

    a. The time of injury and description of the injured area.

    b. Edema, deformities, or other injuries.

    c. Cause of the injury, if known. Report only what you know to be true.

    d. The type of cold pack applied and time.

    e. Response to the cold pack.

---

to the floor. Protect the patient's head from hitting the floor. Guide the patient so that he does not hit hard objects in the area.

■ If the patient is not wearing a gait belt, move close to the patient and wrap your arms around the patient's waist or underarms.

■ Pull the patient close to your body, sliding him down your leg to ease him to the floor. Protect the patient from hitting his head. Guide the patient so that he does not hit any hard objects.

Caring for a Patient with Strains and Bruises

■ **strains:** *injuries to muscles from stretching or overuse*
■ **bruises:** *injuries to the skin caused by hitting or striking; the area turns black and blue in color*

Strains are injuries that occur from overstretching or overusing a muscle. **Bruises** are injuries to the skin caused by hitting, bumping, or striking. The area usually turns black and blue in color. These injuries are painful and edema may occur in the injured area. The purpose of applying a cold pack to a strain or bruise is to decrease pain and swelling. You should apply cold packs only if you are so instructed by your manager. Cold packs are usually left in place for 30 minutes and then removed to avoid tissue damage.

Caring for a Patient with Burns

Burns are commonly caused by hot water or other hot liquids and careless cigarette smoking. Burns can range from minor to severe. Severe burns can lead to loss of skin, damage to the muscle, infection, and death. Even small burns can be very painful. The purpose of burn care is to relieve pain, prevent infection and other complications, and promote healing.

PROCEDURE

7 EMERGENCY CARE FOR A PATIENT WITH BURNS

1. Stay with the patient and call for help. Reassure the patient.

2. Use standard precautions if contact with blood or moist body fluids (except sweat) is likely.

3. Keep the patient's airway open and ensure that the patient is breathing.

4. Remove the source of heat, if present.

5. If the burn is minor and the skin is not broken:

   a. Remove the patient's clothing from the burned area. Do not remove clothing stuck to the skin.

   b. Immerse the burned area in cool water.

6. If the burn is very large or deep, do not get the area wet.

   a. Do not try to remove clothing stuck to the skin.

7. Cover the burned area with a clean pad.

8. Keep the patient as quiet as possible.

9. Cover the patient to maintain body temperature.

10. Check the patient's vital signs as directed. You may be instructed to check the vital signs frequently until the patient is stable. If the patient's upper arms are burned, do not take the blood pressure. Check with the supervisor for further instructions.

11. Do not give the patient food or fluids.

12. Remove gloves, if worn, and dispose of them according to facility policy.

13. Wash your hands.

14. Leave the patient in a position of comfort and safety. Leave the call signal and needed personal items within reach.

15. Observe for and report:

    a. The time the patient was discovered.

    b. The cause of the burn, if known.

    c. Appearance of the burned area.

    d. Emergency measures taken.

    e. Other observations or patient response.

    f. Any witnesses to the incident.

    g. Vital signs.

    h. Any additional information needed by the supervisor to complete the incident report.

Caring for a Patient Who Is Hemorrhaging

■ *hemorrhage: excessive bleeding*
■ *shock: the result of blood loss that causes inadequate blood flow to the vital organs*

Hemorrhage is the medical term for bleeding. Bleeding can occur inside and outside the body. Bleeding inside the body cannot be seen or treated by the patient care technician. This section discusses bleeding on the outside of the body. Many different injuries can cause bleeding. If bleeding is not controlled quickly, serious complications can result. One very serious complication is **shock**, which results from blood loss and causes inadequate blood flow to the heart and brain.

PROCEDURE

8 EMERGENCY CARE FOR CONTROLLING HEMORRHAGE

1. Stay with the patient and call for help.

2. Use standard precautions and select personal protective equipment appropriate to the procedure.

3. If the hemorrhage is visible:

   a. Apply direct pressure over the site of bleeding with a clean pad or towel and your *gloved* hand (Figure 3-17). *continues*

PROCEDURE 8 *continued*

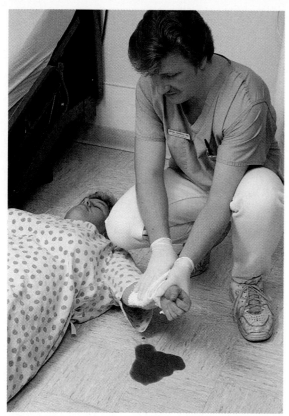

Figure 3-17 Hold pressure on a bleeding area with your gloved hand.

b. Increase the pressure if the bleeding continues.

c. Do not remove the pad to check the injury. If the pad becomes blood-soaked, add extra padding.

d. Continue direct pressure until you are given further instructions by your manager.

4. Keep the patient warm and quiet. Have the patient lie flat.

5. Take the blood pressure, pulse, and respiration as directed. You may be instructed to monitor the vital signs frequently until the patient is stable.

6. Do not give the patient anything to eat or drink. The patient may complain of being very thirsty. Thirst is a sign of shock. Notify the supervisor of this complaint.

7. Leave the patient in a position of comfort and safety. Leave the call signal and needed personal items within reach.

8. Dispose of items containing blood according to facility policy.

9. Remove gloves and dispose of them according to facility policy.

10. Wash your hands.

11. Observe for and report to your supervisor:

   a. The time the bleeding was discovered.
   b. The cause of the bleeding, if known.
   c. The location of the bleeding.
   d. Emergency measures taken.
   e. Blood pressure, pulse, and respiration.
   f. Other information required for the incident report.
   g. Witnesses to the injury.
   h. Other observations and patient response.

If shock is untreated, it can lead to death. The purpose of these procedures is to control bleeding and prevent shock.

Caring for a Patient with Vomiting and Aspiration

Food and air are both taken into the body through the mouth. The passageway by which food and air enter is also shared (Figure 3-18). The passage branches into two divisions in the throat. Food goes into the esophagus, then to the stomach. Air goes into the trachea, then the lungs. A small flap covers the trachea when you are swallowing. This flap prevents food and liquid from running into the lungs and causing choking. Swallowing is made less efficient by some diseases and aging. Occasionally food, water, or other objects accidentally go down the trachea and into the lungs. The medical term for liquids or solids entering the lungs is **aspiration**. Aspiration can occur when a patient is vomiting, bleeding, eating, or drinking. Sometimes thick secretions from the mouth enter the lungs. Aspiration can cause serious complications and should be avoided if possible. The easiest way to prevent aspiration is to turn the patient's body to the

■ **aspiration:** *inhalation of food, fluid, or other objects into the lungs*

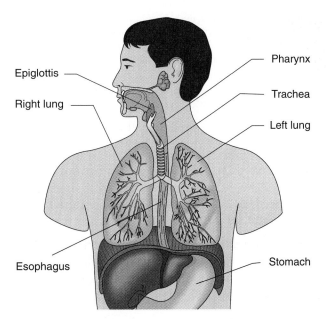

Epiglottis

Right lung

Esophagus

Pharynx

Trachea

Left lung

Stomach

Figure 3-18 The trachea and esophagus share the passage through which food and air move.

side if she is vomiting while lying down. If turning the patient's body is not possible, turn the patient's head to the side. Fluid cannot enter the lungs in this position. The purpose of this procedure is to prevent aspiration of food, fluids, secretions, blood, or vomitus.

PROCEDURE

9 EMERGENCY CARE FOR VOMITING AND ASPIRATION

1. Stay with the patient and call for help.

2. Use standard precautions and select personal protective equipment appropriate to the procedure.

3. Keep the patient's head elevated, if allowed.

4. Keep the patient's body or head turned to the side to allow fluids to drain from the mouth.

5. Provide an emesis basin if the patient is vomiting.

6. Notify your supervisor immediately if the patient:

   a. Is choking or is unable to swallow.

   b. Is unable to spit out the vomitus, blood, or secretions in his mouth.

7. The supervisor may need to suction the patient or notify the doctor.

8. If the patient begins choking and an airway obstruction occurs, follow the procedure for clearing the obstructed airway.

9. After the episode, assist the patient with mouth care.

10. Leave the patient in a position of comfort and safety. Leave the call signal and needed personal items within reach.

11. Dispose of items containing blood or other body secretions according to facility policy.

12. Remove gloves and dispose of them according to facility policy.

13. Wash your hands.

14. Observe for and report to your manager:

    a. If the patient has difficulty swallowing or is bleeding, vomiting, choking, or aspirating.

    b. Observe the vomitus for color, odor, presence of undigested food, blood, or coffee-ground appearance. (Coffee-ground appearance suggests blood in the stomach.)

    c. Measure or estimate the amount of vomitus or blood, and record it on the intake and output record.

    d. Do not discard the vomitus or blood until it is seen by a supervisor and a specimen obtained, if needed.

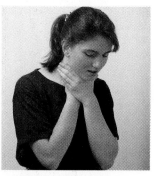

Figure 3-19 The universal choking sign is one or both hands at the patient's throat.

Caring for a Patient with an Obstructed Airway

Sometimes a foreign body (such as food or another object) is aspirated into the windpipe, or trachea. When the airway is blocked, the patient is said to have an **obstructed airway**. This is a serious emergency. The obstruction must be removed immediately or the patient will die. When a person is choking, putting one or both hands about the throat is instinctive. Hands on the throat is called the **universal choking sign** (Figure 3-19). If you see a patient with her hands on her throat, ask if she can speak. If the patient can speak, her airway is not obstructed. Stay with her and see if she can expel the foreign body on her own. If the patient is unable to speak, you must immediately start the obstructed airway procedure. The purpose of this procedure is to remove a foreign object from the airway of an adult. The procedure is different for infants, small children, and pregnant women.

PROCEDURE   OBRA

10 EMERGENCY CARE FOR CLEARING OBSTRUCTED AIRWAY IN A CONSCIOUS ADULT WHO IS SITTING OR STANDING

1. Ask the patient, "Are you choking?" or "Can you speak?"

2. If the patient can speak or cough, leave her alone and see if she can cough the obstruction out. Assist the patient if the cough is weak and ineffective and the patient is in obvious distress.

3. Stay with the patient and call for help.

4. Tell the patient that you will help.

5. Stand behind the patient and wrap your arms around her waist (Figure 3-20A).

6. Make a fist with one hand and place the thumb side of the fist against the abdomen, just above the navel (Figure 3-20B).

7. Grasp your fist with the other hand. Do not put pressure on the ribs or breastbone with your forearms.

8. Squeeze inward and upward five times (Figure 3-20C).

9. If the patient does not expel the foreign body, repeat the inward, upward thrusts. If the patient begins to cough forcefully, wait and see if the object can be expelled.

10. Continue until the foreign body is expelled or the patient loses consciousness.

11. When the foreign body is expelled, stay with the patient and follow your supervisor's directions.

12. Leave the patient in a position of comfort and safety. Leave the call signal and needed personal items within reach. The supervisor may instruct you to monitor the patient's vital signs periodically.

13. Wash your hands.

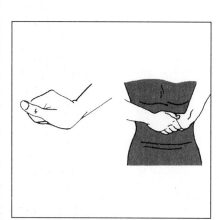

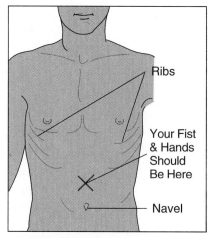

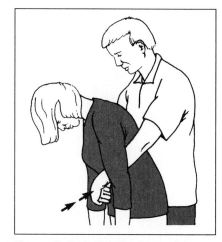

Figure 3-20A Place your hands around the abdomen, slightly above the waist.

Figure 3-20B Turn your thumb inward.

Figure 3-20C Squeeze in and up.

PROCEDURE

11 EMERGENCY CARE FOR CLEARING OBSTRUCTED AIRWAY IN A CONSCIOUS ADULT WHO IS LYING DOWN

Note: This procedure should be done only if the victim is too large for you to wrap your arms around.

1. Place the patient on the floor, face up. In this procedure, do not turn the patient's head to the side.
2. Kneel down and straddle across the patient's hips.
3. Place the heel of one hand on the patient's abdomen, immediately above the navel. Your fingers should be pointing up toward the head.

Do not place your hand on the ribs or breastbone.

4. Place your other hand on top of the first hand. Position your shoulders directly above the patient's abdomen.
5. Press your hands inward and upward five times. Repeat until the foreign body is expelled or the patient becomes unconscious.

PROCEDURE

12 EMERGENCY CARE FOR CLEARING OBSTRUCTED AIRWAY IN AN UNCONSCIOUS ADULT

1. Check to see if the patient responds by gently tapping his shoulder and asking, "Are you OK?"
2. Stay with the patient and call for help.
3. Wear gloves during this procedure and use standard precautions.
4. Position the patient on his back on the floor with his head facing up.
5. Kneel beside the patient and open the airway by tilting the head back with one hand while you gently lift the chin with the other hand. Perform a finger sweep in his mouth with two fingers of your gloved hand to see if a foreign body can be felt or removed.
6. Place your ear close to the patient's nose and mouth. Look at the chest to see if it is rising and falling. Listen and feel for breath sounds on your cheek and ear.
7. If there is no air movement, blow two slow breaths into the patient's mouth through a ventilation barrier device. Remove your mouth and inhale between the two breaths. If the air does not go in, reposition the head and attempt to breathe into the patient's mouth again.

Note: Follow your facility policy for mouth-to-mouth ventilation. To prevent the transmission of disease, standard precautions should be used. This means that a ventilation barrier mask with a valve that prevents the backflow of secretions, or a resuscitation face shield, should be placed between your mouth and the patient's mouth. Familiarize yourself with the devices in your facility. CPR classes are offered to teach you how to use ventilation devices correctly, and are an important component of patient care skills training.

8. If no air enters the patient after the second set of ventilations, straddle the patient's hips.
9. Place the heel of one hand on the patient's abdomen, immediately above the navel. Your fingers should be pointing up toward the head. Do not place your hand on the ribs or breastbone.
10. Place your other hand on top of the first hand. Position your shoulders directly above the patient's abdomen.
11. Press your hands inward and upward five times.

continues

PROCEDURE **12** *continued*

12. Open the airway by doing a tongue/jaw lift. Check the patient's mouth and remove any objects that you can see with your finger.

13. Attempt to ventilate.

14. Repeat steps 6 through 13 until the object is expelled.

15. Assist the supervisor, code team, or EMS as appropriate.

16. Dispose of gloves and face shield according to facility policy.

17. Wash your hands.

18. Observe and report to your manager:

   a. Exact time the choking and unconsciousness started and stopped.

   b. The procedures done and the time that you started and stopped.

   c. The patient's response.

   d. Factors related to the cause of choking.

■ *obstructed airway:* food or a foreign body blocking the trachea or windpipe, making it impossible to breathe
■ *universal choking sign:* one or both hands on the throat
■ *EMS:* Emergency Medical Services; usually an ambulance or fire department

Cardiopulmonary Resuscitation

Cardiopulmonary resuscitation (CPR) is an emergency procedure used in health care facilities if the patient's heart and breathing have stopped. CPR is used to keep the patient alive until more advanced life support can be obtained. It is recommended that you attend a CPR course and learn this valuable lifesaving technique.

KEY POINTS IN CHAPTER

- *Every employee of the health care facility is responsible for keeping the environment safe.*

- *Changes in vision, hearing, blood vessels, and reflexes put some patients at high risk for accidents.*

- *You should correct unsafe conditions, if possible, or report them to the proper person.*

- *Material Safety Data Sheets give instructions for safe use of chemicals, identify health risks of the chemical, and describe first aid and safety precautions.*

- *You should answer the call lights of all patients, whether you are assigned to care for the patient or not.*

- *Identify the patient before giving care.*

- *Before applying a heat or cold application, know the type of application, area to be treated, length of time the application is to be used, proper temperature, safety precautions, and side effects to watch for.*

- *An important responsibility is to know and practice oxygen safety.*

- *Oxygen, fuel, and a spark are necessary to start a fire.*

- *In a fire emergency, the RACE System is used to remove patients from danger, activate the alarm, contain, and extinguish the fire.*

- *Know and follow facility policies for tornado, hurricane, earthquake, and bomb threat emergencies.*

- *The Occupational Safety and Health Administration is a federal agency responsible for overseeing employee safety in the workplace.*

- *If you discover a patient who is having a medical emergency or is injured, stay with the patient and call for help.*

- *The universal sign for choking is one or both hands on the throat.*

REVIEW QUIZ

Multiple Choice Questions

1. Safety is the responsibility of:
   a. the patient care technician.
   b. the housekeeping department.
   c. the maintenance department.
   d. all of the above.

2. Physical changes from aging and disease that increase the risk of incidents are:
   a. changes in vision, hearing, and reflexes.
   b. chest pain and shortness of breath.
   c. nausea, vomiting, and diarrhea.
   d. all of the above.

3. When placing the patient's call signal, you should:
   a. place the call signal by alert patients only when they are in bed.
   b. never place the call signal near confused patients.
   c. place the call signal near all patients at all times.
   d. none of the above.

4. Chemicals:
   a. can be harmful if swallowed.
   b. may irritate the skin and mucous membranes.
   c. should be kept in their original containers.
   d. all of the above.

5. When using heat and cold applications, you should know:
   a. the type of application and area to be treated.
   b. how long the application should stay in place.
   c. the correct temperature and safety precautions to use.
   d. all of the above.

6. The three elements necessary to start a fire are:
   a. oxygen, fuel, and a spark.
   b. oxygen, chemicals, and fuel.
   c. matches, cigarettes, and chemicals.
   d. none of the above.

7. You answer the telephone and the caller advises you that there is a bomb in the facility. You should:
   a. ask the caller to hold while you get your supervisor.
   b. hang up and call the police immediately.
   c. keep the caller on the line and get as much information as you can.
   d. tell the caller not to play silly games.

8. If you find a patient who is ill or injured, you should:
   a. run and get your supervisor.
   b. stay with the patient and call for help.
   c. go to the phone and call an ambulance immediately.
   d. leave the room and pretend that you did not see the patient.

9. If you find a patient who has fallen on the floor next to the bed, you should:
   a. help the patient back to bed.
   b. go to the desk and fill out an incident report.
   c. tell the patient she should have called for help before getting up.
   d. none of the above.

10. You find a patient who is having a seizure. You should do all of the following *except:*
    a. place an object in the patient's mouth so she doesn't swallow her tongue.
    b. stay with the patient and call for help.
    c. loosen tight and restrictive clothing.
    d. move any objects that could harm the patient.

11. A serious complication of hemorrhage is:
    a. bleeding.   c. fractures.
    b. swelling.   d. shock.

12. The universal choking sign is:
    a. waving your hands in the air.
    b. coughing and gagging.
    c. one or both hands on the throat.
    d. none of the above.

True/False Questions

13. ___ Most accidents cannot be prevented.

14. ___ Patients in wheelchairs should be parked across the hall from the linen cart.

15. ___ Changes in vision caused by aging make it difficult to see in dim lighting.

16. ___ When answering a patient's call signal, you should knock on the door before entering the room.

17. ___ Thermal burns are caused by chemicals touching the skin.

18. ___ An example of a generalized cold application is an ice bag placed on a swollen ankle.

19. ___ Heat applications dilate the blood vessels.

20. ___ Oxygen is necessary for life.

21. ___ The first step in the RACE System is to run for help.

22. ___ OSHA is responsible for employee safety in the workplace.

Short Answer/Fill in the Blanks

23. Syncope is the medical word for _____.

24.–26. List three safety precautions to take when a patient is using oxygen.

24. _____

25. _____

26. _____

27. The major cause of fire in a health care facility is _____.

Legal and Ethical Responsibilities

After reading this chapter, you will be able to:

Spell and define key terms.

State the purpose of the legal documents that describe the rights of the health care consumer.

State the purpose of the advance directive.

Describe how to assist patients who are physically or mentally unable to exercise their legal rights.

Define patient abuse and neglect and give an example of each.

List six other legal considerations of concern to the patient care technician.

Describe the purpose of Maslow's hierarchy of needs and explain why understanding this theory is important to the patient care technician.

Explain why understanding the patient's culture is important to the health care provider.

Describe how to promote patient independence and explain why this is important.

▬▬ LEGAL CONSIDERATIONS FOR HEALTH CARE WORKERS

Health care facilities operate under state, federal, and local laws. They also comply with the requirements of their accrediting organization. All health care providers must operate within the scope of these laws. Facilities have policies and procedures governing employee conduct and patient care within their institutions. These policies and procedures are designed to maintain compliance with the various laws governing the agency.

Rights of the Health Care Consumer

The title given to the consumer of health care varies in different settings. Regardless of what the consumer is called, she has certain legal rights to safe care. Institutional policy varies regarding how patients are informed of these rights. Some facilities present a copy of the rights to patients upon admission and have them sign an acknowledgment that they have received the copy. Other agencies post copies of the rights in prominent locations throughout the facility. The bill of rights is written in very simple language that all patients can understand. In some communities with large groups of non-English-speaking residents, the bill of rights has been translated into the language prevalent in the community. Health care workers must be aware of all these patient rights. All health care providers are obligated to uphold and protect these rights. If a patient is mentally confused, the patient care provider may need to assist him to exercise his rights.

■ **Patient's Bill of Rights:**
a list of the rights of patients in hospitals, published by the American Hospital Association

Patient's Bill of Rights

The American Hospital Association has developed the **Patient's Bill of Rights** (Figure 4-1). These rights guarantee all patients safe, considerate, and respectful

A Patient's Bill of Rights

Introduction

Effective health care requires collaboration between patients and physicians and other health care professionals. Open and honest communication, respect for personal and professional values, and sensitivity to differences are integral to optimal patient care. As the setting for the provision of health services, hospitals must provide a foundation for understanding and respecting the rights and responsibilities of patients, their families, physicians, and other caregivers. Hospitals must ensure a health care ethic that respects the role of patients in decision making about treatment choices and other aspects of their care. Hospitals must be sensitive to cultural, racial, linguistic, religious, age, gender, and other differences as well as the needs of persons with disabilities.

The American Hospital Association presents A Patient's Bill of Rights with the expectation that it will contribute to more effective patient care and be supported by the hospital on behalf of the institution, its medical staff, employees, and patients. The American Hospital Association encourages health care institutions to tailor this bill of rights to their patient community by translating and/or simplifying the language of this bill of rights as may be necessary to ensure that the patients and their families understand their rights and responsibilities.

Bill of Rights*

1. The patient has the right to considerate and respectful care.

2. The patient has the right to and is encouraged to obtain from physicians and other direct care givers relevant, current, and understandable information concerning diagnosis, treatment, and prognosis.

   Except in emergencies when the patient lacks decision making capacity and the need for treatment is urgent, the patient is entitled to the opportunity to discuss and request information related to the specific procedures and/or treatments, the risks involved, the possible length of recuperation, and the medically reasonable alternatives and their accompanying risks and benefits.

   Patients have the right to know the identity of physicians, nurses, and others involved in their care, as well as when those involved are students, residents, or other trainees. The patient also has the right to know the immediate and long-term financial implications of treatment choices, insofar as they are known.

3. The patient has the right to make decisions about the plan of care prior to and during the course of treatment and to refuse a recommended treatment or plan of care to the extent permitted by law and hospital policy and to be informed of the medical consequences of this action. In case of such refusal, the patient is entitled to other appropriate care and services that the hospital provides or transfer to another hospital. The hospital should notify patients of any policy that might affect patient choice within the institution.

4. The patient has the right to have an advance directive (such as a living will, health care proxy, or durable power of attorney for health care) concerning treatment or designating a surrogate decision maker with the expectation that the hospital will honor the intent of that directive to the extent permitted by law and hospital policy.

   Health care institutions must advise patients of their rights under state law and hospital policy to make informed medical choices, ask if the patient has an advance directive, and include that information in patient records. The patient has the right to timely information about hospital policy that may limit its ability to implement fully a legally valid advance directive.

5. The patient has the right to every consideration of privacy. Case discussion, consultation, examination, and treatment should be conducted so as to protect each patient's privacy.

*These rights can be exercised on the patient's behalf by a designated surrogate or proxy decision maker if the patient lacks decision-making capacity, is legally incompetent, or is a minor.

A Patient's Bill of Rights was first adopted by the American Hospital Association in 1973. This revision was approved by the AHA Board of Trustees on October 21, 1992.

Figure 4-1 The Patient's Bill of Rights guarantees patients safe, considerate, and respectful care. (Courtesy of American Hospital Association, copyright 1992)

continues

6. The patient has the right to expect that all communications and records pertaining to his/her care will be treated as confidential by the hospital, except in cases such as suspected abuse and public health hazards when reporting is permitted or required by law. The patient has the right to expect that the hospital will emphasize the confidentiality of this information when it releases it to any other parties entitled to review information in these records.

7. The patient has the right to review the records pertaining to his/her medical care and to have the information explained or interpreted as necessary, except when restricted by law.

8. The patient has the right to expect that, within its capacity and policies, a hospital will make reasonable response to the request of a patient for appropriate and medically indicated care and services. The hospital must provide evaluation, service, and/or referral as indicated by the urgency of the case. When medically appropriate and legally permissible, or when a patient has so requested, a patient may be transferred to another facility. The institution to which the patient is to be transferred must first have accepted the patient for transfer. The patient must also have the benefit of complete information and explanation concerning the need for, risks, benefits, and alternatives to such a transfer.

9. The patient has the right to ask and be informed of the existence of business relationships among the hospital, educational institutions, other health care providers, or payers that may influence the patient's treatment and care.

10. The patient has the right to consent to or decline to participate in proposed research studies or human experimentation affecting care and treatment or requiring direct patient involvement, and to have those studies fully explained prior to consent. A patient who declines to participate in research or experimentation is entitled to the most effective care that the hospital can otherwise provide.

11. The patient has the right to expect reasonable continuity of care when appropriate and to be informed by physicians and other caregivers of available and realistic patient care options when hospital care is no longer appropriate.

12. The patient has the right to be informed of hospital policies and practices that relate to patient care, treatment, and responsibilities. The patient has the right to be informed of available resources for resolving disputes, grievances, and conflicts, such as ethics committees, patient representatives, or other mechanisms available in the institution. The patient has the right to be informed of the hospital's charges for services and available payment methods.

The collaborative nature of health care requires that the patients, or their families/surrogates, participate in their care. The effectiveness of care and patient satisfaction with the course of treatment depend, in part, on the patient fulfilling certain responsibilities. Patients are responsible for providing information about past illnesses, hospitalizations, medications, and other matters related to health status. To participate effectively in decision making, patients must be encouraged to take responsibility for requesting additional information or clarification about their health status or treatment when they do not fully understand information and instructions. Patients are also responsible for ensuring that the health care institution has a copy of their written advance directive if they have one. Patients are responsible for informing their physicians and other caregivers if they anticipate problems in following prescribed treatment.

Patients should also be aware of the hospital's obligation to be reasonably efficient and equitable in providing care to other patients and the community. The hospital's rules and regulations are designed to help the hospital meet this obligation. Patients and their families are responsible for making reasonable accommodations to the needs of the hospital, other patients, medical staff, and hospital employees. Patients are responsible for providing necessary information for insurance claims and for working with the hospital to make payment arrangements, when necessary.

A person's health depends on much more than health care services. Patients are responsible for recognizing the impact of their lifestyle on their personal health.

Conclusion

Hospitals have many functions to perform, including the enhancement of health status, health promotion, and the prevention and treatment of injury and disease; the immediate and ongoing care and rehabilitation of patients; the education of health professionals, patients, and the community; and research. All these activities must be conducted with an overriding concern for the values and dignity of patients.

2   *A Patient's Bill of Rights*

Figure 4-1 *continued*

■ **confidential:** *personal, not known to other people*
■ **dignity:** *honor or esteem*
■ **privacy:** *separation from others; alone; personal*
■ **diagnosis:** *the term describing the patient's disease or condition*
■ **prognosis:** *a prediction of the course or outcome of a disease*

■ **Resident's Bill of Rights:** *a legal document listing the rights of residents in long-term care facilities*

care. The rights guarantee that patient information will be kept **confidential** and that the **dignity** and **privacy** of the patient will be respected. Confidentiality and privacy are considered in both patient care procedures and the patient's medical records. The patient is also guaranteed the right to be informed of the **diagnosis**, treatment, and **prognosis**, and may make decisions regarding his or her own care.

Resident's Bill of Rights

Residents in long-term care facilities have the same rights as any other citizen of the United States. The Omnibus Budget Reconciliation Act of 1987 (OBRA) guarantees residents of nursing homes certain legal rights. These rights are listed in the **Resident's Bill of Rights** (Table 4-1). As in the hospital, the patient care technician in the long-term care facility must be familiar with the resident's rights. The patient care technician must respect these rights and assist residents to exercise them. The rights of residents who are mentally confused are no different from the rights of others. The patient care technician must protect the rights of the mentally confused resident.

Table 4-1 Residents' Rights

■ Residents have the right to exercise all their rights as citizens of the state and citizens of the United States, as well as any other rights given them by law.
■ The facility must explain the rights to residents both verbally and in writing in a language that the resident understands.
■ Residents cannot be discriminated against because of age, sex, race, ethnic origin, religion, or disability.

Privacy, Dignity, and Respect
■ Residents have a right to privacy.
■ Residents will be treated with consideration, dignity, and respect.
■ The resident's likes, dislikes, and special needs and preferences must be considered in the services provided by the facility. This is called reasonable accommodation.
■ Personal and clinical records must be kept confidential. The resident has the right to refuse to allow others to see these records unless permission is given in writing.
■ Residents have the right to communicate both verbally and in writing with anyone of their choosing. This includes family members, other visitors, ombudsmen, attorneys, and representatives of governmental agencies.
■ Residents have the right to send and receive personal mail unopened. Residents may request that staff assist them to open and read their mail when it arrives.

Safety and Security
■ Residents have the right to a safe environment.
■ Residents have the right to care that is free from misappropriation of property.

Medical Care and Treatment
■ Residents have the right to choose their own physician. They have the right to be informed

of matters affecting their care and to make decisions regarding their care.
■ Medical problems must be explained to residents in a language they understand.
■ Residents may refuse treatment. If they do refuse treatment, they have the right to be informed of the consequences of their refusal.
■ Residents have a right to voice problems and complaints about their care without fear of reprisal. The facility is required to respond to these complaints.
■ Residents have the right to make choices to withhold life-sustaining treatment in the event of terminal illness.
■ Residents may designate someone else to make treatment decisions for them in the event they become unable to make these decisions themselves.

Freedom from Restraint, Abuse, and Misappropriation of Property
■ Residents have the right to be free from abuse, neglect, and misappropriation of property. The facility is responsible for caring for the resident's health, well-being, and personal possessions.
■ Drugs cannot be given for discipline or convenience to the nursing home staff. Any mood-altering drugs given must be required for the treatment of a medical condition.

continues

Table 4-1, *continued*

- Residents cannot be punished, scolded, or secluded. Their privileges cannot be taken away and they cannot be physically, mentally, or sexually abused.
- Residents cannot be restrained by physical means except for their own safety, the safety of others, in certain medical procedures, or in an emergency.

Financial Matters

- Residents have the right to manage their own financial affairs, or may choose another person to manage their money.
- Facilities must account for and properly manage resident money deposited with them.

Freedom of Association

- Residents have the right to have visitors at any reasonable hour.
- Residents do not have to talk to or see anyone they do not want to visit.
- Residents may make and receive private phone calls.
- Married couples have the right to share a room.
- Residents have the right to organize and participate in resident and family councils.
- Residents may meet with others outside the facility.
- Residents may leave the facility for visits or shopping trips.
- Family members may meet with families of other residents in the nursing home.
- Residents have the right to plan and execute their daily activities.
- Residents have the right to vote in elections.

Work

- Residents may choose to work in the facility as part of their activity plan. They have the right to be paid the prevailing rate for the same type of work in the community. Residents may also perform certain duties without pay, if they choose to do so.

Personal Possessions

- Residents may wear their own clothing.
- Residents may bring in furnishings and personal belongings from their own home.

Grievances

- If the resident has a problem or complaint, she has the right to speak to those in charge. The complaint may be about care or failure to receive expected services. The resident has the right to a response.
- The resident has the right to contact the ombudsman for the facility and the state survey and certification agency.
- The facility may not retaliate against residents who have complained.

Admission, Transfer, and Discharge

- The facility must advise residents about eligibility for Medicaid. If Medicaid or Medicare pays for any items or services, the resident cannot be charged additional money for these services.
- In the event of the resident's death, the facility must give an accounting of money in the resident's personal account to the person responsible for the estate.
- Residents may not be asked to give up their rights to benefits under Medicaid or Medicare.
- The facility is required to have the same policies and practices regarding services, transfer, or discharge for all individuals, regardless of their source of payment.
- The facility may be required to hold the resident's bed for a specified period if the resident is hospitalized or goes on a therapeutic pass.
- The facility cannot make the resident leave or move to another room unless:
  - The health and safety of the resident or others are affected.
  - The facility cannot meet the resident's needs.
  - The resident's condition has improved so that services are no longer required.
  - The resident has not paid the bill and the facility has given the resident reasonable notice of discharge.
- Residents must be given a 30-day written notice before they can be transferred unless there are medical reasons or the life, safety, and health of the resident or others are endangered. The resident may waive the right to the 30-day waiting period if he or she chooses.

Privacy. Patients and residents in all health care agencies have the right to privacy. Always knock on the door and allow time for a response before entering the patient's room. When providing care or performing procedures, close the door to the room, the privacy curtain, and the window curtain. The patient care technician must not unnecessarily expose patients when giving care. Even though the curtains and door are closed, the patient's body should be draped so that only the part you are working on is exposed. This protects the patient's dignity and prevents embarrassment.

Confidentiality. The law guarantees patients confidentiality in their medical care and treatment. This means that unauthorized persons may not read the patients' medical records. It also means that health care workers cannot discuss personal information about the patient or her condition with others. Information about patients should only be discussed in private areas. Do not discuss patients in hallways, on elevators, in the cafeteria, or with others outside the health care agency. If a patient tells you something in confidence, you should not tell anyone else unless the information affects the patient's condition or medical care. For example, a patient tells you something about a private financial matter. You should not tell anyone else. However, if a patient tells you that she is secretly spitting out her medication after the nurse leaves the room, this information should be reported to your supervisor. If a visitor asks you for information about a patient, refer the visitor to the supervisor for information.

Assisting Patients Who Cannot Exercise Their Rights

The patient care technician is responsible for helping patients exercise their rights if they are physically or mentally unable to do so on their own. This involves using a good deal of common sense. For example, a patient with a physical or mental impairment may not be able to cover her body if it is exposed. It is your responsibility to cover the patient. Offer to help patients who cannot do things for themselves. You may notice an unopened card on the patient's table. Offer to open and read the card to the patient.

Give patients as much control over care and daily routines as possible. Always explain what you are going to do and how it will be done. Although the patient may be physically incapable of performing certain tasks, she may be able to tell you how and when she wants them done. Giving the patient control and offering choices about care and routines is an excellent way to help the patient exercise her rights and promotes a healthy self-esteem. It sends a message to the patient that you value her as a person and respect her opinion. Inform patients of facility practices, policies, and procedures that affect them.

Although patients are guaranteed many legal rights, they are not allowed to infringe upon the rights of others. If the rights of one patient are interfering with the rights of another patient, try to find a compromise. If you are unable to resolve the situation quickly, consult your manager.

Abuse and Neglect

■ **abuse:** *the willful infliction of injury, unreasonable confinement, intimidation, or punishment that results in physical harm, pain, or mental anguish*
■ **neglect:** *failing to provide services to patients to prevent physical harm or mental anguish*

Abuse can be physical, verbal, sexual, or mental. **Neglect** can be deliberate or accidental. An example of neglect is forgetting that you are assigned to care for a patient and not providing care. All states have laws concerning abuse and neglect of patients in the health care facility. You are legally responsible for reporting suspected or actual abuse and neglect of patients. The health care agency must always report abuse to law enforcement authorities and state agencies. This is the supervisor's responsibility. There are severe penalties for abusing or neglecting patients. Health care workers who witness abuse or neglect and do not report it may be held equally responsible for the situation. If you suspect a patient has been abused or neglected by a staff member, family, or any other individual, report this information to your supervisor immediately.

Abuse and neglect may occur because the health care worker is feeling stressed. Patients may say things that are hurtful or upsetting to you. Remain calm and do not take a patient's behavior personally. Abuse often occurs when a worker is feeling tired, experiencing personal problems, or losing control. If you feel overwhelmed with your duties or with a patient, discuss it with your supervisor. Arrange to take a break and compose yourself.

Types of Abuse. Abuse can take many different forms. Sometimes the abuser is not even aware that the behavior or action toward a patient is abusive.

- Physical abuse occurs when willful, nonaccidental injury occurs. This can occur by handling a patient roughly or by striking, slapping, or hitting a patient.
- Verbal abuse is swearing, using demeaning terms to talk to a patient, or embarrassing a patient.
- Mental abuse is threatening to harm a patient, or threatening to withhold food, fluid, or care as a form of punishment.
- Sexual abuse occurs when physical force or verbal threats are used to force a patient to perform a sexual act. Touching or fondling a patient inappropriately is also a form of sexual abuse. Any behavior that is seductive, sexually demeaning, harassing, or reasonably interpreted as sexual by the patient may be considered abuse.

Recognizing Signs of Abuse. If you notice new bruises, pain, swelling, or other unexplained injuries on a patient, this may be an indication of abuse and should be reported to your supervisor. Another sign of possible abuse is a patient who responds to the caregiver with fear and anxiety. Patients who have been abused may also show sudden changes in their personality or behavior. You are not required to determine whether the changes in the patient are the result of abuse. Your responsibility is to report the observations to your supervisor for further investigation.

Advance Directives

■ *advance directive: a document that designates the patient's wishes for a time when the patient is unable to speak for himself or herself*
■ *living will: a document that specifies the patient's wishes in the event that the patient is in a terminal condition*
■ *health care proxy: an individual who has been legally designated to make medical decisions on behalf of the patient*
■ *durable power of attorney for health care: a document that designates another individual to make medical decisions on behalf of the patient*
■ *consent: permission to perform care, treatments, and procedures*
■ *negligence: failing to provide services to a patient in the same manner as a reasonably prudent person would do*

Patients and residents of health care facilities have the right to execute an **advance directive**. Advance directives can be in the form of a **living will**, which designates the patient's wishes if he is in a terminal condition and cannot speak for himself. The patient also has the right to designate a surrogate decision maker, often called a **health care proxy**. The document that the patient signs is called a **durable power of attorney for health care**. State laws vary on how advance directives are implemented, but patients in all states have the right to execute these documents. The health care agency informs the patient of this right upon admission to the institution. The agency is obligated to follow the patient's written directions in these documents.

Other Legal Considerations

Consent means to give permission for treatment when a person is conscious and alert. All patients have the right to refuse treatment for any reason. They also have the right to have the consequences of the refusal explained to them. Parents or legal guardians have the right to give consent or refuse treatment for minor children and others who are mentally confused. Report to the supervisor for further directions if a patient or guardian refuses care.

Negligence and Malpractice. **Negligence** involves breaching the standard of care. An example of negligence is telling a patient to get up unsupervised even though you know she is dizzy and weak. The patient falls and is injured. An attorney can argue that the reasonably prudent patient care technician should have known that the patient was at risk of injury. The proper course of action would be to instruct the patient to call for help before getting up, and to remain with her to assist while she is out of bed. To avoid negligence, always perform procedures in the manner in which you were trained, and use good judgment. If you are in doubt about what to do, consult your manager. Follow your facility policies even if you do not agree with them.

■ *malpractice: negligence that results in harm to the patient*

Malpractice is negligence that results in harm to the patient. For example, the care plan states that the patient's side rails are to be up at all times when the patient is in bed. The caregiver forgets to put the rails up and the patient falls from the bed, breaking a hip. The caregiver could be found guilty of malpractice.

■ *defamation of character:* *making false or damaging statements about another person verbally*
■ *slander: making false statements about another person*
■ *libel: making false statements about another person in writing*
■ *abandonment: leaving or walking off the premises before another worker has been assigned to care for your patients*

■ *false imprisonment: holding or restraining a patient against his or her will*

■ *involuntary seclusion: isolation of a patient as a form of punishment*

■ *standards of care: common health care practices based on current information about health care and facility policies*

■ *Good Samaritan laws: laws that protect health care workers who provide emergency care to injured persons outside the place of employment*

Making False Statements. An example of defamation of character is telling others that your neighbor was treated in the hospital for an illegal drug overdose, when the neighbor was actually treated for pneumonia. Slander is a spoken statement. Libel is a written statement. It is best not to discuss patients' conditions with others outside the health care facility. If you need to talk about an upsetting work situation, ask your manager for advice. Discussing patients with others violates the patient's right to confidentiality.

Abandonment. Abandonment means leaving or walking off the premises. If the care provider must leave the facility for any reason, the supervisor should be notified. An equally qualified person must be available to care for the patients. An example of abandonment is leaving the facility before a qualified person has been secured to replace you. You can be accused of abandonment even if other staff members are on duty, if no one else has been assigned to care for your patients.

False Imprisonment and Involuntary Seclusion. False imprisonment means holding or restraining a patient against his will. Use of physical restraints and side rails can be considered methods of false imprisonment. To avoid this situation, follow all facility policies when using restraints. Consult the care plan before using any restraining device. Involuntary seclusion is a form of abuse if used as punishment for the patient. Involuntary seclusion can be used in certain circumstances, though, as part of the therapeutic plan of care.

Standards of Care. Although health care is delivered in many different settings, the legal requirements for health care workers are similar in all settings. Standards of care are based on laws, facility policies, information learned in your basic skills class, and information published in textbooks and journals for health care workers. Standards are defined by community, state, and national practices and are used to measure the worker's performance. They permit you to be judged based on what is expected of a health care worker with your education and experience. All health care agencies have standards of performance that you must follow in your job. In legal situations, you will be held to the same standard of care and judgment as the average worker in your job.

Good Samaritan Laws. All states have Good Samaritan laws to protect health care workers who provide emergency care outside their places of employment. These laws do not apply to workers providing emergency care in the health care facility. If you assist someone at the scene of an emergency, you are protected under these laws if you deliver care that you are trained to provide.

ETHICAL BEHAVIOR WITH PATIENTS AND FAMILIES

Professional boundaries are limits on how a health care worker acts with patients. Compare boundaries to the borders between states on a map. They exist, but you cannot see the boundary lines when you are driving down the highway. Professional boundaries are the same way. They exist, but you do not always know when you cross them. These lines define the best behavior of care providers when caring for patients and meeting their needs. The care provider must act professionally, not personally as a family member or friend. Professional boundaries help the patient care technician act appropriately. You do not want to have too much or too little contact. You must use good judgment and determine the amount of contact that is right for each patient. Consult your manager if you are uncertain.

Patients expect you to act in their best interests and treat them with dignity. This means that you must not take advantage of a patient's situation, and that you should not become inappropriately involved in the patient's personal and family relationships. Sometimes it is difficult to determine where the boundaries are. Some relationships with patients and families are not healthy for the patient or the care provider. Unfortunately, it is not always easy to recognize unhealthy relationships until it is too late. Strive for balance in your relationships with patients and families. If any of the following situations have occurred, you have probably crossed the lines and are operating in a relationship danger zone. Seek help from your supervisor:

- Discussing your personal problems with the patient or family.
- Discussing your feelings of sexual attraction with the patient.
- Keeping secrets with the patient and becoming defensive when someone questions your involvement.
- Thinking you are immune from having a unhealthy or nontherapeutic relationship with a patient.
- Believing that you are the only person who can meet the patient's needs.
- Spending an inappropriate amount of time with the patient, including off-duty visits or trading assignments with others to be with the patient.
- Reporting only partial information about the patient to your supervisor for fear of divulging negative information or secrets the patient has told you.
- Being flirtatious with a patient, including sexual innuendos, jokes that are sexual in nature, or using offensive language.
- Feeling that you must protect the patient from other health care workers and siding with the patient's position regardless of the situation.
- Feeling that you may become involved in a sexual relationship with the patient.

■■■■ BASIC HUMAN NEEDS

The patient care technician has a very important responsibility in helping patients meet their needs. When the patient's needs are not met, you may notice a change in behavior. When needs on a lower level are not met, you will notice physical problems. For example, if the patient needs food and fluids, she may become weak and tired. When needs on a higher level are not met, you may notice anger, withdrawal, or other behavior problems. Your care and observations are important to the success of the patient and all team members in meeting the care plan goals. Understanding the nature of human needs will enable you to assist the patient in meeting these needs.

The care plan is designed to meet the patient's physical and psychological needs. You will be required to assist the patient to meet needs on many different levels. As the patient's condition improves, she will begin to meet more needs on her own. This provides a sense of self-satisfaction and accomplishment, which aids in meeting psychological needs. Patients who are totally dependent on others for their physical care can still derive mental satisfaction from being in control of their care and making decisions about their routines.

■ **self-actualization:** *the realization of one's full potential*

A psychologist named Abraham Maslow proposed a widely accepted theory about human nature. His theory centers around self-actualization and is based on the belief that all human beings are innately good. Normal, healthy development enables people to actualize their own true nature and realize their full potential. Maslow's theory states that self-actualization is the goal of life. If something blocks the path to achieving this goal, the individual becomes frustrated. Aggressive behavior may result from frustration because the individual's needs are not being met.

Maslow's Hierarchy of Needs

■ **Maslow's hierarchy of needs:** *a chart based on a widely accepted theory of physical and psychological needs of all human beings*

Maslow writes that all human beings have the same basic needs. He developed a pyramid, called Maslow's hierarchy of needs (Figure 4-2), to illustrate these needs. The pyramid reads from bottom to top. The needs at one level must be satisfied before the needs at the next level become important. The needs at the bottom of the pyramid are the most urgent. These are the physical needs that are important for survival. As the physical needs at the bottom of the pyramid are met, the psychological needs become important. Psychological needs must

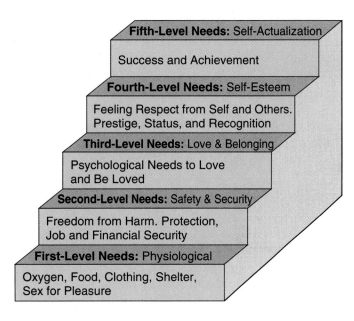

Fifth-Level Needs: Self-Actualization

Success and Achievement

Fourth-Level Needs: Self-Esteem

Feeling Respect from Self and Others. Prestige, Status, and Recognition

Third-Level Needs: Love & Belonging

Psychological Needs to Love and Be Loved

Second-Level Needs: Safety & Security

Freedom from Harm. Protection, Job and Financial Security

First-Level Needs: Physiological

Oxygen, Food, Clothing, Shelter, Sex for Pleasure

Figure 4-2 According to Maslow's theory, the needs on one level must be satisfied before the needs on the next level become important.

be met for a person to be emotionally healthy. The more needs fulfilled, the higher the quality of a person's life.

Physiological Needs. Basic physical needs for survival are at the bottom of the Maslow pyramid. They include the need for food, water, sleep, rest, physical activity, elimination, and oxygen. When these needs are met, needs at the next level become important. We may take these things for granted, but some patients may have diseases or conditions that make it difficult to meet the needs on this level. Think about the patient who is struggling to breathe. The patient is using all of his energy to fulfill this one basic need. Until the patient's breathing problem is resolved, other needs are not important.

Safety and Security Needs. When the patient's basic survival needs are met, safety and security become important. The patient must feel safe and protected from harm in the environment. The patient must also feel personal security in her family, relationships, and job. Financial security is important. If the illness causes the patient to worry about how she will pay the medical bills, or fears she will lose her job because of time lost from work, her security needs are not met. The social worker and other members of the interdisciplinary team may be called to assist her in meeting these needs.

Love and Belonging Needs. Notice that the first two levels of Maslow's hierarchy involve physical needs. After physical needs are satisfied, emotional needs become important. The most basic of the emotional needs is the need to give love and receive love from others. If the patient has a strong family unit, this will help meet the need for love. The patient care technician also helps to meet this need by showing a sincere interest in the patient. Show the patient that you care and accept him, regardless of his disability, condition, appearance, or behavior. Providing privacy during care, treatments, and procedures, and respecting the patient's dignity, will also help you meet this need.

Self-Esteem. Everyone has the need to feel important and worthwhile. Our self-esteem involves the mental image that we believe we project to others. Patients may respond negatively when they feel their self-image is threatened. They may not know or understand why they feel this way. Often they are reacting out of fear. A patient who has had a body part, such as a breast, removed may believe that she is ugly and disfigured. This has a negative effect on self-esteem. She may be angry and complain about your care and many other things. The patient is not mad at you. She is upset about her situation. She is afraid of how she looks, what will happen to her, and how she will manage. This threat to her self-esteem makes her react with anger. Other patients may react in different ways. Assist the patient with her appearance. If she looks attractive, she will feel better about herself. Allow her to talk about what is bothering her. Do not judge her for what she says and does. Be aware of what she is feeling and show that you sincerely care.

Self-Actualization. *Self-actualization* is feeling a sense of accomplishment and success. You can help the patient meet this need by recognizing improvements and assisting him to return to self-care. Sincerely compliment the patient for these accomplishments. This praise helps patients feel that they are overcoming a disease or disability and promotes self-actualization.

■■■ CULTURAL INFLUENCES ON HEALTH CARE DELIVERY

■ **culture:** *the pattern or life-style of an individual or group*

Health care workers will care for patients from many different **cultures**. These patients may come from other countries or communities. Their backgrounds, beliefs, values, religions, and hygiene and health care practices may be very different from your own. Do not judge them for their beliefs. Look at this as an opportunity to learn more about others. If you can learn about the patient's culture, you will be in a better position to meet her needs. Cultural background may influence the patient's beliefs about the illness and preferences in health care. The best way to find out about these preferences is to ask the patient or the family. Asking is not offensive. It shows that you are sensitive, have a sincere desire to learn, and are trying to find ways to help the patient. There is no one good way to meet the needs of an entire cultural group. Trying to place members of a cultural group in a specific category and thinking they are all alike is **stereotyping**. Everyone is an individual with different wants and needs. Different cultural groups have different beliefs and different ways of meeting their needs. Treat all patients as worthwhile human beings and recognize their individuality!

■ **stereotyping:** *fixed images or beliefs that categorize an individual or group*

Language Barriers

Always address each patient in English. Speak slowly, gently, and in a respectful manner. If you determine that the patient does not speak English, ask the patient if she has a bilingual dictionary. If not, try using gestures or writing. Some patients learn to read English before they learn to speak it. Use simple terms. Drawing pictures may be useful. If you must perform a procedure on a patient, use gestures and a demonstration to make the patient understand. Always ask the patient if she understands, or say "Okay?" Do not assume that the patient understands because she smiles. A smile may be only a polite gesture, indicating a lack of understanding. Be prepared to spend extra time with the patient who does not speak English.

■ **personal space:** *a comfortable distance in which to communicate with others*

Cultural Influences on Personal Space. **Personal space** varies in different cultures. In the United States, our personal space is about 18 to 36 inches; for us, this is a comfortable distance from which to communicate with others. People from other cultures may believe that this distance is too close. In other cultures, personal space occupies a much smaller distance. Be sensitive to the patient's discomfort when you are working closely with him. His beliefs about personal space may be different from yours. People from some cultures will not permit members of the opposite sex to care for them. Saudi Arabians, for example, will not permit a male caregiver to enter the room if a female patient is alone.

Use of Gestures and Eye Contact. The use of gestures and eye contact is not universal. In some cultures, making eye contact when you speak is offensive. Gestures that are acceptable to patients in the United States may be offensive to those from other countries. In India, the head motions used for "yes" and "no" are the direct opposites of the nodding or shaking motions used in the United States. Monitor your body language, use of eye contact, and gestures carefully. If something appears to make the patient uncomfortable, stop doing it.

Cultural Influences on Pain. Patients from different cultures react differently to pain. In some cultures, patients are very emotional and react very dramatically to discomfort. In others, the patient will not show any response even to severe pain. In China and Japan, for example, displaying pain in public is unacceptable. In these cultures, pain is considered a sign of weakness.

Cultural Influences on Hygienic Practices. Some countries have different beliefs about bathing, personal hygiene, and the use of deodorants. They may not bathe regularly or use deodorants to eliminate odor. In the United States, it is normal to bathe and use deodorant daily. Women remove hair from their legs and underarms. This is not true of women in some other cultures. Do not be offended if the patient's hygienic practices differ from yours. This may be a difficult problem for you, so consult your supervisor for ways of dealing with this situation.

Cultural Influences on Clothing. Various pieces of clothing may have cultural or religious significance. Some religions require men to keep their heads covered. Others require women to keep their heads covered. In some cultures, women may not show any skin besides their face and hands—all other skin must be covered. Such a patient will be very uncomfortable in a bed wearing only a hospital gown because of the difference in cultural beliefs. Learning about the patient's culture and trying to make accommodations shows that you care and will be greatly appreciated by the patient.

Cultural Influence and Home Remedies. People in some cultures have home remedies that they believe will cure their illness or relieve symptoms. These remedies may consist of wraps, rubs, teas, or inhalants made of herbs and spices. Friends and family members may practice these remedies on patients in the health care facility. In some cases, the remedies may actually interfere with the patient's medical treatment. Report to your supervisor for advice if you observe patients practicing home remedies.

Cultural Influence on Food Preferences. Patients may refuse to eat certain foods or food combinations because of their cultural and religious beliefs. Some patients eat certain foods because they believe the food has a healing effect. People of some religions have days on which they fast and do not eat. The dietitian and supervisor may be able to arrange to have special foods served to these patients to meet their needs.

■■■ PROMOTING INDEPENDENCE

The OBRA legislation requires long-term care facilities to maintain or improve the resident's condition and to promote independence. Being independent also promotes a healthy self-esteem. Restorative care is a very important part of the OBRA philosophy and is used to help the resident attain maximum independence. Restorative care is *simply good patient care!* Regardless of the setting, restorative care is helpful to all patients and makes them feel good about themselves.

There is a common expression, "If you don't use it, you lose it." This is particularly true of self-help skills. We are not doing patients any favors by performing skills that they are able to complete. If the patient does not use the skill, eventually she may lose the ability to perform it. The patient may have low self-esteem because of her inability to care for herself. The sensitive care provider will give the patient every opportunity to perform daily life skills independently. Provide support and encouragement. Set the patient up with the needed materials. Allow the patient as much time as necessary to complete the task. If the patient is unable to complete the task independently, offer to finish it for the patient and provide positive feedback for what the patient was able to accomplish. Do not make the patient feel that she has failed if she is unable to complete the task. Always stress the patient's ability, not the disability.

KEY POINTS IN CHAPTER

Patients and residents in health care facilities have specific legal rights that are guaranteed by accrediting and regulatory agencies.

Health care workers must respect and protect the rights of the health care consumer. If the patient is unable to exercise these rights, the patient care technician should assist.

All human beings have the same basic needs, which are described in Maslow's hierarchy of needs.

The patient's culture and religion influence your ability to provide care.

Restorative care is given to assist the patient to attain and maintain the highest level of independence possible.

REVIEW QUIZ

Multiple Choice Questions

1. An advance directive is a document that:
   a. gives consent for treatment and procedures while the patient is hospitalized.
   b. states the patient's wishes for care if the patient cannot speak for himself.
   c. gives the health care worker the right to act in the patient's best interest.
   d. all of the above.

2. A health care proxy is:
   a. a person who makes health care decisions on behalf of the patient.
   b. the health care worker responsible for diagnostic testing.
   c. the individual who prescribes the patient's medical treatment.
   d. another term for the patient care technician.

3. The Patient's Bill of Rights guarantee patients treatment that is:
   a. private.   c. dignified.
   b. confidential.   d. all of the above.

4. When providing care to a patient:
   a. leave the door open so others will know you are in the room.
   b. closing the door is the only step necessary if the patient is alone in the room.
   c. close the door, privacy curtain, and window curtain.
   d. you may leave the door open if the privacy curtain is pulled.

5. It is acceptable to discuss a patient's condition:
   a. at the nurses station or another private area.
   b. in the elevator.
   c. in the cafeteria.
   d. with your family at home.

6. A visitor asks you what is wrong with Mr. Stone, the patient in room 402. You know that Mr. Stone was recently diagnosed with pneumonia related to AIDS. Your best response is:
   a. "He has AIDS. For further information, consult administration."
   b. "He has pneumonia."
   c. "I'm sorry, but I cannot give you that information."
   d. "Ask the doctor."

7. You are assigned to care for a 24-year-old male patient who is unable to move his arms and legs. He is alert and able to communicate with you. The supervisor has instructed you to bathe and shave the patient. You should:
   a. ask the patient what time he would like the bath.
   b. give the patient as many choices as possible.
   c. provide privacy when bathing and shaving the patient.
   d. all of the above.

8. You care for Mrs. King, a 92-year-old, confused patient on Monday. Mrs. King speaks, but does not make sense. You are off on Tuesday. When you return to work on Wednesday, you are assigned to care for Mrs. King again. When you remove her gown to bathe her, you notice bruises on her upper arms. You should:
   a. Say nothing, as the bruises must have occurred on your day off.
   b. Report your findings to the supervisor of your unit.
   c. Ask Mrs. King why she has bruises.
   d. Tell the supervisor that Mrs. King was neglected on your day off.

9. Mr. Murray is a 72-year-old, confused patient. You are assigned to care for him on the 3 p.m. to 11 p.m. shift. When you make your first round to check your patients, you discover that Mr. Murray is in bed. His sheets are wrinkled and soaking wet. There are brown rings of urine on the bottom sheet, indicating that Mr. Murray's linen has not been changed in quite a while. There is food in the bed, and the patient's face and hands are dirty. It appears as if someone forgot to care for this patient. This may be an example of:
   a. neglect.   c. false imprisonment.
   b. abuse.   d. involuntary seclusion.

10. Signs of abuse may include:
    a. nausea and vomiting.   c. fever.
    b. unexplained injuries.   d. all of the above.

11. Negligence that results in harm to the patient is:
    a. libel.   c. malpractice.
    b. slander.   d. defamation.

12. Walking off duty before a suitable replacement can be obtained is:
    a. involuntary seclusion.   c. neglect.
    b. abandonment.   d. abuse.

13. Good Samaritan laws are designed to protect:
    a. health care workers at the scene of an emergency outside the place of employment.
    b. licensed personnel providing emergency care as part of their job responsibility.
    c. all health care workers on duty in the hospital.
    d. physicians only.

14. Standards of care are based on:
    a. laws.
    b. facility policies and procedures.
    c. information in textbooks and journals.
    d. all of the above.

15. Needs on the lowest level of Maslow's hierarchy include:
    a. love.   c. food.
    b. safety.   d. self-esteem.

16. According to Maslow's theory:
    a. the needs at one level must be satisfied before needs at the next level become important.
    b. the need for self-esteem is the most important of all.
    c. self-actualization is the feeling of love from your family members.
    d. all of the above.

17. People who come from other cultures:
    a. have incorrect beliefs and values.
    b. may have different beliefs than your own.
    c. are all the same.
    d. all of the above.

18. Mrs. Hernandez is a 34-year-old Hispanic female with ovarian cancer. She is in the last stage of her illness and her family members are at her bedside. When you are making the bed, you notice a raw egg in a cup under the bed. You should:
    a. throw the egg away immediately because it is unsanitary.
    b. tell the family to remove the egg.
    c. ask the patient or family the purpose of the egg.
    d. tell the patient she cannot have raw eggs.

19. Personal space is:
    a. a comfortable distance in which to communicate.
    b. a private area used for dressing.
    c. the bathroom.
    d. the patient's room.

20. When caring for patients, you should:
    a. provide all care needed even if the patient can do the care himself.
    b. practice restorative care.
    c. force the patient to do as much as possible.
    d. always consult the doctor for advice.

5 Communication and Interpersonal Skills

OBJECTIVES:

After reading this chapter, you will be able to:

Spell and define key terms.

List five methods of communicating with others and give an example of each.

Describe the four elements of communication.

List eight barriers to communication and give an example of each.

Describe goal-oriented communication.

List six communication styles.

Explain why listening is an important part of communication.

Describe how to communicate with patients with physical disabilities, vision loss, or hearing impairments, patients who are mentally confused, and those who are unable to speak.

■■■■ COMMUNICATION

■ *message: the information the sender wants to communicate*

Communication involves sending and receiving **messages** to exchange information with others. Verbal communication is the most common method used. You will use many forms of communication in health care to interact with patients, families, visitors, coworkers, and supervisors. You will communicate verbally, in writing, through gestures, and through use of your body. To be successful, you must understand and practice effective communication. The messages you send and receive must be interpreted accurately. Communication is more than saying words. It is showing honest concern and caring for other people.

Factors That Influence Communication

■ *barrier: something that interferes with communication*
■ *empathy: understanding how someone else feels*

Sickness, medication, anesthesia, pain, aging, culture, and disease can all affect the patient's ability to communicate. Some patients may have trouble seeing, hearing, or speaking. Sometimes the patient has a language **barrier** and does not speak English. When patients have difficulty communicating, the patient care technician must always practice **empathy**. This involves putting yourself in the patient's shoes and understanding how it feels. Imagine how frustrating it would be if you were unable to make your needs known and communicate with others! Be patient when communicating with patients with physical and mental impairments. Do not assume that patients who are unable to speak are mentally confused. Treat all patients with dignity and respect.

Posture, appearance, and body language also affect communication. All of us use our bodies to communicate. You must become sensitive to the body language of others and monitor your own body language to be sure that it sends the correct message. Your words and body language should both say the same thing.

■■■■ ELEMENTS OF COMMUNICATION

Understanding the elements of communication will help you communicate effectively. Each message has four parts:

■ **sender:** *the person who originates communication*
■ **receiver:** *the person for whom a message is intended*
■ **feedback:** *confirmation that a message was received as intended by the sender*

■ A sender
■ A message
■ A receiver
■ Feedback

Feedback may be verbal or nonverbal. An example of *verbal feedback* is responding with spoken words. An example of *nonverbal feedback* is a nod of the head indicating understanding.

Verbal Communication

Most communication is done verbally, by the spoken word. Although the words that you speak are important, the tone and pitch of your voice can affect and change the meaning of the communication. Choose your words carefully. Avoid using slang or words with more than one meaning. Use words that the receiver is likely to be familiar with. Speak slowly and clearly. Look at the receiver when speaking.

Touch

Touch is a very powerful means of communication. Touch can communicate a calm, caring attitude. It sends a message of compassion, caring, and acceptance (Figure 5-1). All human beings need to be touched. Use touch that is appropriate to the patient's age. For example, holding an adult patient's hand or firmly resting your hand on his or her forearm or shoulder communicates caring. Patting or stroking a child's head communicates caring.

Attending Behavior

■ **attending behavior:** *means and techniques used to improve the transfer of verbal communication*

Attending behavior shows that you are alert and interested in what the other person is saying to you. Five components of attending behavior are:

■ Eye contact
■ Gestures
■ Posture
■ Physical distance from the other person
■ Paraphrasing

Good eye contact is important to communication. The eyes are very powerful messengers. Even if the body is still, a great deal can be learned about how a person is feeling or thinking by looking at the eyes.

Gestures can be movements of your body or movements of your face. We gesture with our facial muscles, eyebrows, mouths, hands, and feet. We may shift restlessly about in a chair. These movements send powerful messages to others.

Posture is how you hold your body when you stand or sit. When you are seated, leaning forward in the chair while another person speaks shows that you are interested. Standing with your hands on your hips suggests anger, disgust, or impatience. Your body should be relaxed for effective communication to occur.

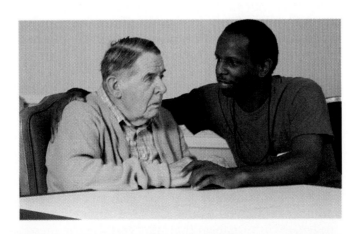

Figure 5-1 Touch sends a powerful message that you care.

Physical distance is important for effective communication. In the United States, a comfortable physical distance from others is about 18 to 36 inches, or one arm's length. If you are closer than this, others may be uncomfortable. If you are farther away, the receiver may be offended, or the message misinterpreted because the receiver could not see or hear you correctly. The patient care technician must realize that comfortable physical distance for communication varies with the culture of the patient and care provider.

■ *paraphrasing: a method of restating the message communicated to you in clear, simple terms*

Paraphrasing is an effective method of showing that you understand what has been said. Listening to the message and paraphrasing provide feedback and show that you are sincerely interested in the conversation.

Barriers to Communication

A barrier to communication can be physical, such as with a patient whose ears are bandaged after surgery. The bandage makes it difficult for the patient to hear. Eliminate barriers whenever possible. If this is not possible, find other means to communicate, such as writing. Barriers can also be mental. Mental barriers occur when you have formed a negative opinion about another person. Enter each communication with an open mind, and try not to form opinions about others based on appearances.

Sometimes other barriers are present, such as mental confusion or inability to speak English. If you are not sure of the patient's ability to communicate, ask the patient his name and speak with him about the season or weather. Provide orienting information if necessary and evaluate the patient's response. Keep your questions simple and ask only one question at a time. If the patient does not understand, rephrase the question. Do not make fun of the patient's lack of understanding. Laugh with the patient, if appropriate. Use the information you have obtained from your evaluation of the patient's understanding to plan your care. Other barriers to communication are:

■ Teasing and kidding. Although these are not always barriers, they may be offensive, so avoid them if you do not know the patient well.

■ Threatening and warning. Never threaten patients that you will withhold care because of something they have said or done. Consult your supervisor.

■ Preaching, moralizing, or passing judgment. Do not judge the patient for what she has said or done. Not expressing your opinion is better. To be successful, you must try to be neutral and objective even if you disagree.

■ Directing and ordering. Your tone of voice and choice of words can turn a request into an order. Select your words carefully to avoid sounding like the patient has no choice.

■ Arguing. This may make the patient defensive and the intent of the original communication will be lost.

■ Interrupting or changing the subject. This sends a message to the patient that what she has to say is not worthwhile, and may inhibit future conversation.

■ Giving brush-offs. Avoid statements such as, "Don't worry about it," which send a message to the patient that her concerns are not important.

Finally, do not talk to the patient about your personal problems. This is never appropriate in the health care setting.

■■■ GUIDELINES FOR COMMUNICATION

Use every contact with a patient as an opportunity for communication. Smile and speak when you are in the patient's room or pass in the hallway. Speak to the patient when giving care. Set aside time to talk to patients. This shows that you like them and are genuinely concerned for their well-being. Communication should be goal-oriented. Before beginning a conversation, set a goal. Think about what you want to accomplish and focus on that topic. Arrange the main points of what you would like to say in logical order. Eliminate unrelated or unnecessary information that may confuse the message.

Communication Styles

After you have set a goal for your conversation, select the style of communication that will help you meet this goal. Six types of conversations and the goal of each are listed in Table 5-1.

Table 5-1

Type of Conversation	Goal
Social conversation	To create a comfortable, relaxed atmosphere. Talk about pleasant things that the patient may be interested in. Do not discuss your problems or complaints with patients.
Interviewing	To obtain information that will help you meet the patient's needs. For example, ask if the patient prefers to take a shower in the morning or evening. Interviewing helps you plan your routine and shows patients you are genuinely interested in their well-being.
Teaching	To show and tell patients something that they will learn, understand, and use. All health care workers are teachers.
Reporting	To communicate accurate information. Reporting is done to your nurse manager or supervisor. Accurate reporting involves communicating factual information.
Problem solving	To help meet the patient's needs. It is different from interviewing because you already know what the patient wants. Your objective is to find a way to do it.
Therapeutic communication	To encourage patients to talk about feelings. This type of communication is particularly sensitive because you must not pass judgment on what the patient thinks or feels. Monitor your body language carefully.

General Guidelines for Having a Conversation

- Knock on the patient's door, introduce yourself by name and title, and address the patient by his preferred name.
- Approach the patient in a friendly, courteous manner.
- If you are in the room to perform a procedure, explain it to the patient before beginning. Allow time for the patient to ask questions and show understanding.
- If your time is limited, prepare the patient in advance by stating how much time you have and when you need to leave.
- Speak in a language that is familiar to the patient.
- Make eye contact during the conversation.
- Be polite.
- Speak clearly and distinctly.
- Listen to what the patient says. Ask questions or make comments to show you are interested.
- Use touch to communicate caring, if appropriate.

General Guidelines to Use When Speaking

These techniques make all types of communication more meaningful.

- Maintain good eye contact during the conversation.
- Sit at the patient's eye level, if possible.
- Speak clearly and directly.
- Use language the patient will understand. Avoid using medical terminology.
- Keep your message brief and concise. This should not be difficult if you have thought about your communication and selected a goal in advance.
- Use nonverbal communication, such as touch, posture, and body language, if appropriate.
- Use open-ended questions to encourage the patient to speak.

Listening

Listening is a very important part of communication. Listening to what someone else is saying may be difficult when you have other things on your mind. Your body language may betray you and send a message that you are not interested in what the other person is saying. Although this may not be the case, it may be what your body is implying, so monitor your movement and expressions closely. Paraphrasing is a good technique to use to show that you are listening. Silence is also a good technique. Silence shows acceptance and respect and encourages the patient to speak. You may be uncomfortable with silence. If so, work to overcome it.

General Guidelines for Listening

- Use open posture. Lean toward the patient. Do not cross your arms in front of your body or place your hands on your hips.
- Give the patient your full attention.
- Maintain eye contact with the patient.
- Show interest in the patient's activities, interests, and concerns.
- Monitor the patient's body language to see if it confirms or conflicts with the verbal message.
- Encourage patients to talk about their feelings and concerns. Allow patients to express anger and negative feelings without passing judgment.
- Use touch to communicate caring, if appropriate.
- Use silence to allow the patient to think and continue the conversation.
- Ask questions if necessary. Use paraphrasing to show interest and understanding. Use noncommittal responses, such as "I see," to show that you are listening.

continues

> ## General Guidelines for Listening, *continued*
>
> - Use responses such as, "I would like to hear more about that," or "Then what happened?" to show that you are interested.
> - Use responses such as, "So you felt bad about that" to show empathetic understanding of the patient's feelings.
> - Wait until the patient is finished speaking before you respond.
> - Request help from your supervisor, if needed, to solve problems.

> ## General Guidelines for Ending a Conversation
>
> - Inform the patient that you have to leave.
> - Tell the patient what time you will be back, and be sure to come back at that time.
> - Tell the patient that you enjoyed the conversation.
> - Ask the patient if she needs anything before you leave.
> - Before leaving the room, make sure that the patient is safe, comfortable, and has the call signal and needed personal items within reach.

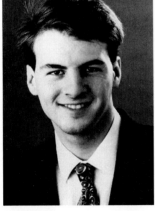

Figure 5-2 John Foppe lives independently and is a successful motivational speaker. John stresses that some people *want* to manage time well, feel confident about themselves, and relate well to others. He *must* do those things to survive. His condition does not give him a different set of problems from other people; he has the same problems as everyone else, but not having arms makes those same problems more difficult. (Courtesy of John Foppe)

■ COMMUNICATING WITH PATIENTS WITH DISABILITIES AND SENSORY IMPAIRMENTS

Sensory impairments can take many forms. Some impairments, such as speech, hearing, or language problems, interfere directly with communication. Other problems, such as physical impairments, may make you uncomfortable and unsure of what to say without offending the patient. People with disabilities are much like you are. They have the same wants and needs. They can do many of the same things you can, but may need to adapt the environment in order to do them. Although the end result may be the same, persons with disabilities may perform the task differently. Their bodies work differently! As a rule, people with disabilities do not want to be treated differently from anyone else. Most are self-sufficient and lead productive lives. People with disabilities are valuable and equal members of society. Although physically challenged, many have developed their talents and qualities using nonphysical skills. John Foppe (Figure 5-2) was born without arms. He overcame his disability, is self-sufficient, and lives independently. He travels throughout the country, without help, telling others that they can overcome adversity! He sets an example that inspires and encourages everyone, whether disabled or non-disabled, whose life he touches. John is an outstanding example of a person with a disability who has overcome tremendous odds and accomplished great things.

Health care providers have a responsibility to emphasize the uniqueness and worth of all persons, rather than the differences between people. Your efforts on behalf of the disabled will do much to eliminate the "them" versus "us" attitude that prevents acceptance of people with disabilities. Treat people with disabilities the way you like to be treated. You will leave the experience feeling fulfilled and richly rewarded.

General Guidelines for Communicating with Patients with Disabilities

■ **paralyzed:** *absence of movement and sensation due to an illness or injury.*

- Avoid referring to the patient as a condition, such as "the paraplegic in 221." Say instead, "the person who is **paralyzed**."
- Use common sense when talking to someone with a disability. Talk to the person with a disability the same way you would anyone else. People with disabilities do not want to be treated differently.
- Do not assume that someone is *not* disabled, or is pretending, because the disability is not visible. Some medical conditions are severely disabling even though the persons who have them may not appear disabled.

■ **prosthesis:** *an artificial body part*

- Shaking hands is appropriate with people who have upper extremity disabilities. Patients with limited movement or a **prosthesis** are able to shake hands. Shake hands gently with a person with arthritis.
- Before helping someone with a disability, ask if you can help. It is all right to offer to help, but unless the patient is struggling, do not assume that someone needs help without asking.
- It is all right to ask patients about their disabilities. Many patients are comfortable and will talk about them, but it is also all right if they do not want to talk about it. Persons who are newly disabled may not have reached a point of mental acceptance and may be uncomfortable speaking about their problem.
- When caring for a patient with a disability, do not assume that the patient can or cannot do something. Assuming can be offensive. Always ask.
- Always stress what patients *can* do and not what they *cannot* do.
- Patients who use wheelchairs, canes, walkers, and crutches because of a disability are not always sick. Many such persons are healthy and strong. They come to the health care agency for therapy, assistance with activities of daily living, tests, and other types of treatment.
- Patients in wheelchairs do not like to be treated as if they are mentally impaired! Most have no mental problem. Talk to the person in the wheelchair, not his or her companion.
- When talking to patients in wheelchairs, position yourself at their eye level.
- Be polite. Show the same manners that you would with anyone else.
- Use good manners, if you walk in front of a patient in a wheelchair, by excusing yourself.
- If you are in a crowded area, such as when attending an activity, do not stand in front of a person in a wheelchair. This blocks the patient's view.
- The wheelchair is an extension of the disabled person's body. Leaning or hanging on the chair is an invasion of the patient's personal space.

continues

General Guidelines for Communicating with Patients with Disabilities, *continued*

- ■ Words such as "see," "hear," "run," and "walk" can be used when speaking with people with disabilities.
- ■ Choose words that are positive and nonjudgmental. Avoid using words like "cripple," "gimp," "spastic," "retard." These terms are demeaning and promote negative perceptions of the physically challenged. Table 5-2 gives examples of acceptable and unacceptable terminology to use in conversation. Remember, always emphasize the person first. Emphasizing the disease is

Table 5-2

Offensive and Unacceptable— Do not use in conversation	Acceptable—Use this instead
Disabled person	A person with a disability
Blind person	A person who is vision impaired
Deaf person	A person who is hearing impaired
A hunchback	A person who has curvature of the spine
The disabled	People who are disabled; the disabled community
He is a cripple	He has a disability
Dumb (or deaf and dumb)	A person who has a speech or hearing impairment
She is nuts [or] crazy	She has an emotional disability or mental illness
Retard	A person who is developmentally disabled [or mentally retarded]
Birth defect	A person who is disabled from birth
Fit	Seizure
Normal person as compared to a person with a disability	A person who is not disabled as compared to a person who is
Confined to a wheelchair	A person who uses a wheelchair

continues

General Guidelines for Communicating with Patients with Disabilities, *continued*

demeaning. Table 5-3 lists phrases to avoid when speaking about persons with disabilities.

- People with disabilities like to laugh and have fun. Do not leave them out!
- Canine companions, such as seeing eye dogs or hearing ear dogs, are on duty. Do not feed or pet them without the owner's permission. This distracts the animals and prevents them from doing their job.
- Do not park in spaces reserved for the disabled (even if you remain in the car)—they need them more than you do!

Table 5-3 Words to Avoid When Speaking to or About the Disabled

abnormal	defect	normal
afflicted	defective	palsied
burden	deformity	poor
cerebral palsied	diseased	spastic
confined to a wheelchair	epileptic	stricken with
courageous	gimp	sufferer
cripple	invalid	suffers with
crippled	imbecile	suffering
deaf and dumb	maimed	unfortunate
deaf mute	moron	victim

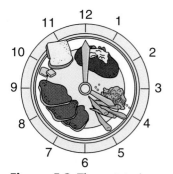

Figure 5-3 The potato is between 12 and 2 o'clock. The vegetables are between 3 and 5 o'clock. The meat is between 6 and 9 o'clock. The bread is between 10 and 12 o'clock.

Communicating with Patients with Vision Loss

Vision loss can range from problems that can be corrected with glasses to complete blindness. Some people are legally blind but still have very limited vision. Do not assume that the patient can see because he is wearing glasses. Some who wear glasses are still severely impaired. Blind people are like patients with other disabilities. They have a loss in one area of life, but they have developed other areas. Most are self-sufficient, even if they need environmental adaptations. Do not rearrange furniture, equipment, or supplies in the room without the patient's approval. People with visual impairments memorize the location of items. Moving things could result in accidents, injuries, or frustration because the patient is unable to find a needed item. When serving a meal tray to a visually impaired or blind patient, describe the location of food items as though they were on a clock face (Figure 5-3). Say "The bread is at 10:00 and the milk is

General Guidelines for Communicating with Patients Who Have Vision Loss

- Knock on the door and identify yourself by name and title before entering the room. Call the patient by the preferred name.
- Assist patients to clean their glasses and encourage wearing them.
- When speaking, sit in a good light where the patient can see your face. The light source should not be behind your back, as it will shine in the patient's eyes from this location.
- Speak clearly and directly in a normal tone of voice. Blindness does not interfere with the patient's ability to hear.
- Use touch to communicate, if appropriate, but do so slowly and gently so the patient is not startled.
- When you are performing tasks in the room, tell the patient what you are doing. It is acceptable to discuss new things you see, interesting changes, and what various people are doing. You are the patient's eyes!
- Tell the patient when you are finished.
- Replace everything in its original location.
- Tell the patient when you are leaving the room. Make sure the patient is comfortable and safe, with the call signal and needed personal items within reach.
- If you must assist the patient to walk, have the patient hold your upper arm (Figure 5-4). Walk alongside and slightly ahead of the patient. The patient can tell a great deal from your body movement. Walk naturally at the patient's pace. Tell the patient when there are steps, obstacles, turns, doors, and so forth. Be very specific when giving directions. Pause slightly before taking a step up or down or making a turn. Avoid revolving doors (and escalators if you are in a public place). If you are walking and are interrupted by someone, let the patient know you will be stopping.
- When using stairs, guide the patient's hand to the railing. Stop on each step before proceeding to the next one.
- When seating the patient, place the patient's hand on the back or arm of the chair.
- Do not leave a blind patient in an open area. Lead him to the side of a room, chair, or landmark from which he can obtain a direction for travel.

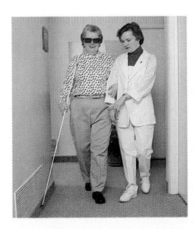

Figure 5-4 The patient who is vision impaired walks slightly to the side of the PCT, gently holding the upper arm.

at 2:00." When you are providing care or would like the patient to assist with a procedure, provide detailed, step-by-step directions.

Communicating with Patients Who Have Hearing Loss

Hearing loss can mean that a patient has difficulty hearing. It may also mean the patient is completely deaf. There are many causes of hearing loss. Some hearing loss can be corrected with hearing aids. Other types can be corrected with surgery. Some people have uncorrected hearing loss. People who are deaf communicate in many different ways. Some use sign language, which is a combination of hand signals and facial expressions. Others read lips. Some people use reading and writing as their primary form of communication. Special telephone and television communication systems and amplifiers are available for people who are deaf and

General Guidelines for Communicating with Patients Who Have Hearing Loss

- Approach the patient from the front or side. Lightly touch the patient's arm or shoulder. Avoid startling the patient.
- Eliminate as much background noise and activity as possible.
- Assist patients to use their hearing aids, if appropriate.
- If the patient hears better in one ear, position yourself on that side when speaking.
- Sit in a good light where the patient can see your face. The light source should not be behind your back, as it will shine in the patient's eyes from this location.
- Do not chew gum, eat, or put your hands in front of your mouth when speaking.
- Be considerate and try to make the patient feel confident in you.
- Look directly at the patient when speaking.
- Speak slowly, clearly, and distinctly. Use your lips to emphasize words.
- Choose short, simple words. Use short sentences.
- Speak in a lower pitched voice than normal. You may need to raise the loudness of your voice, but do not shout.
- Tell the patient what you are going to talk about.
- Write down key words, if necessary. Use communication boards or other adaptive equipment, if available.
- If the patient does not understand a word, use a different word instead of repeating what you said more loudly.
- Keep the conversation brief. Limit the conversation to a single topic.
- Do not convey impatience by your body language.
- If you do not understand what a person who is deaf or has a speech impairment says, asking her to repeat it is acceptable.
- If an interpreter is helping you, speak to the patient, not the interpreter.
- Tell the patient when you are leaving the room. Make sure the patient is comfortable and safe, with the call signal and needed personal items within reach.

hearing impaired. Patients with hearing loss can function independently but, as with other disabilities, may need environmental adaptations.

Caring for Patients with Hearing Aids. Some patients use hearing aids to help them hear more clearly. The hearing aid amplifies sound and improves communication. However, the patient may still be unable to hear normally, even with the hearing aid in place. Many types of hearing aids are available, but they all work on the same principle. The aid contains a tiny microphone that changes sound and increases the strength of electrical signals. A tiny speaker converts the signal to a sound wave and sends the message to the patient's ear.

General Guidelines for Caring for Hearing Aids

- The hearing aid is fragile. Avoid dropping it. Always hold the hearing aid over a soft surface or table when cleaning or caring for it.
- Keep the hearing aid clean. Remove it daily and wipe off any dust, ear wax, or body oil with a tissue.
- If the hearing aid is the cannula type, remove ear wax from the speaker opening with a pipe cleaner or special appliance cleaner. Ask the patient if he has a tool called a wax loop, and use it if available. Never use a toothpick, paper clip, or other sharp object.
- When caring for a female patient, do not spray hairspray when the hearing aid is in place.
- Avoid getting the hearing aid wet. If it has an outer ear mold, the ear piece may be washed with mild soap and warm water. The part of the hearing aid containing the batteries should never get wet. Allow the mold to dry thoroughly before reattaching it to the unit.
- Remove the aid when bathing the patient or washing the hair.
- Turn the hearing aid off when it is not in the patient's ear. Opening the battery case when the aid is stored prevents unnecessary drain on the battery.
- Remove the battery at night and check it for leaks. Replace worn out or leaking batteries. Wipe the battery gently with a clean cloth before reinserting it.
- Avoid temperature extremes. Do not store the aid in a cold area, on a radiator, or in direct sunlight.
- If the hearing aid has a cord, check it for cracks or breaks.
- Insert the hearing aid properly. Sometimes the shape of the ear changes with aging and the hearing aid may need to be refitted. If the patient complains of pain, this may be the problem. Advise the supervisor if this occurs.
- When communicating with the patient, follow the same guidelines that you use when communicating with a person with a hearing impairment.
- Check bed linen carefully before placing it in the soiled linen hamper. A hearing aid is small, expensive, and easily lost. It will not survive a trip through the washer and dryer!

General Guidelines for Troubleshooting Hearing Aid Problems

Never try to repair a hearing aid yourself. However, if the patient has problems with the aid, there are several things you can do that may resolve them.

- Check the aid to see if it is turned on. Some models have settings marked on them: "M" for microphone, "T" for telephone, and "O" for off. Set the switch to the "M" setting.
- Check the volume of the aid to be sure it is turned up loud enough for the patient to hear.
- Hold the hearing aid in the palm of your hand. Turn the volume up all the way. Cup the aid between your hands. You should hear a loud whistle. Weak or absent sound indicates that the battery is low.
- Before changing the battery, check the position of the old battery so you can put the new one in the same way. When inserting a new battery, place it in the unit gently. If you meet resistance, do not force it. Consult the supervisor.
- Check the ear mold for wax. If present, remove it.
- Ask the supervisor to check the patient's ears with an otoscope for wax buildup.
- If the hearing aid is in the patient's ear and makes a loud, whistling sound, check the position. The aid should be securely in the ear. Make sure that hair, ear wax, or clothing are not interfering with the position. Check the tubing for cracks. Whistling usually indicates an air leak.
- If the hearing aid works only intermittently, or makes a scratchy sound, check for dirt under and around the battery. Also check the volume control and connections. If the hearing aid has a connecting wire, make sure it is plugged in tightly and is not cracked or bent.

Communicating with Patients Who Have Problems with Language and Understanding

Some patients' illnesses or injuries affect their ability to speak and understand spoken communication. These patients may be able to understand some things, but not others. You must assume that they understand you. Try to communicate with them as you would other patients. Do not make the mistake of being silent while you are caring for them. Your silence may be received as a negative message by the patient.

These patients may be able to speak, but what they say does not make sense. They may use certain words or phrases that have meaning to them but not to you. Sincerely try to understand what they are saying. Be empathetic and do not show frustration. If you learn what they are saying, share this information with other members of the interdisciplinary team. This will enable all team members to help meet the patient's needs. Some patients are unable to speak correctly, but can understand you. Do not assume that the patient with a speech problem is mentally confused. Test the patient's ability to answer yes-or-no questions, or to follow simple directions, to determine the patient's mental status.

General Guidelines for Caring for Patients Who Have Problems with Language and Understanding

- Knock on the door and identify yourself by name and title before entering the room. Call the patient by the preferred name.
- Approach the patient in a friendly, courteous manner.
- Assist the patient with the use of glasses and hearing aids, if used.
- Explain what will be done.
- Use short, simple words. Pronounce them clearly and slowly.
- Focus on one topic and use short sentences.
- Use gentle touch to show that you care.
- Keep conversations short but frequent.
- Use facial expressions and gestures to convey your message.
- Allow adequate time for the patient to respond. Do not be tempted to complete a sentence for the patient.
- Listen carefully to the response. Pay close attention to what the patient is saying.
- If you think you understand what the patient is saying, use paraphrasing to give the patient feedback.
- Allow the patient time to finish speaking. Do not cut him off.
- Monitor your body language. Do not convey frustration due to your lack of understanding of the patient.
- Assume that the patient understands you if you are not sure and cannot get a response.
- Encourage the patient to point to things and use gestures.
- Use adaptive devices, such as picture boards (Figure 5-5) if available. A speech-language pathologist often provides these devices and teaches the patient to use them.
- Tell the patient when you are leaving the room. Make sure the patient is comfortable and safe, with the call signal and needed personal items within reach.

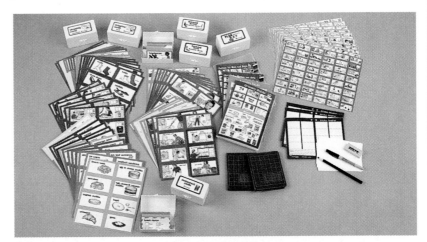

Figure 5-5 Pictures and similar communication devices allow patients to communicate by pointing to convey a message. (Picture Communication Package is provided by Sammons Preston, Inc., a BISSELL® Healthcare Company. Reprinted with permission)

General Guidelines for Communicating with Patients Who Have Problems Speaking

- Knock on the door and identify yourself by name and title before entering the room. Call the patient by the preferred name.
- Approach the patient in a friendly, courteous manner.
- Assist the patient with the use of glasses and hearing aids, if used.
- Keep conversations short but frequent.
- Use questions that can be answered with yes or no. Tell the patient to nod her head in response. If the patient is unable to nod the head, tell her to blink her eyes once for yes and twice for no.
- Allow adequate time for the patient to respond.
- Give the patient a pen and paper to write with, if able, or use assistive communication devices such as picture or word boards.
- Listen carefully to the response.
- If you think you understand what the patient is saying, use paraphrasing to give the patient feedback.
- Do not pretend to understand the patient if you don't.
- Emphasize the positive aspects of the message, such as words and gestures you do understand.
- Allow time to complete the conversation, to avoid sending the message that you are impatient with the patient.
- Assume that the patient understands you if you are not sure and cannot get a response.
- Use appropriate body language. Do not convey frustration at your inability to understand.
- Encourage the patient to point to things and use gestures.
- Tell the patient when you are leaving the room. Make sure the patient is comfortable and safe, with the call signal and needed personal items within reach.

Communicating with Patients Who Have Problems Speaking

Some diseases and injuries leave the patient unable to speak. These patients may be able to make noise, but not form words. However, they often understand what is being said to them. Do not make the mistake of thinking that the patient has a mental impairment because she is unable to speak. Over time, some patients are able to regain their speech with aggressive therapy. Some develop other methods of communication. These patients are often able to make themselves understood by gestures, writing, or other adaptive communication devices.

Communicating with Patients Who Are Mentally Retarded

Mental retardation affects about 3% of the population in the United States. A person who is mentally retarded is one who has experienced difficulty learning since childhood. Mental retardation is like any other disability. The patient did not cause it. The condition developed before birth or in early childhood. There are many levels of retardation, ranging from profound to mild. Patients with profound retardation function at the level of a newborn. People with mild re-

General Guidelines for Communicating with Patients Who Are Mentally Retarded

- Keep your words and sentences short and simple.
- Give clear, concise instructions.
- Do not "talk down" to the patient. Treat adults as adults.
- Listen to what patients say. Often they know more than you think.
- People who are mentally retarded are very sensitive to the moods of others. If you are upset, they will be too; if you are happy and relaxed, they will be too. Ask yourself how you look to them.
- If making decisions is upsetting to the patient, limit choices to no more than two.
- If you notice the patient becoming frustrated, slow down. Do not push.
- Praise and compliment the patient for even small accomplishments.
- Treat people who are mentally retarded with the same respect that you would give others.

tardation function at about the fourth-grade level. Most persons with a diagnosis of mental retardation (89%) are mildly retarded. People who are mentally retarded have the same needs as you, but learn more slowly and are limited in what they can learn. Most are able to live productive lives.

Individuals who are mentally retarded need acceptance and attention. Like all other patients, they must be treated with dignity and respect. They must be allowed to express themselves and relieve stress. They are able to make simple choices, but may become confused and frustrated if given too many options. If making decisions overwhelms the patient, limit choices to no more than two. Patients with mental retardation respond well to consistent treatment and expectations. When caring for these patients, use of the care plan by all staff is very important because this ensures consistent care. It is important for people who are mentally retarded to feel worthwhile. They like to help and feel like they are contributing. Most are happy and loving.

People who are mentally retarded should not be pressured to learn things or perform new tasks. They can be taught, but teaching them requires great patience. They often do not function well in high-pressure situations, and may not function well in large, loud groups unless someone is there to support them. They know if others are ridiculing them, and feel hurt and rejection.

Communicating with the Patient's Family, Friends, and Visitors

You are a representative of the health care facility to visitors. Speak to and smile at visitors in the hallway. If someone looks lost, ask if you can be of assistance. Maintain an open, friendly, and supportive attitude with visitors. Show them where the lounges, vending machines, cafeteria, restrooms, and smoking areas are. Answer any questions they have about your facility's policies and procedures. However, you must protect patient confidentiality, even with family members. If they ask you questions about the patient's condition, refer them to your supervisor. You may tell them something about the patient's activities, such as "He ate a good lunch."

Families may react in different ways to the patient's illness. They may show anxiety or anger. Be patient and understanding. Do not argue with them. Listen carefully and be empathetic. If family members have a complaint, report it to your supervisor immediately. If you notice a patient becoming upset when visitors are in the room, report this to your supervisor.

Sometimes you must perform a procedure on a patient when visitors are in the room. Ask the visitors to step out until you have completed the procedure. Show them where they can wait. When you are done with the procedure, inform them they can return to the room.

Answering the Telephone. Patient care technicians are required to answer the telephone in many health care facilities. If this is your responsibility, answer the phone by stating the name of your facility or unit. Identify yourself by name and title. Be courteous and polite. If a physician is on the line to give orders for a patient, you must get a supervisor to take the call. Unlicensed personnel cannot legally take orders from the physician. If the caller is not a physician, determine what is requested and provide the information, if possible. If not, obtain the information or transfer the caller to the proper person. If the person being called cannot come to the telephone, take a clear message. Write down the date and time of the call, the name of the caller, and a brief message. Sign your name and title to the message. Inform the caller that you will deliver the message. Thank the person for calling.

KEY POINTS IN CHAPTER

- *Many factors influence communication.*
- *Health care workers communicate with many people verbally, in writing, and through gestures, touch, and body language.*
- *The four elements of communication are the sender, the message, the receiver, and feedback.*
- *Using goal-oriented communication means deciding what you want to accomplish and focusing on a topic.*
- *Persons with disabilities should be treated the way you like to be treated. Some persons with disabilities have special communication needs.*
- *Courtesy is important when answering the telephone in the health care facility.*

REVIEW QUIZ

Multiple Choice Questions

1. Communication may be influenced by:
   a. sickness.
   b. medication.
   c. aging.
   d. all of the above.

2. Empathy means:
   a. understanding how the patient feels.
   b. feeling sorry for the patient.
   c. understanding emotional needs.
   d. solving problems for the patient.

3. The sender is the person who:
   a. gets the message.
   b. initiates a communication.
   c. interprets the message.
   d. relays communication to another person.

4. Feedback is:
   a. your interpretation of what the supervisor said.
   b. your interpretation of what the patient said.
   c. confirmation that a message was received as intended.
   d. all of the above.

5. Which of the following are components of attending behavior?
   a. eye contact and gestures.
   b. thinking and feeling.
   c. crossing your arms and legs.
   d. all of the above.

6. Comfortable personal space in the United States is:
   a. 8 inches.
   b. 18 inches.
   c. 42 inches.
   d. 48 inches.

7. Paraphrasing is:
   a. repeating what the speaker says word for word.
   b. interpreting the message for another person.

c. using sign language for a patient who is hearing impaired.

d. restating a message in clear, simple terms.

8. Something that interferes with communication is a:
   a. gesture.
   b. barrier.
   c. suggestion.
   d. symptom.

9. Thinking about what you want to accomplish in a conversation and focusing on a topic is an example of using:
   a. goal-oriented communication.
   b. paraphrasing.
   c. empathy.
   d. feedback communication.

10. A communication style in which you want to obtain information to meet the patient's needs is:
    a. therapeutic communication.
    b. problem solving.
    c. interviewing.
    d. social conversation.

11. When communicating with a patient in a wheelchair, you should avoid using the word:
    a. see.
    b. run.
    c. walk.
    d. none of the above.

12. When caring for patients with vision or hearing loss, you should:
    a. be as quiet as possible when you are in the room so the patient is not disturbed.

b. make as much noise as possible when you are in the room so the patient knows what you are doing.

c. announce yourself by name and title when entering the room.

d. none of the above.

13. When caring for patients who have problems with speech or understanding, you should:
    a. explain the care you will be giving in medical terms.
    b. choose short, simple words and use short sentences.
    c. use sign language.
    d. all of the above.

14. When caring for a person who is mentally retarded, you should:
    a. treat the patient with courtesy and respect.
    b. not explain procedures.
    c. never smile, because this is upsetting to the patient.
    d. all of the above.

15. You answer the telephone on your unit. The caller identifies herself as Dr. Gonzales and states that she wants to give orders for Mrs. Keene. You should:
    a. ask the doctor to hold while you get the nurse.
    b. write down the orders the doctor gives you.
    c. tell the doctor to call back later.
    d. none of the above.

Observations, Recording, and Reporting

After reading this chapter, you will be able to:

- *Spell and define key terms.*
- *Differentiate between signs and symptoms and between subjective and objective observations.*
- *Describe how to report and record patient information.*
- *List 10 guidelines for documenting in the medical record.*
- *Correctly use medical terminology and abbreviations.*

■■■■ COMMUNICATING WITH OTHER MEMBERS OF THE HEALTH CARE TEAM

You will communicate with other members of the health care team frequently throughout your shift. Some communication is written. Some is verbal. Reporting and recording your observations and care are a very important part of your job. Remember the principles of goal-oriented communication.

Observing the Patient

The patient care technician is responsible for making observations about the patient and reporting those observations to the supervisor. This is a very important responsibility. Because you spend more time with the patient than other health care workers do, you are in a position to notice changes immediately.

Use your senses to make observations. Many changes that you detect will be things that you can see. You may notice changes in movement, position, facial expression, or color. These changes may indicate pain or another problem. Use your ears to observe changes you can hear, such as noisy breathing or things the patient tells you. Your sense of smell is useful to detect unusual odors that may indicate a problem. You will note temperature changes or moisture on the skin with your sense of touch.

Observation of the patient is a continuous process. Bath time gives you the perfect opportunity to make observations of the patient's entire body and note changes. If you see, feel, hear, or smell anything that seems abnormal, report your observations to the supervisor. Even changes that seem insignificant may indicate a problem. For example, a red area on the skin may seem minor, but the area can quickly turn into a serious pressure sore. Report your observations to the supervisor, who will decide on the course of action.

Reporting Your Observations

Signs are seen or observed. For example, the red area you noticed on the patient's skin during the bath is a sign. **Symptoms** cannot be detected by using your senses. **Objective observations** are factual. **Subjective observations** may or may not be factual. For example, reporting that the patient did not eat lunch is an Objective observation. Reporting that the patient probably was not hungry is subjective, because it reflects what you think—it is your interpretation of a

■ ***sign:*** *observation about the patient that can be observed by others*
■ ***symptom:*** *something the patient reports about his or her condition*
■ ***objective observations:*** *factual observations that you make by seeing, hearing, feeling, touching, and smelling*
■ ***subjective observations:*** *observations based on what you think or what the patient tells you; may or may not be factual*

fact. Actually, the patient may have felt nauseated, or had another reason for not eating. Information reported to the supervisor should be objective.

Recording Your Observations

■ *chart:* the notebook or binder containing the patient's medical record
■ *medical record:* written documentation of the patient's true condition and a record of progress and care

The patient's **chart** (Figure 6-1), or **medical record**, is a legal document. It can be subpoenaed and used in court. It is a record of the patient's true condition and a record of progress and care. Policies vary regarding who is responsible for recording information on the chart. You may be responsible for documenting information. A common rule in health care is, "If it is not charted, it was not done." Documentation of care given is very important and should be taken seriously. Documentation on the medical record should be objective. It should also be clear, concise, and easy to read. Some facilities use flow-sheet charting (Figure 6-2). This is common for vital statistics, such as vital signs, height, and weight. Routine care, such as bathing, and noting of bowel movements, may also be charted on flow sheets. Other charting is done by narrative note. Know and follow your facility policy.

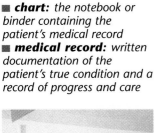

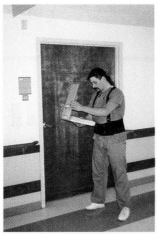

Figure 6-1 The medical record provides information about the patient's progress and care.

Name _Cedrone, Paul_   Room _311_

Activities of Daily Living

DATE		7/14								
		7-3	3-11	11-7	7-3	3-11	11-7	7-3	3-11	11-7
I.	DIET:									
	A. MEALS-AMT. EATEN	all / all								
	B. NOURISHMENTS									
II.	PERSONAL HYGIENE									
	A. Complete bath									
	B. Assist									
	C. Self	✓								
	D. Shower/tub bath									
	E. Mouth care	X2								
	F. Peri care									
	G. Back care									
III.	ACTIVITY									
	A. Bed rest	✓								
	B. Dangle									
	C. C&B									
	D. BRP									
	E. Ambulate									
	F. ROM									
IV.	Elimination									
	A. Bowels	X1								
	1. Amount	small								
	2. Consistency	liq.								
	3. Enema and results									
	4. Incontinent									
	B. Bladder									
	1. Voided	X3								
	2. Catheterized									
	3. Catheter care									
	4. Incontinent									
V.	TREATMENTS									
	1. Leg exercised TCDB									
	2. Antiembol. stockings - removed and replaced									
	3. Dressing changes									
	4. Irrigations									
	5. Soaks - hot packs, cold packs									
VI.	SPECIMENS (Specify)									
VII.	DIAGNOSTIC TESTS									
VIII.	OTHER	stool gu. neg								
IX.	SIDE RAILS UP	↑↓								
X.	SLEEP (naps, well, poorly)	naps								
XI.	Signature	S. Lopez NA								

Figure 6-2 The ADL flow sheet provides a record of personal care given on each shift.

Table 6-1

Standard Clock	24-Hour Clock	Standard Clock	24-Hour Clock
12:00 midnight	2400 or 0000	12:00 noon	1200
1:00 A.M.	0100	1:00 P.M.	1300
2:00 A.M.	0200	2:00 P.M.	1400
3:00 A.M.	0300	3:00 P.M.	1500
4:00 A.M.	0400	4:00 P.M.	1600
5:00 A.M.	0500	5:00 P.M.	1700
6:00 A.M.	0600	6:00 P.M.	1800
7:00 A.M.	0700	7:00 P.M.	1900
8:00 A.M.	0800	8:00 P.M.	2000
9:00 A.M.	0900	9:00 P.M.	2100
10:00 A.M.	1000	10:00 P.M.	2200
11:00 A.M.	1100	11:00 P.M.	2300

Charting Time. Entries in the chart are made in chronological order, by date and time. Some facilities color-code the charts to identify the shift. For example, blue ink is used for the day shift, green for the second shift, and red for the night shift. A more common practice is for all shifts to record in black ink. When this is done, the time of the entry must be made by using the 24-hour clock (Table 6-1). When this system is used, indicating times by noting A.M. or P.M. is not necessary. The day starts at midnight, or 2400 hours. This is the same as 12:00 A.M. For the first hour, only minutes are recorded. 12:25 A.M. is recorded as 0025. After the first hour, each hour increases by one until 24 hours are reached.

Computers in Health Care Facilities. Use of computers has become common in health care facilities, because the computer can store, process, and retrieve a large amount of information easily. Departments can communicate with each other by computer. The information is legible and easy to read, and patient information is readily available and easy to find. Statistics and data can be collected by computer and used to spot problems and trends. Patient care units in health care facilities do not use standard word processing programs for recording patient information. Special health care programs are available. These programs are usually simple to use, even for those with no computer experience. If you will be working with the computer, your facility will provide training on the programs you will be using. Don't be afraid of the computer. Becoming computer literate may be frustrating at first, but it can make your job much easier. Look at it as an opportunity to learn something new that will benefit you and allow you to spend more time with the patients.

General Guidelines for Charting

- Charting must be accurate and legible. Follow your facility policy for printing or charting in script. Make sure the entry can be easily read.
- Know the meaning and correct spelling of words before you write them on the chart.
- Chart the facts. Be specific. Do not make judgments or chart your personal opinions.
- Use the correct color pen with permanent ink. Never chart in pencil.
- Use short, concise phrases.
- Chart after an event occurs or care is given (Figure 6-3). Never chart in advance.
- Chart the exact time of the event.
- Leave no blank lines or spaces.
- If you make a mistake, do not erase or use correction fluid. Draw a single line through the entry and write "error" and your initials.
- Sign your first initial, last name, and title immediately after your entry.

DAILY NURSES' NOTES

DATE	TIME	
3-2-XX	0900	Dangled at bedside + tolerated well. Transferred to w/c c̄ gait belt + ÷ assist. *Ellen Stacy*, PCT
3-2-XX	0945	c/o pain in (L̶)(R) foot. Nurse notified. *Ellen Stacy*, PCT
3-2-XX	1030	Transferred back to bed c̄ gait belt + ÷ assist. Resting quietly @ present. *Ellen Stacy*, PCT

PATIENT	BED NO.	PHYSICIAN
Martin, Frank	412-A	Clark

Figure 6-3 Follow your facility policy for documenting on the medical record.

■■■ MEDICAL TERMINOLOGY

Medicine has a language of its own. This language is used to describe the diagnosis, body parts, procedures, orders, measurements, treatments, activities, time, and place. Each chapter in this book presents and defines new vocabulary. Learning these terms will help you master medical terminology. You will use medical terms to communicate with other members of the interdisciplinary team and to document on the patient's medical record.

Word Elements

Medical terms are a combination of word elements. You cannot expect to remember every medical term. You can, however, use your knowledge of the language of medicine to understand what unfamiliar terms mean.

■ **prefix:** the word element at the beginning of a word
■ **suffix:** the word element at the end of a word
■ **root:** the element that gives meaning to a medical word

The three elements of medical words are the prefix, suffix, and root. The prefix is the beginning of the word. A suffix is the ending of the word. The root provides the basic meaning of the word. For example, the root "arth" means joint. The suffix "algia" means pain. If you see the word *arthralgia*, you will know that it means pain in the joints. The letters "i" or "o" are sometimes added to the root word to make the word easier to connect and pronounce. Medical words can consist of a prefix and a suffix, a prefix and a root, a root and a suffix, or two roots.

■ *Word roots.* The word root (or root word) provides the basic meaning of the word. Table 6-2 contains a list of common root words.

■ *Prefixes.* The prefix is found at the beginning of a medical term. It does not stand alone. It is always accompanied by a root, a suffix, or both. Table 6-3 lists common prefixes.

Table 6-2 Common Word Roots

Root	Meaning	Root	Meaning
abdomin (o)	abdomen	cyst (o)	bladder, cyst
aden (o)	gland	cyt (o)	cell
angi (o)	vessel	dent (i) (o)	tooth
arteri (o)	artery	dermat (o)	skin
arth (o)	joint	encephal (o)	brain
bronch (i) (o)	bronchus	enter (o)	small intestine
cardi (o)	heart	erythr (o)	red
cephal (o)	head	fibr (o)	fiber
cerebr (o)	brain	gastr (o)	stomach
chol (e)	bile	geront (o)	elderly
col (o)	colon	gloss (o)	tongue
crani (o)	skull	glyc (o)	sugar *continues*

Table 6-2, continued

Root	Meaning	Root	Meaning
gynec (o)	female	pharyng (o)	throat
hem (o)	blood	phleb (o)	vein
hemat (o)	blood	pneum (o)	lung, air
hepat (o)	liver	proct (o)	rectum
hydr (o)	water	psych (o)	mind
hyster (o)	uterus	pulm (o)	lung
lapar (o)	abdomen, flank, loin	py (o)	pus
laryng (o)	larynx	rect (o)	rectum
lith (o)	stone	rhin (o)	nose
mamm (o)	breast	splen (o)	spleen
mast (o)	breast	stern (o)	sternum
men (o)	menstruation	thorac (o)	chest
my (o)	muscle	thromb (o)	clot
myel (o)	bone marrow, spinal cord	tox (o)	poison
nephr (o)	kidney	trache (i) (o)	trachea
neur (o)	nerve	ur (o)	urine
ocul (o)	eye	urethr (o)	urethra
ophthalm (o)	eye	urin (o)	urine
oste (o)	bone	uter (i) (o)	uterus
ped (i) (o)	child	ven (o)	vein

Table 6-3 Common Prefixes

Prefix	Meaning	Prefix	Meaning
a, an	without, not	ante	before
ab	away from	anti	against
ad	toward		*continues*

Table 6-3, *continued*

Prefix	Meaning	Prefix	Meaning
bi	double, two	neo	new
bio	life	non	not
brady	slow	pan	all
circum	around	per	by, through
dys	difficult, abnormal	peri	around
epi	on, over	poly	many
hemi	half	post	after
hyper	high, above, excessive	pre	before
hypo	low, below normal	pseud	false
inter	between	retro	backward
intra	inside, within	semi	half
leuk	white	septic	infection
micro	small	sub	under, below
		tachy	fast

- *Suffixes.* The suffix is found at the end of the medical term. Like the prefix, it does not stand alone, but is combined with a root, a prefix, or both. Table 6-4 lists common suffixes.
- *Word combinations.* Table 6-5 shows some examples of how different elements are combined to form words.

Table 6-4 Common Suffixes

Suffix	Meaning	Suffix	Meaning
algia	pain	itis	inflammation of
alysis	analyze	logy	study of
ectomy	surgical removal	lysis	destruction of
emia	blood	megaly	enlargement
gram	record		*continues*

Table 6-4, *continued*

Suffix	Meaning	Suffix	Meaning
meter	instrument that measures	*ptosis*	sagging, falling
ostomy	surgical opening	*rrhagia*	excessive flow
otomy	surgical opening	*rrhea*	discharge
pathy	disease	*scope*	instrument that examines
penia	deficiency	*stasis*	constant
phasia	speaking	*therapy*	treatment
plegia	paralysis	*uria*	condition of urine
pnea	breathing		

Table 6-5 Word Combinations

Medical Term	Prefix	Root	Suffix	Meaning
antiseptic	*anti*	*septic*	—	against infection
arthritis	—	*arthr*	*itis*	inflammation of joints
cardiology	—	*cardi*	*ology*	study of the heart
colostomy	—	*col*	*ostomy*	surgical opening into the colon
dyspnea	*dys*	—	*pnea*	difficult breathing
hemiplegia	*hemi*	—	*plegia*	paralysis in one-half of the body
hypoglycemia	*hypo*	*glyc*	*emia*	low blood sugar
glycosuria	—	*glyc*	*uria*	sugar in urine
leukemia	*leuk*	—	*emia*	condition of white blood cells
urinalysis	*urin*	—	*alysis*	analysis of the urine

ABBREVIATIONS

■ **abbreviation:** *a shortened form of a word*

In health care, abbreviations are used frequently to save space and time. Sometimes medical abbreviations represent Latin terms for a word. Other medical abbreviations are a combination of the letters used to form the word. For example, AIDS is the abbreviation for acquired immune deficiency syndrome. Learning common medical abbreviations is important for you. Abbreviations are used in conversation, in documentation, in the care plan, and on your assignment sheet. Some abbreviations are facility-specific. Each facility will have a list of abbreviations approved for use in charting. Refer to this list if you do not understand the meaning of an abbreviation. Sometimes an abbreviation can mean more than one thing. For example, D/C is the abbreviation for *discontinue*, but it can also be used to mean *discharge*. The context of the sentence in which an abbreviation is used should give you a clue to its meaning. Table 6-6 lists common medical abbreviations.

Table 6-6 Common Medical Abbreviations

Abbreviation	Meaning	Abbreviation	Meaning
abd.	abdomen	BRP	bathroom privileges
$\overline{ac}$	before meals	BS	blood sugar
ad lib	as desired	BSC	bedside commode
ADLs	activities of daily living	BSE	breast self-examination
adm	admission	C	Celsius, centigrade
AIDS	acquired immune deficiency syndrome	$\overline{c}$	with
aka	above-the-knee amputation	c	centimeter
am	morning	cc	cubic centimeter
AMA	against medical advice	CA	cancer
amb	ambulate	CAD	coronary artery disease
amt	amount	cal	calorie
ant	anterior	cath	catheter
AROM	active range of motion	CBC	complete blood count
ASAP	as soon as possible	CC	chief complaint
as tol	as tolerated	CHF	congestive heart failure
ax	axillary (under the arm)	ck or ✓	check
bid	twice a day	cl liq	clear liquid
bilat	bilateral	cm	centimeter
BKA	below the knee amputation	CNA	certified nursing assistant
BM	bowel movement	c/o	complains of
BP or B/P	blood pressure	COLD, COPD	chronic obstructive lung (pulmonary) disease
BR	bedrest, bathroom		*continues*

Table 6-6, *continued*

Abbreviation	Meaning	Abbreviation	Meaning
CPR	cardiopulmonary resuscitation	Fx	fracture
C & S	culture and sensitivity	GI	gastrointestinal
cu	cubic	gtt	drop
CVA	cerebrovascular accident, stroke	GU	genitourinary
CXR	chest x-ray	Gyn	gynecology
d	day	h	hour
D/C, DC	discontinue, discharge	H	hydrogen
DNR	do not resuscitate	HAV, HBV, HCV, etc.	hepatitis A virus, hepatitis B virus, hepatitis C virus, etc.
DOA	dead on arrival	Hg	mercury
DOB	date of birth	HIV	human immunodeficiency virus
DSD	dry sterile dressing	H_2O	water
Dx	diagnosis	H_2O_2	hydrogen peroxide
E	enema	HOB	head of bed
ECG, EKG	electrocardiogram	HOH	hard of hearing
EENT	eye, ear, nose, and throat	H & P	history and physical
ENT	ear, nose, and throat	hr	hour
et	and	hs	bedtime (hour of sleep)
exam	examination	ht	height
F	Fahrenheit	Hx	history
FB	foreign body	IDDM	insulin-dependent diabetes mellitus
FBS	fasting blood sugar	IM	intramuscular
FE	Fleet's enema	I & O	intake and output
FS	frozen section, finger stick	IPPB	intermittent positive pressure breathing
FSBS	finger stick blood sugar	isol	isolation
FU or F/U	follow up		
FUO	fever of unknown origin		*continues*

Table 6-6, *continued*

Abbreviation	Meaning	Abbreviation	Meaning
IV	intravenous	*neg* or −	negative
K or *K+*	potassium	*NG*	nasogastric
L	liter, left	*NIDDM*	non-insulin-dependent diabetes mellitus
lat	lateral		
lb	pound	*NKA*	no known allergies
LE	lower extremity	*noc*	night
LLE	left lower extremity	*NPO*	nothing by mouth
lg	large	*N/S*	normal saline
liq	liquid	*N & V*	nausea and vomiting
LLQ	left lower quadrant	*NVD*	nausea, vomiting, and diarrhea
L/min or *LPM*	liters per minute	*OBS*	organic brain syndrome
LOC	level of consciousness, level of care	*occ*	occasional
		O₂	oxygen
LPN	licensed practical nurse	*OOB*	out of bed
LTC	long-term care	*os*	mouth
LUQ	left upper quadrant	*OT*	occupational therapy
LVN	licensed vocational nurse	*oz* or ℥	ounce
M	meter	$\bar{p}$	after
meds	medications	*P*	pulse
MI	myocardial infarction (heart attack)	$\overline{pc}$	after meals
mL or *ml*	milliliter	*PE*	physical examination
mm	millimeter	*peds* or *pedi*	pediatrics
MRSA	methicillin-resistant *staphylococcus aureus*	*per*	by, through
		pm	afternoon or evening
NA or *N/A*	not applicable, Nursing Assistant (meaning determined by context)	*po*	by mouth
N/C	no complaints	*pos* or +	positive

continues

Table 6-6, continued

Abbreviation	Meaning	Abbreviation	Meaning
preop	preoperative	R/O	rule out
prep	prepare	ROM	range of motion
prn	as needed	rt	right
prog	prognosis	RUE	right upper extremity
PROM	passive range of motion	RUQ	right upper quadrant
pt or Pt	patient	Rx	prescription, therapy, treatment
PT	physical therapy	s̄	without
PVD	peripheral vascular disease	semi	half
q̄	each, every	sm	small
q̄d	every day	SOB	shortness of breath
q̄h	every hour	spec	specimen
q̄2h, q̄3h, q̄4h, etc.	every 2 hours, every 3 hours, every 4 hours, etc.	S/S, S & S	signs and symptoms
q̄hs	every night at bedtime	SSE	soapsuds enema
qid	4 times a day	stat	immediately
q̄m or q̄am	every morning	Std. prec.	standard precautions
q̄od̄	every other day	supp	suppository
q̄s̄	sufficient quantity	Sx	symptoms
qt	quart	T, temp	temperature
quad	quadrant	TB	tuberculosis
R	rectal, respiration, right	TID	three times a day
reg	regular	TKO	to keep open
rehab	rehabilitation	TLC	tender loving care
resp	respirations	TPN	total parenteral nutrition
RLE	right lower extremity	TPR	temperature, pulse, respiration
RLQ	right lower quadrant	trach	tracheostomy
RN	registered nurse		

continues

Table 6-6, continued

Abbreviation	Meaning	Abbreviation	Meaning
TWE	tap water enema	WA or W/A	while awake
Tx	traction, treatment	w/c	wheelchair
UA or U/A	urinalysis	WNL	within normal limits
UE	upper extremity	wt	weight
URI	upper respiratory infection	XR or X/R	x-ray
UTI	urinary tract infection	y/o	years old
vag	vaginal	yr	year
VRE	vancomycin-resistant enterococcus	↑	up
VS	vital signs	↓	down

KEY POINTS IN CHAPTER

- *The patient care technician communicates with other members of the health care team verbally and in writing.*

- *Observations about the patient are reported to the supervisor for assessment and action.*

- *The patient care technician records information about the patient in the medical record in writing or by using the computer.*

- *The patient care technician uses sight, hearing, smell, and touch to make valuable observations.*

- *Signs can be seen or observed. Symptoms are things the patient tells you.*

- *Objective observations are factual. Subjective observations are based on what you think or what the patient tells you.*

- *The medical record is a factual, permanent record of the patient's progress and care.*

- *The medical record is a legal document. Entries in it must be accurate and complete.*

- *Understanding medical terminology and medical abbreviations is important in communicating with other members of the health care team.*

REVIEW QUIZ

Multiple Choice Questions

1. A sign is an observation that you:
   a. detect with your senses.
   b. think.
   c. believe.
   d. all of the above.

2. A symptom is:
   a. something you know to be true.
   b. what the patient tells you.
   c. what you think.
   d. none of the above.

3. Objective means:
   a. something you think and feel.
   b. a complaint of pain.
   c. something you observe.
   d. none of the above.

4. The medical record:
   a. is a legal document.
   b. can be used in court.
   c. contains factual information.
   d. all of the above.

5. When using the 24-hour clock, 5:15 P.M. is:
   a. 0515 hours.
   b. 1515 hours.
   c. 1715 hours.
   d. 2015 hours.

6. The following is true about documenting in the patient's chart:
   a. correction fluid should be used if you make a mistake.
   b. factual information should be written on the chart.
   c. charting is always done before care is given.
   d. all of the above.

7. The prefix is found:
   a. at the beginning of a word.
   b. at the end of a word.
   c. in the middle of a word.
   d. in the root of the word.

8. A suffix is found:
   a. at the beginning of a word.
   b. at the end of a word.
   c. in the middle of a word.
   d. in the root of the word.

9. The root:
   a. introduces the word.
   b. describes the suffix.
   c. provides depth.
   d. provides meaning.

10. The term *myalgia* means:
    a. heart attack.
    b. infection of the bone.
    c. pain in the muscles.
    d. inflammation of the throat.

11. The term *colectomy* means:
    a. removal of the colon.
    b. removal of a cyst.
    c. pain in the small intestine.
    d. irritation of the gallbladder.

12. The term *phlebitis* means:
    a. infection of the lungs.
    b. inflammation of a vein.
    c. irritation of the throat.
    d. pus in a wound.

13. *Hydrotherapy* is:
    a. a disease of the lungs.
    b. removal of the uterus.
    c. water therapy.
    d. oxygen therapy.

14. The supervisor writes on your assignment sheet, "Mr. Dominguez, room 611-B/P at H.S." You know this means:
    a. to take the blood pressure at bedtime.
    b. to give Mr. Dominguez the bedpan at his side.
    c. that the patient should have big portions for his supper.
    d. that Mr. Dominguez has a blood problem with his system.

15. Mrs. Shane is to ambulate in the hallway TID. You know this means:
    a. every other day.
    b. twice a day.
    c. three times a day.
    d. ten times a day.

Short Answer/Fill in the Blanks

Define the following words based on your knowledge of medical terminology.

16. tachycardia _____

17. bradycardia _____

18. gastritis _____

19. ophthalmology _____

20. nephrectomy _____

21. pyuria _____

22. dyspnea _____

23. hemolysis _____

24. dysuria _____

25. mastectomy _____

26. intraabdominal _____

PERSONAL CARE SKILLS

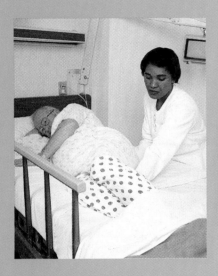
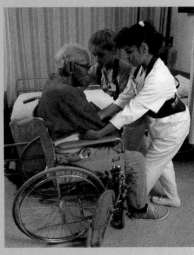
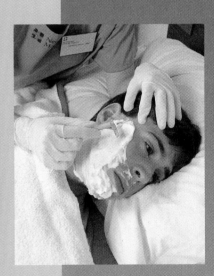

Body Mechanics and Lifting, Moving, and Positioning Patients

After reading this chapter, you will be able to:

Spell and define key terms.

Demonstrate good body mechanics when lifting and moving patients and other heavy objects.

Describe why positioning the patient in good body alignment is important.

Demonstrate proper positioning in the supine, prone, lateral, Fowler's, semisupine, and semiprone positions.

Describe the cause of pressure sores and list 10 methods of preventing pressure sore development.

Demonstrate how to assist patients with ambulation.

NOTE TO THE STUDENT

The direct care procedures begin in this chapter and continue through the remainder of the text. The beginning and ending steps of all procedures are the same. This text instructs you to "Perform your beginning procedure actions" or "Perform your procedure completion actions" before and after each procedure. These steps have been printed inside the front cover of your textbook for easy reference. Eventually, the steps will be committed to memory and you will not have to refer to them. However, in the initial stages of your training, refer to them often, because they are very important. Tables 7-1 and 7-2 summarize these important actions.

BODY MECHANICS

body mechanics: *correct use of the body to lift or move heavy objects or patients*

The patient care technician routinely lifts, moves, and positions patients and other heavy objects. Good body mechanics should be used any time you lift or move patients or heavy objects. Using your body correctly when picking up items from the floor, and when bending and lifting, is also important. Good body mechanics involve using the largest, strongest muscles to do the job. Your strongest muscles are in your legs and arms. Your weakest muscles are in your back and abdomen.

Practice the principles of good body mechanics until they become a habit. They will make your job easier and prevent fatigue by making the best use of your strength and energy. Use of proper body mechanics helps prevent injury to both care provider and patient.

Posture

Good posture is the foundation on which proper body mechanics is built. Good posture is the same whether you are standing, sitting, or lying down. Keep your back straight with your feet flat on the floor. Your weight should be distributed evenly on both feet. The feet should be at least 12 inches apart to maintain a

Table 7-1 Beginning a Procedure

Beginning Procedure Action	Rationale
1. Assemble equipment and take to patient's room.	Improves efficiency of the procedure. Ensures that you do not have to leave the room.
2. Knock on patient's door and identify yourself by name and title.	Respects patient's right to privacy. Notifies patient who is giving care.
3. Identify patient by checking his or her identification bracelet.	Ensures that you are caring for the correct patient.
4. Ask visitors to leave the room and advise where they may wait.	Respects patient's right to privacy. Shows hospitality to visitors.
5. Explain what you are going to do and how patient can assist. Answer questions about the procedure.	Informs patient of what is going to be done and what is expected. Gives patient an opportunity to get information about the procedure and the extent of patient participation.
6. Provide privacy by closing the door, privacy curtain, and window curtain.	Respects patient's right to privacy. All three should be closed even if the patient is alone in the room.
7. Wash your hands.	Applies the principles of standard precautions. Prevents the spread of microorganisms.
8. Put on gloves if contact with blood, moist body fluids, secretions, excretions, mucous membranes, or nonintact skin is likely.	Applies the principles of standard precautions. Protects PCT and patient from transmission of pathogens.
9. Put on a gown if your uniform will have substantial contact with linen or other articles contaminated with blood, moist body fluid (except sweat), secretions, or excretions.	Applies the principles of standard precautions. Protects uniform from contamination with bloodborne pathogens.
10. Put on a gown, mask, and eye protection if splashing of blood or moist body fluid is likely.	Applies the principles of standard precautions. Protects PCT's mucous membranes, uniform, and skin from accidental splashing of bloodborne pathogens.
11. Raise the bed to a comfortable working height.	Prevents back strain and injury caused by bending at the waist.
12. Lower the side rail on the side where you are working.	Provides an obstacle-free area in which to work.

Table 7-2 Ending a Procedure

Procedure Completion Actions	Rationale
1. Check to make sure patient is in good alignment.	All body systems function better when the body is correctly aligned. Patient is more comfortable when the body is in good alignment. *continues*

Table 7-2, *continued*

Procedure Completion Actions	Rationale
2. Remove gloves.	Prevents contamination of environmental surfaces.
3. Raise the side rail.	Prevents contamination of the side rail by gloves. Preserves patient's right to a safe environment. Prevents accidents and injuries.
4. Remove other personal protective equipment, if worn, and discard according to facility policy.	Prevents unnecessary environmental contamination.
5. Wash your hands.	Applies the principles of standard precautions. Prevents the spread of microorganisms.
6. Return bed to the lowest horizontal position.	Preserves patient's right to a safe environment. Prevents accidents and injuries.
7. Open the privacy and window curtains.	Privacy is no longer necessary unless preferred by patient.
8. Leave patient in a position of comfort and safety, with the call signal and needed personal items within reach.	Prevents accidents and injuries. Ensures that help is available. Eliminates need to call or reach for personal items.
9. Wash your hands.	Although PCT's hands were washed previously, they have contacted the patient and other items in the room. Wash them again before leaving to prevent potential transfer of microorganisms to areas outside the patient's unit.
10. Inform visitors that they may return to the room.	Shows courtesy to visitors and patient.
11. Report completion of the procedure and any abnormalities or other observations.	Informs supervisor that your assigned task has been completed so that further patient care can be planned and you can be assigned to other duties. Notifies supervisor of abnormalities and changes in patient's condition for further assessment.
12. Document the procedure and your observations.	Ongoing progress and care given are documented. Provides a legal record and a record of what has been done for other members of the interdisciplinary team.

wide base of support. Your knees should be bent slightly and your arms should hang at your sides (Figure 7-1).

Back Support Belts. Use a back support belt (lifting belt) (Figure 7-2) if this is your preference or the policy of your facility. Back injuries are very common in health care workers. Several studies have shown that workers using back support have fewer back injuries, though other studies have found no difference in the rate of injuries. Many care providers feel better if they are wearing the belt for support. The belt also reminds you to keep your back straight and to use good body mechanics. Using improper body mechanics when wearing the belt is difficult. For this reason alone, the belt may prove beneficial. You are less likely to be injured if you are using good body mechanics.

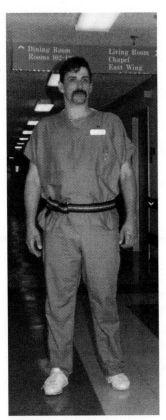

Figure 7-1 Good posture is the foundation for good body mechanics and prevention of injury.

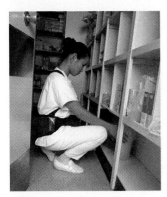

Figure 7-2 The back support reminds you to use your muscles correctly when lifting and moving patients and heavy objects.

■ **pressure sore (pressure ulcer, bedsore, decubitus ulcer):** *an ulcer that forms on the skin over a bony prominence as the result of pressure*
■ **decubiti:** *more than one pressure sore or decubitus ulcer*
■ **bony prominences:** *places where the bones are close to the surface of the skin*

General Guidelines for Using Good Body Mechanics

■ Keep your back straight.
■ Position your feet at least 12 inches apart.
■ Use the large muscles in your legs when lifting patients or heavy objects.
■ Bend from the hips and knees, never from the waist.
■ Face your work. Avoid twisting at the waist. If you must turn, pivot instead.
■ Squat when lifting heavy objects from the floor.
■ Keep heavy objects as close to your body as possible when lifting, moving, and carrying.
■ Use both hands when lifting and moving heavy objects.
■ Push, pull, or slide heavy objects instead of lifting them, whenever possible. Use your body weight to help you.
■ Use smooth, even movements instead of quick, jerking motions.
■ Avoid unnecessary bending and reaching.
■ Always use a transfer belt to move patients from one place to another, unless contraindicated.
■ Ask for help from others if you are not sure you can move a patient or lift an object.
■ Use mechanical lifting devices for moving heavy patients.
■ When giving bedside care, raise the height of the bed to a comfortable height for your body so you will not have to bend at the waist. When finished, remember to lower the bed to the lowest horizontal position.

■ PRESSURE SORES

The skin is the largest organ of the body, and it performs many vital functions. The skin protects the body from infection and injury. If the skin is broken, pain results and there is an increased risk of infection. The skin also removes waste products, water, and salt through sweat. At certain places the skin joins with mucous membranes that line openings into body cavities. Some of these areas are covered with hair. The hair is a natural defense of the body to trap invading microbes and prevent them from entering the system. The hair and nails are considered part of the skin system.

One of the primary purposes of moving and positioning patients is to prevent **pressure sores**. Pressure sores may also be called *pressure ulcers, bedsores, decubitus ulcers,* or **decubiti**. These areas usually develop as the result of pressure over **bony prominences**. Figure 7-3 shows common sites for pressure sore development. Pressure sores can also develop in other areas if tubing or clothing is constricting or rubbing on the skin. Sores are the result of inadequate blood and oxygen flow to an area of the body. They can form in a short time and can quickly cause tissue destruction. Patients can develop pressure sores while lying in bed or sitting in a chair. Pressure sores are painful and heal slowly. Infections and other complications may develop. They are much easier to prevent than they are to treat.

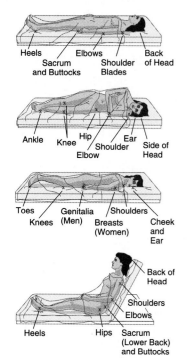

Figure 7-3 Pressure sores can develop in many areas.

Stages of Pressure Sore Development

Pressure sores are staged according to their severity. If a pressure sore is detected in the early stages of development, it can be prevented from worsening.

- Stage I pressure sores (Figure 7-4) begin as red areas. The redness does not go away within 30 minutes after pressure has been relieved. In a dark-skinned person, a Stage I pressure sore appears as a dark blue or black area on the skin. The skin is not broken in a Stage 1 area.
- Stage II pressure sores (Figure 7-5) are blistered or open areas. They are shallow and involve part of the top layer of skin.
- Stage III pressure sores (Figure 7-6) are areas in which the entire layer of skin has been lost and the subcutaneous fat and muscle are exposed.
- Stage IV pressure sores (Figure 7-7) involve destruction of the entire top layer of skin. Damage extends through the fat into the muscle, tendon, and bone.

Prevention of Pressure Sores

The best way to prevent pressure sores is to keep pressure off the skin covering bony prominences. This can be done by proper positioning and padding and by moving the patient frequently. Good nutrition and hydration play an important role in keeping the body healthy and preventing skin breakdown, as discussed in more detail in Chapter 10. Remember that the patient care technician has a very important responsibility for the prevention of pressure sores. Take this responsibility seriously!

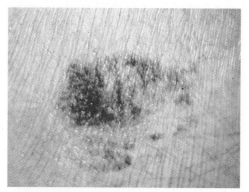

Figure 7-4 A Stage I pressure sore can worsen rapidly. (Permission to reproduce this copyrighted material has been granted by the owner, Hollister Incorporated)

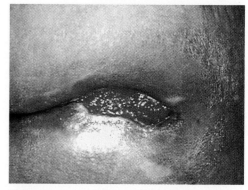

Figure 7-6 In a Stage III pressure sore, fat and muscle are exposed. (Permission to reproduce this copyrighted material has been granted by the owner, Hollister Incorporated)

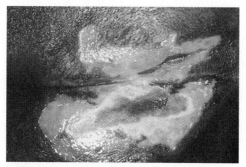

Figure 7-5 Stage II pressure sore. (Permission to reproduce this copyrighted material has been granted by the owner, Hollister Incorporated)

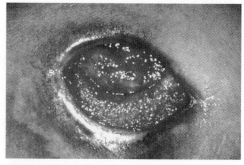

Figure 7-7 A Stage IV pressure sore severely damages the skin and extends into muscle, tendon, and bone. (Permission to reproduce this copyrighted material has been granted by the owner, Hollister Incorporated)

General Guidelines for Prevention of Pressure Sores

- Turn the patient at least every two hours, and more often if necessary.
- Teach patients who are physically able to shift their weight every 15 minutes to relieve pressure.
- Patients who are sitting in chairs should also be moved every two hours. Encourage patients to shift their weight frequently.
- Keep the skin clean and dry. Excessive moisture promotes skin breakdown.
- Rinse the skin well after using soap. Soap residue promotes irritation and skin breakdown.
- Avoid using powders and corn starch, which can irritate the skin.
- If the patient does not have control of bowel or bladder, wash the patient well with soap and water or a facility-approved cleansing agent after each episode of incontinence. Rinse the skin well. Urine and bowel products are very irritating to the skin.
- Use facility-approved moisturizing lotions if the patient has dry skin. Skin that is supple and well hydrated is not as easily damaged as dry skin.
- Keep bed linens free of crumbs and wrinkles. The pressure from wrinkles and crumbs can cause skin breakdown.
- Use lifting sheets to move patients in bed, whenever possible, to avoid friction and shearing.
- Use pressure-relieving pads in bed and chair.
- Pad areas of the patient's body where the skin or bones rub together.
- Inspect the patient's skin daily for red or open areas.
- Check the skin folds under the breasts, abdomen, and groin for signs of redness or irritation. Dry these areas well after bathing.
- Follow the directions on the care plan for preventive skin care.
- Avoid elevating the head of the bed more than 45 degrees, to prevent shearing.

■ **friction:** *rubbing, usually of the skin against bed linen*
■ **shearing:** *skin damage caused by stretching of a patient's skin between the bone inside and the sheet outside*

Observation and Reporting. Early detection and treatment of pressure sores will prevent the areas from worsening. A patient who presently has, or has previously had, a pressure sore is at high risk for further breakdown, so use aggressive preventive measures. Immediately report to the supervisor if you discover a red area that does not go away after the pressure has been removed for 30 minutes. Also report blisters, abrasions (scrapes), open areas, bruises, areas of pain, and areas that appear discolored.

■ **abrasion:** *a scrape or injury that rubs off the surface of the skin*

■ POSITIONING PATIENTS

The patient care technician positions patients frequently throughout the day. Use good posture and good body mechanics when performing these procedures. In addition, positioning the patient in good alignment is very important. This means

■ **alignment:** *placement; anatomical position*

that the spine is straight and other parts of the body are in good position. When the patient is positioned correctly, function of the body systems is improved.

Moving and Positioning Devices for Comfort and Pressure Relief

Sometimes common devices are used to help you move and position patients. These devices make your job easier and the patient more comfortable. Some devices are used to help you physically turn the patient. These include the **draw sheet** and turning pads (Figure 7-8). Pulling the fabric on the sheet or pad is easier for you than pulling the patient. Using these devices prevents accidental injury to the patient's skin and trauma to muscles, bones, and joints. The turning pad can be secured to the side rails after the move is completed to maintain the patient's position

Foam wedges (Figure 7-9) are used to keep the patient in good alignment in bed. Sometimes patients will slip, move, or turn themselves after you have positioned them. Use of the foam wedge as a prop will help maintain the patient's position. They are also useful in preventing pressure sores.

Pillows may also be used to position patients. They are sometimes used when the patient is in a side-lying position, to prevent rolling over to the back. Small, flat pillows or a bath blanket may also be used as pads to prevent the knees and ankles from rubbing together when the patient is lying on the side. Commercial devices (Figure 7-10) are also available for this purpose. Pillows are also used to support the forearms and may be placed under the knees when the patient is lying on his or her back. Using pillows for positioning helps the patient feel more comfortable and secure. *Sheepskins* (Figure 7-11) are synthetic devices that can be used for padding bony areas. They may also be placed on the bed to promote patient comfort and prevent friction and shearing.

■ *draw sheet:* a small sheet placed horizontally across the center of the hospital bed

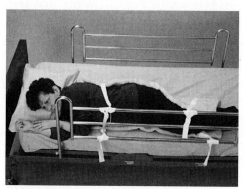

Figure 7-8 The turn holder is used to turn the patient and hold her on the side. (Courtesy of Skil-Care Corp.)

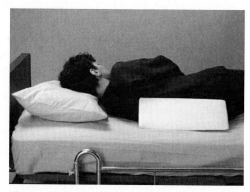

Figure 7-9 The foam wedge can be used for positioning and pressure sore prevention. (Courtesy of Skil-Care Corp.)

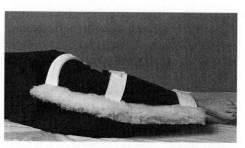

Figure 7-10 The knees and ankles must be separated to prevent pressure sores. (Courtesy of Skil-Care Corp.)

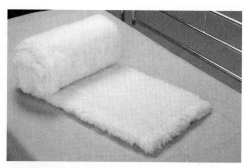

Figure 7-11 Sheepskins come in many different sizes. It relieves pressure on the skin and prevents shearing when the patient is moved. (Courtesy of Skil-Care Corp.)

A patient who is using a pressure-relieving pad or device still requires turning. Although some pressure is relieved, the devices do not remove it entirely, so further breakdown is possible. Some commonly used pressure-relieving devices include:

- Heel and elbow protectors (Figure 7-12)
- Foam heel elevators (Figure 7-13)
- Foam wedges, squares, and other foam pads
- Special foam, gel, air, and water mattresses, cushions, and overlays
- Low air loss and other therapeutic beds (Figure 7-14)

Side rail pads (Figure 7-15) may be used for patients who are restless, have seizures, or have diseases that cause involuntary arm and leg movements. These pads prevent the patient from striking or slipping through the rails and being injured.

A foot cradle is used to keep the weight of bedding off the patient's feet and lower legs. This device fastens to the foot of the bed and provides a frame over the patient's feet. When the patient is in bed, the sheet and blanket are placed over the top of the cradle.

A footboard may be used at the end of the mattress to prevent pressure on the heels and to keep the feet upright so deformities do not develop. When a

■ **foot cradle:** *a metal or plastic frame suspended over the foot of the hospital bed to keep the weight of the linen off the patient's feet*

■ **footboard:** *a piece of wood or plastic placed at the end of the hospital bed for positioning the patient's feet*

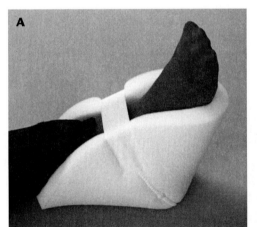
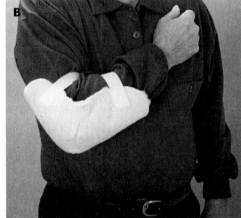

Figure 7-12 Many types of pads are available to protect the A. heels and B. elbows. (Courtesy of Skil-Care Corp.)

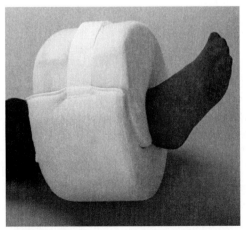

Figure 7-13 This foam ring keeps the heel elevated off the bed. (Courtesy of Skil-Care Corp.)

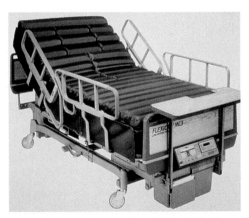

Figure 7-14 A low air loss therapy bed. (Courtesy of Hill-Rom, Charleston, SC)

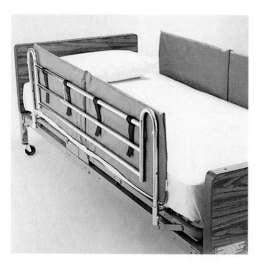

Figure 7-15 Padded side rails. (Courtesy of Skil-Care Corp.)

footboard is used, the heels hang over the end of the mattress and the sole of the foot rests against the board. Other devices that perform the same function as the footboard are applied directly to the patient's foot. Supportive devices to prevent deformities are discussed in more detail in Chapter 15.

General Guidelines for Positioning Patients

- Evaluate the patient's ability to participate in the procedure. This involves the ability to follow directions and the patient's ability to move, considering physical limitations.
- Ask another care provider to help you if the patient is heavy, combative, unable to follow directions, unable to assist with the move, or larger than you, or if you are unsure of your ability to move the patient alone.
- Know and follow your facility policies for positioning. In some facilities, a doctor's order is required to use certain positions. Consult the care plan or your supervisor for specific turning and positioning instructions.
- Some facilities use "turn schedules," which specify positioning the patient in designated positions at certain times. Follow the individual turn schedule for the patient.
- Use good body mechanics.
- Use smooth, easy motions. Do not tug or jerk the patient over quickly.
- Avoid trauma and injury to the patient during the procedure.
- Encourage the patient to assist to the extent he or she is able. Make sure the patient understands what is expected and how to do it.
- Use draw sheets, lifting sheets, and similar devices whenever possible, to avoid friction, shearing, and pulling on the patient's skin. Using a lift sheet to move patients also helps prevent back strain for the care provider.
- Use mechanical lifting devices, if needed.

continues

■ **combative:** *hitting or fighting the care provider*

General Guidelines for Positioning Patients, *continued*

- Use pillows or props to maintain the patient's position, if necessary.
- Pad bony areas, such as between the knees and ankles, to prevent discomfort and skin breakdown caused by the skin surfaces rubbing together.
- Position the patient in good body alignment.
- If you are using a new position with a patient for the first time, check the patient frequently to be sure the position will be well tolerated.
- Monitor the location of catheters and tubing and avoid pulling them or accidentally dislodging them. After the move, position them correctly so they are not obstructed and do not put pressure on skin.
- Change the patient's position at least every two hours, and more often if indicated.

PROCEDURE

13 MOVING THE PATIENT TO THE SIDE OF THE BED

1. Perform your beginning procedure actions.
2. Cross the patient's arms over the chest.
3. Place your upper hand, palm side up, under the patient's shoulders.
4. Place your lower hand, palm side up, under the mid back.
5. Lift the upper part of the body toward the near side of the bed.
6. Place your hands under the patient's waist and thighs.
7. Lift the middle section of the body toward the near side of the bed.
8. Place your hands under the thighs and lower legs and lift them toward the near side of the bed.
9. Perform your procedure completion actions.

PROCEDURE

14 TURNING THE PATIENT ON THE SIDE TOWARD YOU

1. Perform your beginning procedure actions.
2. Move the patient to the side of the bed, if necessary (see Procedure 13).
3. Cross the patient's arms over the chest.
4. Cross the leg farthest away from you over the near leg.
5. Place your top hand behind the patient's far shoulder. Place your bottom hand on the patient's hip (Figure 7-16A).
6. Roll the patient toward you.
7. Raise the side rail and move to the opposite side of the bed.

continues

PROCEDURE **14** *continued*

8. Lower the side rail.

9. Place your hands under the patient's bottom shoulder and pull back slightly toward the center of the bed. The patient should not be lying directly on the shoulder. Repeat this action for the patient's hips (Figure 7-16B).

10. Roll a pillow or place a positioning device behind the patient's back to maintain the position, if necessary.

11. Raise the side rail and return to the opposite side of the bed.

12. Lower the rail.

13. Bend the knees slightly. The upper leg should be positioned slightly ahead of the lower leg. Place a pillow or folded bath blanket from the knees to the ankles to keep the legs from rubbing together (Figure 7-16C).

14. Place a pillow under the patient's upper arm, if necessary, for support.

15. Check the lower arm to be sure it is not under the patient. If the patient is not able to move the arm, place it in a position of comfort at the side of the body, or bent at the elbow with the hand by the head.

16. Perform your procedure completion actions.

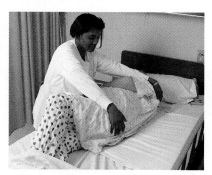

Figure 7-16A Place your hands on the patient's shoulder and hip and roll the patient toward you.

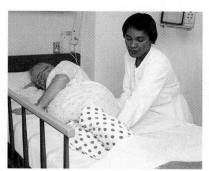

Figure 7-16B Pull the patient's hips toward the center of the bed.

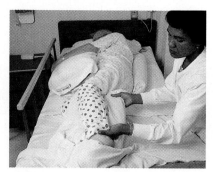

Figure 7-16C Use pillows for comfort, pressure sore prevention, and to maintain position.

PROCEDURE

15 TURNING THE PATIENT ON THE SIDE AWAY FROM YOU

1. Perform your beginning procedure actions.

2. Move the patient to the side of the bed, if necessary (see Procedure 13).

3. Bend the patient's far arm at the elbow, so the hand is near the head. Cross the near arm over the chest.

4. Cross the near leg over the far leg.

5. Place your top hand on the patient's shoulder and your bottom hand on the hip. Turn the patient on the side facing away from you.

6. Roll a pillow or place a positioning device behind the patient's back to maintain the position, if necessary.

7. Raise the side rail and move to the opposite side of the bed.

8. Lower the side rail.

9. Bend the knees slightly. The upper leg should be positioned slightly ahead of the lower leg. Place a pillow or folded bath blanket between the knees, calves, and ankles to keep them from rubbing together.

10. Place a pillow under the patient's upper arm, if necessary, for support.

11. Check the lower arm to be sure it is not under the patient.

12. Perform your procedure completion actions.

PROCEDURE

16 ASSISTING THE PATIENT TO MOVE TO THE HEAD OF THE BED

1. Perform your beginning procedure actions.
2. Lower the head of the bed.
3. Remove the pillow and place it against the headboard.
4. Instruct the patient to bend the knees and place the feet flat on the bed. The arms should be at the sides with elbows bent.
5. Place your top arm under the shoulders.
6. Place your bottom arm under the hips.
7. On the count of three, instruct the patient to push up with the elbows and feet while you lift.
8. Replace the pillow and straighten the bed linen.
9. Perform your procedure completion actions.

PROCEDURE

17 MOVING THE PATIENT TO THE HEAD OF THE BED WITH A LIFTING (DRAW) SHEET

1. Ask another care provider to assist you.
2. Perform your beginning procedure actions.
3. Lower the head of the bed.
4. Lower the side rails.
5. Remove the pillow and place it against the headboard.
6. Roll the lift sheet inward until it touches the patient's body (Figure 7-17).
7. Grasp the lift sheet with your top hand at the level of the patient's shoulder and your bottom hand at the hip.
8. Face the head of the bed. On the count of three, shift your weight from the rear foot to the front foot and lift the patient toward the head of the bed.

9. Replace the pillow.
10. Straighten the lift sheet.
11. Perform your procedure completion actions.

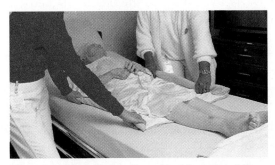

Figure 7-17 Roll the draw sheet in toward the patient's body, then hold it with an overhand grasp.

PROCEDURE

18 MOVING THE PATIENT UP IN BED WITH ONE ASSISTANT

1. Ask another care provider to assist you.
2. Perform your beginning procedure actions.
3. Lower the head of the bed.
4. Lower the side rails.
5. Remove the pillow and place it against the headboard.

continues

PROCEDURE 18 continued

6. Place your top arm under the patient's shoulders and your bottom arm under the patient's hips. Your assistant should do the same.

7. Grasp arms with your assistant.

8. Face the head of the bed. On the count of three, shift your weight from the rear foot to the front foot and lift the patient toward the head of the bed.

9. Replace the pillow.

10. Perform your procedure completion actions.

PROCEDURE

OBRA

19 LOGROLLING A PATIENT

1. Ask two other care providers to assist you.

2. Perform your beginning procedure actions.

3. Place a pillow between the patient's legs to keep them apart.

4. Two care providers stand on one side of the bed. One care provider stands on the opposite side.

5. Lower the side rails.

6. Move the patient to the side of the bed where two care providers are standing (see Procedure 13).

7. Have one of the care providers (on the side where two are standing) go to the other side of the bed.

8. Roll the patient as a unit in a single, smooth motion onto the side facing the two care providers. The care provider at the head of the bed makes sure that the patient's head and neck stay in a straight line during the turn.

9. Position pillows for comfort (see Procedure 14).

10. Perform your procedure completion actions.

PROCEDURE

20 MOVING A DEPENDENT PATIENT FROM BED TO STRETCHER

1. Ask three other care providers to assist you.

2. Perform your beginning procedure actions.

3. Two care providers stand on each side of the bed and lower the side rails.

4. The bed and stretcher should be the same height. Push the stretcher against the side of the bed and lock the wheels.

5. Roll the bottom sheet of the bed close to the patient's body.

6. On the count of three, all care providers lift the sheet and move the patient from the bed to stretcher.

7. Roll the patient to one side and push the bed sheets under the body.

8. Roll the patient to the other side and pull the bed sheets out and remove them.

9. Cover the patient, secure the safety straps of the stretcher, and raise the side rails.
Note: The patient on a stretcher should never be left unattended.

10. Perform your procedure completion actions.

11. Reverse the procedure to return the patient to bed.

▉▉ BASIC BODY POSITIONS

Four basic body positions are used when positioning patients in bed: the supine, lateral, Fowler's, and prone positions. The semiprone and semisupine positions are variations of the basic positions and are used to relieve pressure and prevent pressure sores. Fowler's position also has several variations, which are determined by the height of the head of the bed. Special positions may be used if the patient has special medical needs. The care plan and your supervisor will provide specific instructions if special positioning is necessary.

The Supine Position

■ ***supine position:*** *lying on the back face up*

The patient in the supine position (Figure 7-18) is lying on his or her back. This position may be preferred for sleeping. When the body is in good alignment, the patient's head and shoulders are supported on a pillow. The spine is straight. The arms are at the sides, and may be supported on pillows for comfort. The legs are straight. A pillow may be placed behind the knees for comfort. The feet are upright. A footboard or other supportive device may be used at the end of the bed.

The Semisupine Position

■ ***semisupine (tilt) position:*** *a modified side lying position in which the body is supported on pillows to relieve pressure from most of the bony prominences*

The semisupine position (Figure 7-19) is also called the *tilt position*. It should not be confused with the lateral position. The patient in this position is not lying directly on the side. The spine is straight and the patient is positioned so that he is leaning against a pillow for support. Both legs are straight. The top leg is slightly behind the bottom leg. A pillow is placed under the top leg to keep it even with the hip joint. The lower shoulder is pulled slightly forward so that pressure is distributed over the back, not the shoulder joint. The arms can be at the sides or folded across the abdomen.

The Prone Position

■ ***prone position:*** *lying on the abdomen with the head turned to one side*

The patient in the prone position (Figure 7-20) is lying on the abdomen. The head is turned to one side. A small, flat pillow is used under the head. Additional padding may be used under the shoulders if they roll forward. The arms should be along the sides, or one arm bent so the hand is next to the head. Both arms should not be up, as this strains the shoulder muscles. Another flat pillow may be placed under the abdomen for comfort. The spine and the legs are straight. The feet may be positioned so the toes are between the mattress and end of the bed. A pillow or small pad may be placed under the ankles to keep pressure off the toes.

Some facilities do not use the prone position without a physician's order. Know and follow your facility policy. If you have placed the patient in the prone position, check every 15 minutes to be sure the patient can tolerate the position and is not having difficulty breathing.

The Semiprone Position

■ ***semiprone position:*** *a modified prone position in which the body is supported on pillows to relieve pressure from most of the bony prominences*

The semiprone position (Figure 7-21) is the opposite of the semisupine position. It is usually very comfortable for the patient. Like the semisupine position,

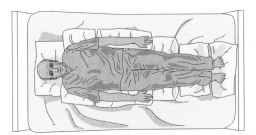

Figure 7-18 The patient in the supine position is supported with pillows for comfort.

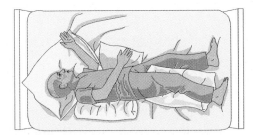

Figure 7-19 The semisupine position relieves pressure from the major pressure points.

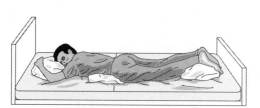

Figure 7-20 The patient in the prone position has a pillow under the abdomen and ankles for comfort.

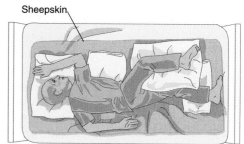

Sheepskin

Figure 7-21 The semiprone position is a comfortable, pressure-relieving position.

it eliminates pressure on the major areas at risk of pressure sore formation. To place the patient in the semiprone position, begin by placing the patient prone. Lift the patient's chest and shoulder closest to you and place a pillow under them. The opposite arm is positioned behind the patient. A second pillow is folded in half and placed under the top leg. The legs and spine are straight. The patient's head is turned to either side and a small pillow is used.

Follow your facility policy for use of the semiprone position. Like the prone position, some facilities require a doctor's order. Check the patient in the semiprone position every 15 minutes to be sure he can tolerate the position and is not having difficulty breathing.

The Lateral Position

■ *lateral position:* lying on the left or right side

A patient in the lateral position (Figure 7-22) is lying on one of his sides. The spine is straight. The bottom shoulder and hip are pulled slightly forward so pressure is not directly on the joints. A pillow may be rolled behind the back to hold the patient in this position. The arms can be positioned where they are most comfortable for the patient. Usually, the elbow of the bottom arm is flexed and the hand is placed near the head. The upper arm is folded across the abdomen and supported on a pillow. The upper leg is flexed and pulled slightly ahead of the bottom leg. A pillow is used to support the upper leg and keep the knees from rubbing together.

Fowler's Position

■ *Fowler's position:* a position that places the patient in a semi-sitting position in bed

A patient in Fowler's position is lying on the back with the head elevated. This position is used for patients who are receiving tube feedings or are having difficulty breathing. The knee of the bed may also be elevated slightly for comfort. This position places extra pressure on the patient's buttocks and spine and increases the risk of pressure sore formation, so careful attention must be paid to skin care. You may be directed to position patients in three different Fowler's positions. In the high Fowler's position, the head of the bed is elevated 90 degrees (Figure 7-23A). For

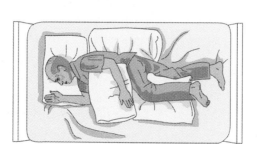

Figure 7-22 The patient in the lateral position is supported on pillows. This position can be used for either the left or right side.

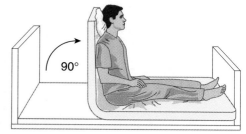

90°

Figure 7-23A High Fowler's position may be used for eating or for patients with breathing difficulty.

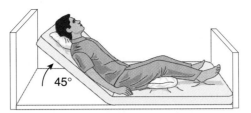

Figure 7-23B Fowler's position may be used for patients receiving tube feedings and those with breathing problems. A pillow is placed under the knees for comfort.

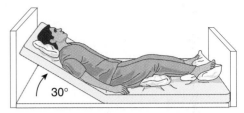

Figure 7-23C Semi-Fowler's position is a comfortable position for most patients. Pillows are placed under the knees for comfort and at the feet to prevent deformity.

Fowler's position, the head is elevated 45 degrees (Figure 7-23B). Patients positioned in the semi-Fowler's position have the head elevated 30 degrees (Figure 7-23C).

ASSISTING PATIENTS WITH MOBILITY

The patient care technician frequently helps transfer patients. The procedures in this section involve helping patients to get out of bed. Make sure that your uniforms fit loosely enough to allow you to lift and move patients without tearing or binding. As with other procedures, use of good body mechanics for yourself and helping patients maintain proper body alignment in both bed and chair are very important.

Assisting Patients to Sit on the Side of the Bed

■ *dangling: sitting on the side of the bed with the legs over the edge of the mattress*

Sitting on the side of the bed, or **dangling**, is the first step for getting out of bed. Sitting on the side of the bed for a few minutes helps patients who have been lying down to balance before getting up. The patient may become dizzy or faint after lying down for a long time. Dangling also helps to equalize the system before the patient is transferred to the chair or begins to walk. Stay with the patient while dangling. Monitor the skin for perspiration or pale color. If these changes occur, return the patient to the supine position and notify the nurse.

PROCEDURE   OBRA

21 ASSISTING THE PATIENT TO SIT ON THE SIDE OF THE BED

1. Perform your beginning procedure actions.

2. Place the bed in the lowest horizontal position.

3. Elevate the head of the bed, if permitted by facility policy.

4. Assist the patient to move to the side of the bed closest to you.

5. Place your arm closest to the head under the patient's shoulders, palm side up.

6. Place your other arm under the patient's knees, palm side up.

7. Lift the back and knees up and pivot the patient so the legs are hanging over the side of the bed and the back is straight.

8. Help the patient maintain balance, if necessary.

9. If the patient will be getting out of bed, assist the patient to put on robe and nonslip footwear.

10. Stay with the patient and observe for changes in color and moisture of the skin.

11. To return the patient to bed, reverse the procedure and pivot the patient back to the supine position.

12. Perform your procedure completion actions.

transfer: *to move patients from one place to another*

Assisting Patients to Get Out of Bed

If the patient tolerates dangling without difficulty, the next step is to assist the patient to get out of bed. The patient care technician should evaluate the patient and check the care plan before moving him or her. Follow the directions for **transfer** on the care plan. If the patient is larger than you are, cannot follow directions, or is otherwise unable to help with the transfer, ask another care provider to help you.

The Transfer Belt

A heavy canvas belt is called a *transfer belt* when it is used to move patients from one place to another. It is called a *gait belt* when it is used to help patients walk. In some facilities, each patient is assigned a belt that is used only for that patient. Other facilities require the patient care technician to wear the belt and use it for all patients. Use of the transfer belt is safer for both you and the patient. It prevents pulling and tugging on the patient's skin. The belt makes it easier for you to move the patient and gives you control if the patient starts to slip or fall. The belt should be used for most routine transfers. Never use just a regular belt or the belt on a pair of pants in place of a transfer belt.

General Guidelines for Assisting Patients with Mobility

- Wear a back support belt if this is your preference or facility policy.
- Refer to the care plan or supervisor for specific instructions.
- Explain the procedure to the patient. Before beginning the move, make sure the patient understands what is to be done and what is expected.
- Use a transfer belt to prevent injury to you or the patient.
- Adjust the bed to the lowest horizontal position.
- Lock the brakes on beds, wheelchairs, lifts, stretchers, and other equipment before beginning the move.
- Use lifting devices, if needed.
- Make sure that mechanical lifts and other moving devices are in good working condition.
- When transferring a patient with a weak or paralyzed side, always move the patient toward the stronger side. Support the patient's weaker side during transfers.
- Be alert to catheters and other tubes so that they are not accidentally pulled or removed.
- Have the patient wear nonskid footwear if standing during the transfer.
- Apply artificial limbs and braces correctly before transferring the patient.
- Avoid lifting the patient under the arms. This can cause pain, dislocation, and other injuries.
- The patient should never place hands around your neck during the transfer.
- When ambulating patients, look for hazards on the floor and approach corners slowly, watching for approaching traffic.
- Check the tips of canes, crutches, and walkers. If they are worn through, do not use them.

■ *contraindicated:* not indicated, inappropriate
■ *colostomy:* a surgical procedure in which the colon is attached to the outside of the body and waste is eliminated into a plastic bag attached to the skin
■ *gastrostomy:* a surgical procedure in which a feeding tube is placed directly into the patient's stomach, with the end extending through the abdominal skin
■ *incision:* a cut in the skin made with a knife

Contraindications for Use of the Transfer Belt. The transfer belt may be contraindicated for patients with some conditions. Facilities have different policies for use of the transfer belt. Know and follow your facility policy. Check with your supervisor or the patient's care plan for specific instructions. In general, contraindications to use of the transfer belt are:

■ Colostomy
■ A gastrostomy tube
■ Recent abdominal surgery or a fresh incision
■ Severe cardiac or respiratory disease
■ Fractured ribs
■ Pregnancy

General Guidelines for Using the Transfer Belt

■ The patient should be dressed before the belt is applied. Do not apply it over bare skin.
■ The belt is placed around the waist and buckled in front.
■ Be sure a female patient's breasts are not under the belt.
■ Thread the belt through the teeth side, then back through the opening on the other side so it is double-locked (Figure 7-24).
■ Check the fit of the belt by placing three fingers under it. The belt should be snug, but there should be enough space for your fingers to fit comfortably.
■ Before attempting to move the patient, be sure her feet are flat on the floor. If they are not, use the belt to move the patient to the edge of the bed until her feet are resting firmly on the floor.
■ If you are transferring a patient into or out of a wheelchair, keep the footrests out of the way during the transfer. After the patient is seated, the legs should not dangle. The feet are supported on the floor or on the wheelchair footrests.
■ Teach the patient to assist by pushing off the bed with her hands when you count to three.
■ Always hold the belt with an underhand grasp. For transfers, one hand should be on each side of the buckle in front.
■ When the patient is standing, pivot to transfer.
■ The chair should be close enough so the patient can feel the back of the chair with her hands after you pivot.
■ Remove the belt after the patient is seated.

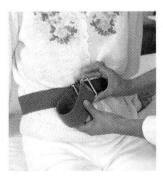

Figure 7-24 Threading the belt through the teeth, then back through the buckle, double-locks the belt for security.

PROCEDURE

22 ASSISTING THE PATIENT TO TRANSFER TO CHAIR OR WHEELCHAIR, ONE PERSON, WITH TRANSFER BELT

1. Perform your beginning procedure actions.

2. Assist the patient to dress and put on nonslip footwear.

3. Apply the transfer belt snugly around the patient's waist and check it with three fingers for tightness.

4. Stand in front of the patient. Keep your feet apart, knees bent, and back straight. Place one hand under each side of the belt, using an underhand grasp.

5. Move the patient so his feet are touching the floor. The patient's knees should be separated to provide a wide base of support.

6. Instruct the patient on the count of three to lean forward and push up from the bed with his hands while you lift up on the belt. Support the patient's knees and feet by placing your knees and feet firmly against them.

7. Assist the patient to pivot until his knees touch the back of the chair and he can reach the armrests with his hands.

8. Bend your knees and assist the patient to lower himself into the chair.

9. Remove the transfer belt.

10. Adjust the wheelchair legs and footrests.

11. Perform your procedure completion actions.

12. Reverse the procedure to return the patient to bed.

PROCEDURE

23 ASSISTING THE PATIENT TO TRANSFER TO CHAIR OR WHEELCHAIR, TWO PERSONS, WITH TRANSFER BELT

1. Perform your beginning procedure actions.

2. Assist the patient to dress and put on nonslip footwear.

3. Apply the transfer belt snugly around the patient's waist and check it with three fingers for tightness.

4. Stand in front of the patient. Keep your feet apart, knees bent, and back straight. Each care provider places one hand under the front of the belt and one hand under the back of the belt, using an underhand grasp.

5. Move the patient so his feet are touching the floor. The patient's knees should be separated to provide a wide base of support (Figure 7-25).

6. On the count of three, both care providers move the patient at the same time. Coordination of movement is very important.

7. The care provider on the side closest to the chair stands so that she can pivot and move away, allowing the patient unobstructed access to the chair. This care provider should stand with one leg behind the other, so that stepping back quickly is easy.

8. The other care provider uses one knee to support the patient's weak leg. This care provider's other leg is positioned further back.

9. Instruct the patient to lean forward and push off the bed, using the palms of his hands, on the count of three.

10. The patient's knees should be spread apart. Instruct him to put both feet down with the stronger foot behind the weaker foot.

continues

PROCEDURE **23** *continued*

11. Both care providers bend their knees, squat slightly, and spread their feet to provide a wide base of support.

12. On the count of three, lift the patient to a standing position. The care providers pivot slowly and smoothly by moving their feet, legs, and hips toward the chair until the patient can feel the back of the wheelchair with his legs.

13. Instruct the patient to place his hands on the armrests of the chair and lean forward slightly.

14. Both care providers bend their knees and lower the patient into the chair (Figure 7-26).

15. Remove the transfer belt.

16. Adjust the wheelchair legs and footrests.

17. Perform your procedure completion actions.

18. Reverse the procedure to return the patient to bed.

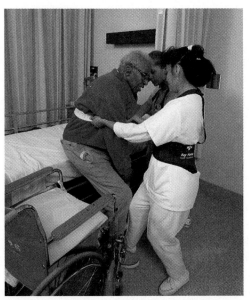

Figure 7-25 One PCT stands on each side of the patient with one hand in front and one hand in back of the belt. The hands are placed at the sides of the belt in preparation for transfer. The PCTs support the patient's knees and feet while lifting.

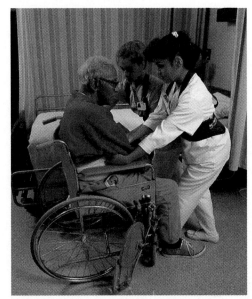

Figure 7-26 The PCTs bend their knees and lower the patient to the chair.

PROCEDURE

OBRA

24 ASSISTING THE PATIENT TO TRANSFER FROM BED TO CHAIR OR WHEELCHAIR, ONE ASSISTANT

Note: For the safety of both the PCT and the patient, use this procedure only if use of the transfer belt is contraindicated.

1. Perform your beginning procedure actions.

2. Assist the patient to dress and put on nonslip footwear.

3. Bring the patient to the edge of the bed so her feet touch the floor. The patient's knees should be separated to provide a wide base of support.

4. Place your hands under the patient's arms and around the back of her shoulders.

continues

PROCEDURE **24** *continued*

5. Brace the patient's knees and feet with your knees and feet.

6. On the count of three, pull the patient to a standing position.

7. Pivot the patient until her knees touch the back of the chair and she can reach the armrests with her hands.

8. Bend your knees and assist the patient to lower herself into the chair.

9. Adjust the wheelchair legs and footrests.

10. Perform your procedure completion actions.

11. Reverse the procedure to return the patient to bed.

Moving the Patient with a Mechanical Lift

Several types of mechanical lifts are available. Some are hydraulic. Others are electric. The most commonly used lift is the hydraulic lift. It is used when a patient is heavy, unable to assist, unbalanced, or has an amputation or other condition that makes transfer with a belt difficult or impossible. For safety reasons, the hydraulic lift should be operated by two or more care providers. Never attempt to operate it alone. Some electric and battery-operated lifts can safely be used by one person. Know and follow your facility policy for use of mechanical lifts.

Because the mechanical lift is a hydraulic unit, check the floor by the lift each time you use it. If you see an oily substance on the floor, do not use the lift until it has been checked and repaired. The fluid may be hydraulic fluid. If hydraulic fluid is leaking, the lift may slip, causing injury to both the patient and the care provider. Check the sling, release mechanisms, attachment straps, and chains for safety before using the lift. If anything is in need of repair, do not use it. Follow your facility policy for tagging the lift out of service. Obtain safe equipment before attempting to move the patient.

PROCEDURE

25 TRANSFERRING THE PATIENT USING A MECHANICAL LIFT

1. Perform your beginning procedure actions.

2. Place the chair at right angles to the foot of the bed, facing the head.

3. Lower the side rail on the side nearest you.

4. Roll the patient onto his side.

5. Position the sling under the patient's body so it supports the shoulders, buttocks, and thighs. Straighten the sling.

6. Roll the patient onto the sling and properly position it on the other side (Figure 7-27A).

7. Position the lift over the bed (Figure 7-27B). Spread the legs of the lift to the widest open position to maintain a broad base of support.

8. Attach the suspension straps or chains to the sling. The "S" hook should face *away* from the patient to prevent injury (Figure 7-27C).

9. Position the patient's arms comfortably inside the sling.

10. Attach the straps or chains to the lift frame.

11. Reassure the patient, lock the hydraulic mechanism, and slowly raise the boom of the lift until the patient is suspended over the bed.

12. Slowly guide the lift away from the bed.

13. Position the lift above the chair.

14. Your assistant holds the sling back and helps lower the patient slowly into the chair, keeping

continues

PROCEDURE **25** *continued*

the hips back while you slowly release the hydraulics and lower the lift.

15. When lowering the lift, watch placement of the patient's feet and arms to prevent injury (Figure 7-27D).

16. Unhook the straps or chains and remove the lift. The lift seat remains under the patient.

17. Position the footrests to support the patient's feet.

18. Perform your procedure completion actions.

19. Reverse the procedure to return the patient to bed. When raising the patient from the chair, monitor the position of the "S" hooks, which sometimes catch under the arms of the chair.

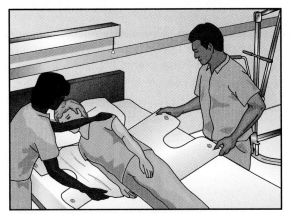

Figure 7-27A The lift seat is placed between the shoulders and mid-thigh.

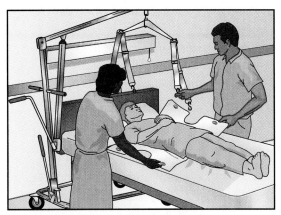

Figure 7-27B Move the frame over the bed and lower the boom to attach the straps.

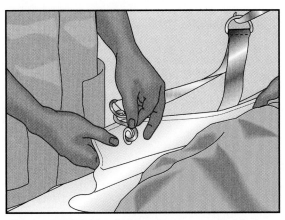

Figure 7-27C The "S" hooks are attached facing away from the patient.

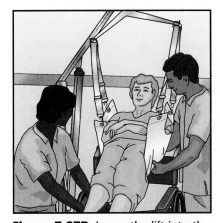

Figure 7-27D Lower the lift into the chair.

◼ ASSISTING PATIENTS WITH AMBULATION

◼ **ambulation:** *the act of walking or moving from one place to another*

Ambulation is an excellent form of exercise. The body functions more efficiently in an upright position. Patients may have difficulty walking because of illness, injury, surgery, or weakness. In the initial stages of ambulation, the patient care technician will assist patients until they regain strength and become more independent. Some patients may never become independent. However, walking them is important so that they do not lose the use of their legs. You will be assigned to walk the patient for a specified distance each day. If the patient is in a physical therapy program, the care plan will contain specific instructions for ambulation.

PROCEDURE

26 AMBULATING THE PATIENT WITH A GAIT BELT

1. Perform your beginning procedure actions.

2. Lower the bed to the lowest horizontal position.

3. Assist the patient to dangle.

4. Assist the patient to dress and put on nonslip footwear.

5. If the patient is not familiar with the gait belt, explain how and why it will be used.

6. Check the fit of the belt with three fingers.

7. Using an underhand grasp, place your hands under the belt on each side and bring the patient to a standing position.

8. Walk behind and slightly to one side of the patient. Maintain a firm, underhand grasp at the center back of the gait belt (Figure 7-28).

9. Encourage the patient to use handrails in the hallway.

10. Walk the distance specified by the care plan, physical therapist, or supervisor's instructions.

11. Monitor the patient for signs of fatigue. If this occurs, assist the patient to sit in a chair.

12. If the patient starts to fall, pull her close to your body. Using good body mechanics, hold the belt securely and ease the patient down your leg to the floor (Figure 7-29). Bend your knees as you lower the patient. Do not attempt to hold the patient up. This may injure both the patient and the PCT. Use of the belt gives you control of the fall and helps prevent head injuries.

13. After the ambulation, return to the patient's room.

14. Assist the patient to sit in the chair or return to bed.

15. Remove the gait belt.

16. Perform your procedure completion actions.

17. Upon completion of this procedure, you may be asked to record the distance the patient walked and her vital signs.

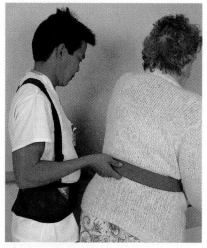

Figure 7-28 Hold the center of the belt securely with an underhand grasp.

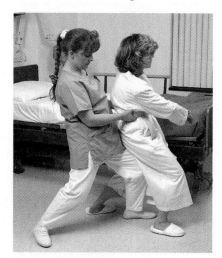

Figure 7-29 Hold the belt securely and pull the patient close to your body. Ease the patient down your leg to the floor.

Assisting the Patient to Walk with a Cane, Walker, or Crutches

Canes, crutches, and walkers are assistive devices used for ambulation. Usually the physical or occupational therapist provides the device and teaches the patient how to use it correctly. Use of these devices enables patients who are weak or unsteady to ambulate independently. Check the rubber tips on any assistive device before the patient uses it. If the rubber is worn through, the tip must be

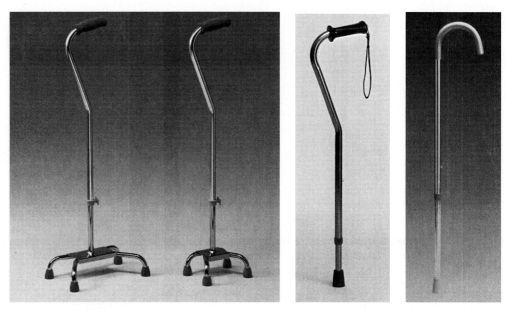

Figure 7-30 Different types of canes are used to meet the patient's need. (Courtesy of Lumex Medical Products)

replaced before the patient gets up. If you feel that a patient is not using an assistive device correctly, notify your supervisor, who will contact the therapy department.

Canes. Canes are usually used when only one side of the body is weak. Many different types of canes are available (Figure 7-30). The cane is held in the strong hand. A cane should "fit" correctly. The top of the cane should be at the panty line level. If the cane is the proper height, the patient's shoulders will be even and not raised. The physical therapist may teach the patient a special gait pattern to use. Most patients move the cane forward simultaneously with the weak leg. This provides extra support and balance.

Walkers. Walkers are commonly used for patients who have weakness in both legs or have difficulty balancing. Patients who have broken a hip often use walkers. The walker provides a sturdy base of support. Like the cane, several different types of walkers are available (Figure 7-31). The therapist will select the one that best meets the patient's needs. The walker should be adjusted so the handgrip is at panty line height. When the patient walks, the walker is moved forward first

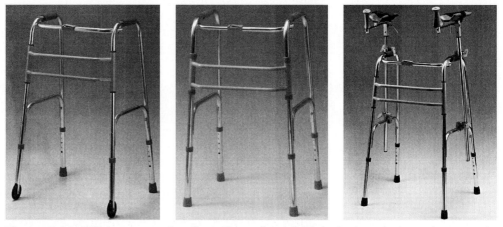

Figure 7-31 Different types of walkers. The walker wheels lock when downward pressure is applied to the top of the walker. (Courtesy of Lumex Medical Products)

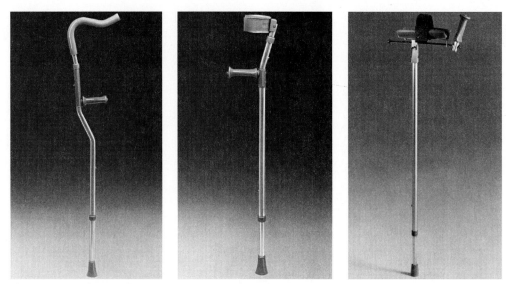

Figure 7-32 Different types of crutches. (Courtesy of Lumex Medical Products)

and placed on the floor. The patient steps into the walker with the weak leg, then the strong leg.

The patient care technician must be aware of safety at all times. Teach your patients safety as well. Many patients want to use the walker as a transfer device. They may try to hold the walker while they get out of a chair. This is unsafe, as the walker is not stable and may tip, causing a fall. The patient should be taught to push against the arms of the chair when rising.

Crutches. Crutches (Figure 7-32) are used by patients who have only one leg or have an injury to one leg. The correct height of the crutch is three finger widths below the armpit. Several different gaits are used in crutch walking, depending on the patient's medical problem. The therapist will teach the patient the correct gait for his or her condition.

KEY POINTS IN CHAPTER

■ *Use good body mechanics when lifting and moving patients and other heavy objects.*

■ *Patients must always be positioned in good body alignment.*

■ *The primary cause of pressure sores is lack of oxygen and circulation to the skin, caused by pressure.*

■ *Pressure sores are easier to prevent than to treat.*

■ *A transfer belt should always be used when moving patients, unless contraindicated.*

REVIEW QUIZ

Multiple Choice Questions

1. Using your body correctly to do the job is good body:
  a. maintenance.
  b. mechanisms.
  c. muscles.
  d. mechanics.

2. Your strongest muscles are in the:
  a. back.
  b. abdomen.
  c. legs.
  d. chest.

3. Using your body correctly involves:
  a. keeping your feet eight inches apart.
  b. using the strong muscles in your legs when lifting.
  c. lifting heavy objects instead of pushing them.
  d. all of the above.

4. Which of the following is true about pressure sores?
   a. They are the result of inadequate blood and oxygen to the skin.
   b. They take a long time to develop.
   c. Infections are not a consideration regarding pressure sores.
   d. All of the above.

5. A Stage II pressure sore may:
   a. be a large red area with intact skin.
   b. look like a blister or abrasion.
   c. involve the subcutaneous fat.
   d. involve muscle, tendon, and bone.

6. A Stage IV pressure sore:
   a. is a large red area with intact skin.
   b. looks like a blister or abrasion.
   c. involves only the top layer of skin.
   d. involves muscle, tendon, and bone.

7. A pressure sore in the early stages of development on a person with dark skin may appear:
   a. black.   c. red.
   b. pink.   d. gray.

8. Which of the following measures prevent pressure sores?
   a. Turning the patient every four hours.
   b. Padding areas where bones and skin rub together.
   c. Using Fowler's position.
   d. All of the above.

9. When moving and positioning patients, the care provider should:
   a. use pillows and props to maintain the position.
   b. use good body mechanics.
   c. avoid friction and shearing.
   d. all of the above.

10. Patients should be repositioned every:
    a. two hours.   c. four hours.
    b. three hours.   d. shift.

11. Millie Davis is an obese, dependent patient. You are assigned to move her up in bed. Mrs. Davis has a pressure sore on her left hip. The best way to move her is:
    a. lift her by yourself.
    b. lift her on a draw sheet with one or more other care providers assisting.
    c. to ask another care provider to lift the hips while you lift the feet.
    d. use a mechanical lift.

12. A patient in the supine position is lying:
    a. face up.
    b. face down.

c. on the abdomen with the head turned to the side.
d. on the side.

13. A patient in the prone position is lying:
    a. on the back.   c. on the left side.
    b. on the abdomen.   d. on the right side.

14. The supervisor asks you to place Mr. Kay in semi-Fowler's position while his tube feeding is running. You know his head should be elevated:
    a. 15 degrees.   c. 45 degrees.
    b. 30 degrees.   d. 90 degrees.

15. Sitting a patient on the side of the bed is called:
    a. proning.   c. semisitting.
    b. supining.   d. dangling.

16. When transferring patients from one place to another, you should:
    a. lock the brakes of the bed, wheelchair, or stretcher.
    b. adjust the bed to the lowest possible height.
    c. use a transfer belt unless contraindicated.
    d. all of the above.

17. Contraindications for using the transfer belt include patients who have:
    a. had a stroke.   c. a gastrostomy.
    b. head injuries.   d. all of the above.

18. When moving a patient (by yourself) with a transfer belt:
    a. use an underhand grasp.
    b. use an overhand grasp.
    c. stand behind the patient.
    d. lift from the side.

19. When using the mechanical (hydraulic) lift:
    a. ask another care provider to assist you.
    b. check the floor for leaky hydraulic fluid.
    c. reassure the patient during the procedure.
    d. all of the above.

20. You are assigned to ambulate Mr. Wells using a transfer belt. You are in the middle of the hallway when he starts to fall. You should:
    a. let go of the belt.
    b. hold Mr. Wells up and call for help.
    c. ease the patient down your leg.
    d. tell the patient to grab the handrail.

21. The correct height for the hands on a walker or cane is at the:
    a. waist level.   c. mid-thigh level.
    b. panty line level. d. none of the above.

Short Answer/Fill in the Blanks

22–26. List five methods the patient care technician can use to prevent pressure sores.

22. _____   25. _____

23. _____   26. _____

24. _____

27–36. List 10 rules of good body mechanics.

27. _____   32. _____

28. _____   33. _____

29. _____   34. _____

30. _____   35. _____

31. _____   36. _____

THE PATIENT'S UNIT

The patient's unit is the area for the patient's personal use (Figure 8-1). Most of the personal care you deliver is done in the patient's unit. Caring for the patient includes caring for the unit. Some health care facilities also provide a telephone, television set, or radio as part of the unit.

The patient has a right to be treated with respect and dignity. Showing respect includes knocking on closed doors and providing privacy when visitors are present. When providing personal care in the room, you must close the door, pull the privacy curtain, and close the drapes on the window, even if no one else is present in the room.

Safety and Infection Control

Think safety when you enter and leave the room. The patient care technician is responsible for keeping the unit safe.

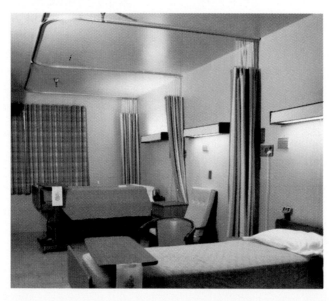

Figure 8-1 The patient's unit. Each unit is surrounded by a cubicle curtain for privacy.

General Guidelines for Caring for the Patient's Unit

- Know your facility policy for use of side rails. Check the care plan to see if side rail use is indicated for the patient for whom you are caring. If so, check side rails to be sure they are secure.

- Keep the bed in the lowest horizontal position unless you are at the bedside giving direct care.

- The bed wheels should be locked unless the bed is being moved.

- Check the call signal daily. The call signal should be within the patient's reach at all times, even if the patient is mentally confused.

- When the patient is in bed or in a chair, place the call signal, water, tissues, and other needed personal items within reach. This reduces the risk that the patient will overreach for an item and fall.

- Cleaning the unit is usually the job of another department. The patient care technician is responsible for caring for the patient's personal items. You are expected to wipe tabletops after care, when food is spilled, or when soiling occurs.

- Controlling odors is very important. The best way to do this is to eliminate them by removing the source.

- The top of the **overbed table** is cleaned several times a day. The overbed table is used to hold clean supplies when giving personal care. The height of the table can be adjusted. The table is also used to hold drinking water and meal trays. You may need to wipe this table frequently throughout the shift so that it is kept clean at all times. The patient care technician may provide fresh drinking water one or more times during each shift.

- Follow all infection control guidelines for separation of clean and soiled items in the patient's unit. Know which surfaces can be used to hold clean and soiled items.

- Follow your facility policy for disposing of gloves. Many facilities require that gloves be discarded in a closed container, not the open wastebasket in the room.

- Always respect the patient's choices about arrangement of personal items. This shows you care about the patient as a person.

- Know and follow your facility policy for storage of food, hygienic products, chemicals, and over-the-counter medications in the room.

- Some long-term care facilities allow residents to self-administer medication. These medications may be kept in the room. If this is the case, be sure they are stored in a secure location.

- Respect the patient's right to privacy when you are performing a procedure that exposes the body. Even if all the curtains are closed, use of a bath blanket is necessary to preserve the patient's dignity.

- Check the floor for items and equipment that could cause the patient to fall.

- Clean spills on the floor immediately and place a "wet floor" sign until the floor dries. Follow your facility policies for cleaning and disinfecting blood and body fluid spills.

continues

■ **overbed table:** *a narrow table on wheels used to hold the patient's water, meal trays, and clean items*

General Guidelines
for Caring for the Patient's Unit, *continued*

■ If you think that an electrical or mechanical safety hazard exists, follow your facility policy for having the equipment locked and tagged out until it can be removed or repaired.

■ Check bed linen for lost items, such as dentures and hearing aids, before placing it in the soiled linen hamper. These items are expensive and will be ruined in the washer.

■ If the patient uses the bathroom at night, leave a night light on.

■ The gatch handles on manually operated beds must be kept under the bed when not in use (Figure 8-2A). This helps prevent injury and falls to both patients and staff. The gatch handles, at the foot of the bed, are turned clockwise to elevate the bed and counterclockwise to lower the bed. The handle on the left raises the head of the bed (Figure 8-2B). The handle on the right elevates the knee area (Figure 8-2C). Adjusting the position of the bed assists in maintaining patient position and comfort. The center handle raises or lowers the height of the bed (Figure 8-2D). When you are providing care or making the bed, raise the bed with the center handle until it is at a comfortable working height for you. This helps prevent fatigue and back injuries. If the bed is elevated, the side rails should be kept up unless you are directly next to the bed.

■ Most facilities use electric beds. The position is changed by an electrical control box that is used to elevate the head, knee, or height of the bed. Many different types of beds are used in health care facilities. Become familiar with how to operate the beds used in your facility.

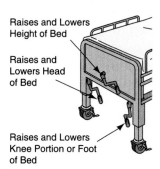

Raises and Lowers
Height of Bed

Raises and
Lowers Head
of Bed

Raises and Lowers
Knee Portion or Foot
of Bed

Figure 8-2A A mechanical bed

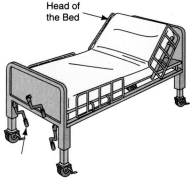

Head of
the Bed

Figure 8-2B This handle raises and lowers the head of the bed.

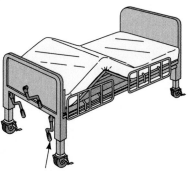

Figure 8-2C This handle raises and lowers the knee of the bed.

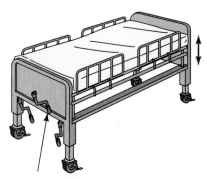

Figure 8-2D This handle raises and lowers the height of the bed.

■ **bedside stand:** *the nightstand used to store personal possessions and grooming and hygiene items*

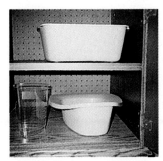

Figure 8-3 Clean items are stored on the top shelf and dirty items on the bottom shelf of the bedside stand.

■ **bath blanket:** *a soft cotton or flannel blanket used to protect patient privacy and provide warmth during procedures in which the body is exposed*

The Bedside Stand

The bedside stand is an important piece of furniture. It is used to store personal items and articles used to deliver care. Bedside stands vary in design. Most have at least one drawer. The lower part of the stand may have a cupboard-type door or several drawers. Clean and soiled items must be kept separate in the cupboard and drawers. For example, the drawer in the top of the bedside stand is often used to store personal hygiene items, such as a toothbrush, brush, and comb. These items should not come into contact with each other. The lower part of the bedside stand usually stores the washbasin, bedpan, and urinal. The washbasin is considered a clean item. It should not be stored next to the bedpan or urinal, which are considered soiled. The inside of the cupboard-type bedside stand is divided by a shelf. Most facilities store the washbasin on the top shelf and the bedpan and urinal on the bottom shelf (Figure 8-3). In bedside stands with drawers, keep these items in separate drawers.

Making the Bed

The patient care technician is responsible for making the bed each day. A clean, wrinkle-free bed promotes patient comfort and prevents skin breakdown. If the patient is out of bed, the unoccupied bedmaking procedure is used. A wide variety of linen is available for bed making. Flat sheets may be used on both the top and bottom, though many facilities use fitted sheets on the bottom. Most facilities place draw sheets (lift sheets) under patients who must be turned by the staff. Disposable or reusable underpads are placed under the buttocks if the patient is incontinent or uses the bedpan or urinal in bed. A plastic or rubber draw sheet covered with a cotton sheet may also be used, but many facilities have eliminated these in favor of large underpads. A thin flannel bath blanket is used to cover and drape the patient when personal care is given. Only the part of the body you are working on is exposed. Thermal blankets are usually used for warmth. Many different types of bedspreads are available.

Methods of Making the Bed. You may be instructed to make beds in several different ways. Table 8-1 describes different bedmaking methods.

Table 8-1		
Method of Bedmaking	**Procedure Variations**	**Rationale**
Unoccupied bed	■ Most common type of bedmaking procedure. ■ Used for making all types of beds.	■ Making the unoccupied bed is easier and faster for the PCT. It is more comfortable for the patient.
Occupied bed	■ Used when the patient is confined to bed.	■ Changes wet or soiled linen for patient comfort and prevention of skin breakdown. Provides fresh, clean linen for a feeling of comfort and security.
Closed bed	■ The bed is made with the top sheet, blanket, and spread pulled all the way to the top. ■ The pillow may be covered or placed on top of the spread, depending on agency policy. ■ The open end of the pillow case faces away from the door.	■ Used when the patient is expected to be out of bed all day or when making a bed after the patient has been discharged. Presents a neat, tidy appearance.

continues

Table 8-1, *continued*

Method of Bedmaking	Procedure Variations	Rationale
Open bed	■ The bed is made in the normal manner. ■ The top sheet and spread are fan-folded to the foot of the bed.	■ This procedure is used when the patient is temporarily out of bed. The patient can easily and quickly be covered upon return to bed.
Surgical bed	■ The bed is made in the normal manner, but the top linen is not tucked in at the foot of the bed. ■ The top linen is fanfolded to the side of the bed. ■ An extra pad may be placed at the head of the bed to contain secretions. A disposable or reusable underpad may be placed on the bed.	■ One side of the bed is left open to receive the patient on a stretcher upon return from surgery. The fanfolded linen can easily and quickly be unfolded to cover the patient.

Planning Your Work. Plan your work before making the bed. Bring all necessary linen into the room and stack it in the order of use. Before making the bed, elevate it to a comfortable working height for you. Avoid walking around the bed many times. Make one side of the bed at a time, then go to the other side to complete the bedmaking procedure. It may take a little practice to learn to make the bed this way, but it saves your strength and energy and reduces fatigue and injury to your back.

General Guidelines for Handling Clean and Soiled Linen

■ Wash your hands before handling clean linen.

■ Carry all linen away from your uniform.

■ Bring only the necessary amount of linen to the room. Extra linen cannot be removed and used for other patients until it has been washed.

■ Do not shake linen. Unfold clean linen.

■ Check bed linen for lost articles before removing it from the bed.

■ Roll soiled linen with the soiled side in.

■ Wash your hands immediately after handling used linen, even if it is not visibly soiled.

■ Follow your facility policy for placement of clean and soiled linen in the patient's room.

■ Soiled linen is never placed on the floor. Some facilities allow the soiled linen hamper in the room and some do not. If you cannot bring the hamper into the room, you may be able to place soiled linen in a plastic bag or pillowcase draped over the back of the chair. Follow your facility policy.

continues

General Guidelines for Handling Clean and Soiled Linen, *continued*

- Linen contaminated with blood or body fluids may be placed in plastic bags that are tied or secured at the top. If the outside of the bag accidentally becomes contaminated during the bagging process, the first bag should be placed in a clean outer bag. If the outside is not contaminated, double-bagging is not necessary.

- Some facilities use water-soluble bags that dissolve in the washer for linen contaminated with blood or body fluids. Water-soluble bags must always be double-bagged inside a regular plastic bag. Wet linen may cause a water-soluble bag to dissolve before it reaches the laundry.

- Keep the lids on soiled linen hampers. Soiled linen should not overflow under the lid.

- Clean and soiled linen should never touch each other.

- If you are handling linen contaminated with blood, body fluids, secretions, or excretions, you must wear gloves. Wear a gown if your uniform will have substantial contact with soiled linen.

- After you have discarded the soiled linen, remove the personal protective equipment and wash your hands. Doing so will prevent contamination of clean linen and other environmental surfaces.

- Follow your facility policy for separation of clean linen carts and soiled linen hampers in the hallways. Most facilities require one room's width separation of clean and soiled equipment.

- Follow your facility policy for removal of linen hampers from the hallways when food carts are on the unit.

PROCEDURE

27 MAKING THE UNOCCUPIED BED

1. Perform your beginning procedure actions.
2. Gather supplies needed: disposable gloves, two large sheets (or one flat and one fitted sheet), a linen draw sheet (if used), underpad (if used), pillowcase, laundry bag or hamper, and blanket or bedspread, if needed. Stack the linen in the order of use.
3. Carry clean linen away from your uniform (Figure 8-4).
4. Stack the linens on a clean area near the bed in the order of use, from bottom to top.
5. Lower the head so the bed is flat.
6. Remove and fold the bedspread if you are reusing it.

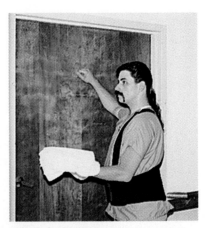

Figure 8-4 Clean linen is carried away from your uniform.

continues

PROCEDURE 27 *continued*

7. Apply gloves if linen is wet or soiled.

8. Remove the soiled linen from the bed by rolling it in a ball, soiled side facing in. Follow your facility policy for wiping the mattress. If the mattress is soiled with excretions or secretions, it should be wiped with disinfectant.

9. Place soiled linens in the hamper or laundry bag.

10. Remove gloves and discard them according to facility policy.

11. Wash your hands.

12. Center the lengthwise middle fold of the bottom sheet in the middle of the bed.

13. Open the sheet.

14. Place the end with the small hem even with the foot of the mattress (Figure 8-5).

15. Tuck the top of the sheet under the mattress.

16. Miter the corner (Figure 8-6) or pull the corners of the fitted sheet over the edge of the mattress.

17. Beginning at the head of the bed, tuck in the sheet, working from head to foot.

18. Place the draw sheet across the center of the bed.

19. Tuck the edge of the sheet under the mattress.

20. Center the lengthwise middle fold of the top sheet in the center of the bed.

21. Open the sheet and position it so the top edge is even with the top of the mattress.

22. Place the blanket or bedspread on the bed.

23. Miter linens at the foot of the bed.

24. Move to the other side of the bed.

25. Pull and straighten the bottom sheet.

26. Pull the sheet tight and tuck the bottom sheet under the mattress at the head of the bed.

27. Miter the corner of the sheet at the head of the bed or tuck in the corners of the fitted sheet.

28. Pull the bottom sheet tight and tuck it under the mattress.

29. Pull the linen draw sheet tight and tuck it under the mattress. Tuck the center of the sheet first, then the edges.

30. Check to be sure the bed is smooth and wrinkle free.

31. Straighten the top sheet.

32. Straighten the blanket or spread.

33. Tuck the sheet and blanket or spread under the foot of the mattress.

34. Miter the top linens at the foot of the bed.

35. Fold the spread back about 30 inches.

36. Fold the top sheet back about 4 inches at the top edge of the sheet.

37. Place the pillow on the bed.

38. Grab the center end of the pillowcase with your dominant hand. Fold it up over your arm (Figure 8-7A). Grab the pillow with this hand (Figure 8-7B). Unfold the pillowcase over the pillow (Figure 8-7C).

39. Straighten the pillowcase.

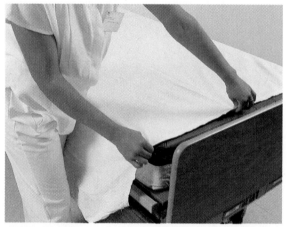

Figure 8-5 The small hem of the sheet is placed at the lower edge of the mattress.

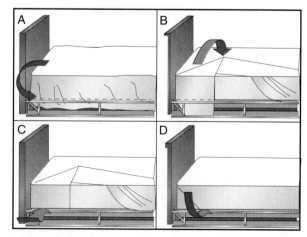

Figure 8-6 Miter the corner following steps A through D.

continues

PROCEDURE 27 *continued*

40. Place the pillow at the head of the bed with the open end facing away from the door.

41. Cover the pillow with the bedspread.

42. Perform your procedure completion actions.

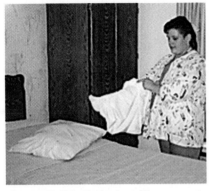
Figure 8-7A Grab the pillowcase at the seam and fold it over your wrist.

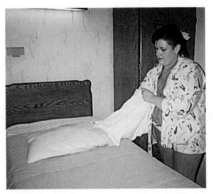
Figure 8-7B Grab the pillow with your pillowcase-covered hand.

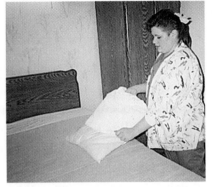
Figure 8-7C Unfold the pillowcase over the pillow.

■ *miter:* tuck a sheet in by forming a 45-degree angle perpendicular to the mattress
■ *occupied bed:* a bed with a patient in it

Making the Occupied Bed

Sometimes patients have conditions that require them to stay in bed all the time. When patients are confined to bed, you must make the bed using the occupied bed procedure. Sometimes only part of the linen is changed while the patient is in bed. Always apply the principles of standard precautions when changing a bed. Wear gloves if contact with blood, body fluids (except sweat), secretions, or excretions is likely. Wear a gown if you anticipate that your uniform will have substantial contact with linen contaminated by these substances.

PROCEDURE

28 MAKING THE OCCUPIED BED

1. Perform your beginning procedure actions.

2. Gather supplies needed: disposable gloves, two large sheets (or one flat and one fitted sheet), a linen draw sheet (if used), underpad (if used), pillowcase, laundry bag or hamper, and blanket or bedspread, if needed. Stack the linen in the order of use.

3. Carry clean linen away from your uniform.

4. Stack the linens on a clean area near the bed in the order of use, from bottom to top.

5. Lower the head so the bed is flat.

6. Remove the bedspread and blanket. Fold them and place them on the chair.

7. Apply gloves if linen is wet or soiled.

8. Cover the top sheet with a bath blanket. Remove the sheet by sliding it out underneath without exposing the patient. Dispose of it according to facility policy.

9. Turn the patient on the side away from you (following the guidelines in Procedure 15).

10. Loosen the bottom sheet.

11. Roll the soiled bottom sheet(s) inward and tuck along patient's back.

12. Center the lengthwise middle fold of the bottom sheet in the middle of the bed.

continues

PROCEDURE **28** *continued*

13. Open one-half of the sheet lengthwise.

14. Place the end with the small hem even with the foot of the mattress or fit the corner of the fitted sheet.

15. Tuck the top of the sheet under the head of the mattress on the side where you are working.

16. Miter the corner.

17. Beginning at the head of the bed, tuck in the sheet, working from head to foot.

18. Place the draw sheet across the center of the bed.

19. Tuck the edge of the draw sheet under the mattress.

20. Roll the remaining half of the sheets and tuck them under the soiled sheet.

21. If an underpad is used, place it on top of the draw sheet and roll it inside.

22. Help the patient roll over the linen onto the side facing you.

23. Raise the side rail.

24. Go to the other side of the bed.

25. Lower the side rail.

26. Loosen the soiled linens.

27. Dispose of linens according to facility policy. *Do not put soiled linen on the floor.* Raise the side rail if leaving the bedside.

28. Remove gloves and discard according to facility policy.

29. Wash your hands.

30. Return to the bedside and lower the side rail.

31. Pull the bottom sheet over the mattress.

32. Tuck the bottom sheet tightly under the head of the mattress.

33. Miter the corner of the sheet at the head or fit the corner of the fitted sheet.

34. Pull the bottom sheet tight and tuck it under the mattress.

35. Pull the draw sheet tight and tuck it in. If an underpad is used, smooth and straighten it.

36. Help the patient roll on her back. Cover the patient with the bath blanket.

37. Place the top sheet over the bath blanket, centering the center fold.

38. Pull the bath blanket from under the clean sheet without exposing the patient.

39. Place the blanket and bedspread over the sheet.

40. Fold the top sheet over the edge of the blanket.

41. Tuck the top linens under the foot of the mattress, allowing room for the patient's toes.

42. Miter the corner of top linens at the foot of the bed.

43. Raise the side rail.

44. Go to the other side of the bed.

45. Lower the side rail.

46. Miter the corner of the top linens at the foot of the bed.

47. Remove the pillow and soiled pillowcase.

48. Place a clean pillowcase on the pillow.

49. Fold and store the bath blanket or put it in the soiled linen hamper, according to facility policy.

50. Perform your procedure completion actions.

KEY POINTS IN CHAPTER

- *The patient's unit is an area for the patient's personal use.*
- *Respect the patient's rights when giving care and handling the patient's belongings.*
- *Think safety when you enter and leave the room.*
- *Follow your facility infection control policies for separation of clean and soiled items.*
- *Follow your facility policies for handling soiled linen.*
- *Practice the principles of standard precautions when making a bed if contact with blood, body fluids (except sweat), secretions, or excretions is likely.*
- *Personal protective equipment is removed after soiled linen is disposed of. The hands are washed before handling clean linen and touching other environmental surfaces.*

REVIEW QUIZ

Multiple Choice Questions

1. When giving personal care to the patient, close the:
   a. door.
   b. window curtain.
   c. privacy curtain.
   d. all of the above.

2. The following is true about the use of side rails:
   a. Side rails should be kept up for all patients.
   b. Side rails should be kept down for all patients.
   c. Consult the care plan to see if use of side rails is indicated.
   d. The patient always determines if side rails are used.

3. The overbed table is used for:
   a. clean items, food, and water.
   b. holding soiled linen and toilet articles.
   c. storing the bedpan and urinal.
   d. medical procedures only.

4. When caring for a patient in a bed with gatch handles, which handle elevates the head of the bed?
   a. right.
   b. left.
   c. center.
   d. it varies with the bed.

5. Which of the following is true about storing items in the bedside stand?
   a. The hairbrush and urinal are stored on the top shelf.
   b. The washbasin and bedpan are stored on the bottom shelf.
   c. The washbasin and urinal are stored on the top shelf.
   d. The bedpan and urinal are stored on the bottom shelf.

6. Which of the following is true about handling linen?
   a. Clean and soiled linen are always carried away from your uniform.
   b. Extra linen in a room cannot be removed and used for another patient.
   c. Soiled linen is never placed on the floor.
   d. All of the above.

7. You are assigned to make an unoccupied bed in room 931. The linen is saturated with fresh blood. The correct personal protective equipment to wear includes:
   a. mask, gown, gloves.
   b. gown, gloves.
   c. gloves, mask, face shield.
   d. mask, face shield.

True/False Questions

8. ___ Shake soiled linen before placing it in the hamper to check for lost items.

9. ___ The call signal is placed close to alert patients only because the mentally confused do not know how to use it.

10. ___ A bath blanket is used to drape the patient when providing personal care.

Personal Care Skills

After reading this chapter, you will be able to:

Spell and define key terms.

Describe how personal care affects self-esteem.

List four daily care routines and describe the type of care given in each.

Demonstrate routine oral hygiene, special oral hygiene, and care of dentures.

List the general guidelines for assisting patients with bathing and perineal care.

Demonstrate the backrub procedure.

List the guidelines for assisting patients with personal grooming.

List the guidelines for hand, foot, and nail care.

Demonstrate correct application of anti-embolism stockings.

Demonstrate dressing and undressing a dependent patient.

PERSONAL CARE OF THE PATIENT

■ **hygiene:** *personal cleanliness*

Good personal **hygiene** is essential to maintaining or restoring the patient's health. Good hygiene prevents infection, eliminates odors, promotes relaxation, stimulates circulation, and enhances self-esteem. Hygienic habits and practices are developed over a person's lifetime. They may be influenced by culture or religion. Some adaptation of routine and customary practices may be necessary in the health care facility. Even minor changes can be upsetting to the patient. Personal care and hygiene are very private matters for most people.

Providing personal care is a major responsibility of the patient care technician. It is also an area in which you must be sensitive to the needs, emotions, and cultural practices of individuals. Most personal care involves exposing and touching the patient's body. Often you are bathing and caring for private areas. Think how you would feel if someone else had to do these things for you. Remember, the patient feels this way, too. The patient may feel embarrassment or shame because she is unable to care for herself. Be kind, compassionate, and sensitive to the patient's feelings. Do not show disgust if you must care for the patient who has lost control of the bowels or bladder. If you react negatively, this will further lower the patient's self-esteem.

Activities of Daily Living

■ **activities of daily living (ADLs):** *personal care activities that people do each day to meet their human needs*

Activities of daily living (ADLs) are things that people do every day to meet their personal hygiene and basic human needs. Examples of activities of daily living are bathing, shaving, caring for the hair, mouth, and nails, and applying makeup. Dressing, eating, and toileting are also activities of daily living. These activities are on lower levels of Maslow's hierarchy of needs, so they are very important. If the patient cannot fulfill these needs independently, the care provider must assist. Personal care of the patient includes care of the mouth, teeth, skin, hair, nails, and feet. It may involve cleaning up body excretions if a patient is **incontinent**. Incontinence is often the result of a medical problem that the

■ **incontinent:** *unable to control the bladder, bowel, or both*

patient cannot control. It may be temporary. Patients who become incontinent may feel guilty and embarrassed, so you must be sensitive to the patient's feelings. Personal care also involves bathing, dressing, and grooming the patient. Good personal hygiene prevents skin breakdown, provides security and comfort to the patient, and improves self-esteem.

The patient has taken care of her activities of daily living throughout her life. Sometimes she is able to do all or part of these skills. If so, she should be encouraged to continue. You must provide the supplies needed and arrange them conveniently so the patient can use them. It may take longer, but you will enhance the patient's feelings of self-worth by allowing her to do these things. Organize your time so that you can do something else while the patient is performing self-care skills. This makes good use of your time. If the patient is unable to complete the task, you will finish it for her. This is part of providing restorative nursing care.

Daily Care Routines

Personal care is given as often as necessary to maintain comfort and keep the patient clean. Patients who can be out of bed may be able to continue with their regular routines, but you must assist patients who are weak or bedfast.

Routine care is given at certain times. You may be assigned to give AM care, morning care, afternoon care, or HS care. Staff on duty in the early morning are responsible for providing AM care. Patients are prepared for breakfast or special tests done in the morning. Routine bathing and skin care are usually done during morning care. Many patients like to have afternoon care before visitors arrive. HS care may also be called *evening care.* This care makes the patient comfortable and improves the ability to rest and relax. Table 9-1 summarizes the routine hygienic measures.

Changing the Patient's Gown. The hospital gown may need to be changed frequently. Avoid exposing the patient during this procedure.

■ **AM care:** *routine care given to prepare the patient for breakfast*
■ **morning care:** *routine care given after breakfast*
■ **afternoon care:** *routine care given after lunch*
■ **HS care:** *routine care given at bedtime to prepare the patient for sleep*

Table 9-1

Type of Care	Responsibilities
AM care (may also be called early AM care)	1. Assisting with using the bathroom, bedpan, or urinal. 2. Cleansing incontinent patients and changing wet or soiled linen. 3. Assisting the patient to wash face and hands for breakfast. 4. Providing oral care or assisting the patient to brush teeth. 5. Straightening the bed. 6. Assisting the patient to dress, or put on robe and slippers if getting out of bed for breakfast. 7. Transferring the patient to the chair, or assisting the patient to a comfortable position for eating in bed, if necessary. 8. Tidying the unit and removing unnecessary articles before breakfast. 9. Passing fresh drinking water and assisting the patient to drink, if necessary. 10. Cleaning and wiping the overbed table in preparation to receive the breakfast tray.
Morning care (may also be called AM care)	1. Assisting with using the bathroom, bedpan, or urinal. 2. Cleansing incontinent patients and changing wet or soiled linen. 3. Assisting the patient to wash face and hands after breakfast. 4. Providing oral care or assisting the patient to brush teeth after breakfast. 5. Providing bed baths, tub baths, and showers. 6. Shaving male patients. 7. Assisting female patients with makeup.

continues

Table 9-1, *continued*

Type of Care	Responsibilities
Morning care (may also be called AM care), *continued*	8. Performing range of motion exercises, if indicated on the care plan. 9. Assisting patients to change pajamas or dress in street clothes, according to preference and facility policy. 10. Brushing and caring for the hair and nails. 11. Assisting patients with walking and other activity. 12. Transporting patients to other areas for treatments and tests. 13. Changing the bed linen or making the bed, according to facility policy. 14. Tidying the unit.
Afternoon care (may also be called PM care)	1. Assisting with using the bathroom, bedpan, or urinal. 2. Cleansing incontinent patients and changing wet or soiled linen. 3. Assisting the patient to wash face and hands after lunch. 4. Providing oral care or assisting the patient to brush teeth after lunch. 5. Changing the patient's gown, if necessary. 6. Assisting patients to return to bed for a nap. 7. Assisting patients out of bed after they have rested. 8. Assisting patients to brush hair or freshen makeup, if desired. 9. Assisting patients with ambulation. 10. Performing range of motion exercises, if indicated on the care plan. 11. Straightening the bed linen. 12. Passing fresh drinking water and assisting the patient to drink, if necessary.
HS care (may also be called evening care)	1. Assisting with using the bathroom, bedpan, or urinal. 2. Cleansing incontinent patients and changing wet or soiled linen. 3. Assisting with a bedtime supplement or nourishment, if ordered. 4. Assisting the patient to wash face and hands before bedtime. 5. Providing oral care or assisting the patient to brush teeth at bedtime. 6. Assisting patients with a partial bath before bedtime. 7. Assisting patients into gowns or pajamas for bed (or change, if necessary or desired). 8. Giving backrubs. 9. Straightening the bed linen. 11. Tidying the unit. 12. Passing fresh drinking water and assisting the patient to drink, if necessary.

PROCEDURE

29 CHANGING THE PATIENT'S GOWN

1. Perform your beginning procedure actions.

2. Reach behind the patient and untie the gown strings.

3. Remove and loosen the gown under the patient's body.

4. Unfold the clean gown and drape it across the patient's chest, on top of the bath blanket or top sheet.

5. Remove the patient's arms from the sleeves of the gown, but keep the chest covered. If the patient cannot pull his arms from the sleeves, insert your hand into the sleeve to support the patient's hand, and pull the sleeve down and off.

6. Assist the patient to insert his arms into the sleeves of the clean gown. If the patient

continues

PROCEDURE **29** *continued*

cannot place his arms in the sleeves, put your hand in the sleeve of the gown. Grab the patient's hand. Slide the gown off your hand, then up over the patient's hand and arm.

7. After both arms are in the sleeves, remove the soiled gown by pulling it under the clean gown, without exposing the patient.

8. Tie the strings and straighten the clean gown under the bedding.

9. Perform your procedure completion actions.

ORAL HYGIENE

Oral hygiene involves cleaning of the mouth, teeth, gums, and tongue. A person who is ill may have a bad taste in the mouth, caused by illness or medication. The tongue may be coated with a substance that spoils the appetite. The purpose of oral hygiene is to remove food particles and make the mouth feel fresh and clean. Oral care also benefits the teeth and gums and prevents tooth decay and other serious dental problems from developing. A clean mouth helps prevent mouth odor and creates a feeling of well-being. Another purpose of providing oral hygiene is observation. While assisting with oral care, you have an opportunity to observe the mouth. One of your responsibilities is to provide good mouth care for the patient.

> ## General Guidelines for Giving Oral Hygiene
>
> - Encourage the patient to do as much self-care as possible.
> - Allow the patient to brush her own teeth. Take her to the bathroom sink, if possible.
> - Always wear gloves when performing oral hygiene. Avoid contaminating environmental surfaces and clean supplies with your gloves.
> - Observe and report any signs of irritation, sores, loose teeth, pain, swelling, or other abnormalities to your supervisor.

■ *emesis basin: a kidney-shaped basin used for oral care procedures*

PROCEDURE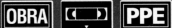

30 BRUSHING THE PATIENT'S TEETH

1. Perform your beginning procedure actions.

2. Gather supplies needed: disposable gloves, fresh water, disposable drinking cup, straw, toothbrush, toothpaste, mouthwash, emesis basin, towel.

3. Drape the towel across the patient's chest.

4. Mix equal parts of water and mouthwash in the cup.

5. Let the patient rinse her mouth.

6. Hold the emesis basin under the chin so the patient can spit out the mouthwash.

continues

PROCEDURE **30** *continued*

7. Wet the toothbrush and apply toothpaste.

8. Gently insert the toothbrush into the mouth with the bristles pointing down. Then rotate the toothbrush so the bristles face the teeth. Brush all surfaces of the teeth (Figure 9-1), using an up-and-down motion. Brush the tongue gently, avoiding the back of the tongue, which may cause the patient to gag.

9. Hold the emesis basin under the chin and allow the patient to spit out the toothpaste.

10. Let the patient rinse her mouth with the mouthwash solution.

11. Hold the emesis basin under the chin and allow the patient to spit out the mouthwash.

12. Wipe the mouth with a towel.

13. Perform your procedure completion actions.

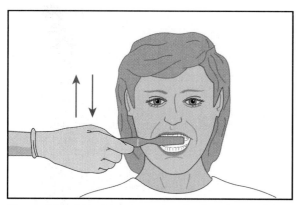 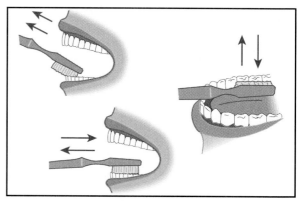

Figure 9-1 Wearing gloves, brush all surfaces of the teeth thoroughly.

Special Oral Hygiene

■ *NPO: nothing by mouth*

Patients who are NPO, unconscious, receiving tube feeing, or using oxygen require more frequent mouth care. The mucous membranes of the mouth dry out quickly and become coated with mucus. Sometimes they crack and bleed. The purpose of providing special oral hygiene is to keep the mucous membranes and lips moist.

General Guidelines for Giving Special Oral Hygiene

■ Always wear gloves when performing this procedure.

■ Explain the procedure to the patient even if she is confused or unresponsive.

■ Turn the patient's head to the side when cleaning the mouth to avoid getting liquids into the lungs.

■ Moisten the lips with lip balm or other lubricant according to facility policy. If oxygen is in use, use a water-soluble lubricant.

PROCEDURE

31 SPECIAL ORAL HYGIENE

1. Perform your beginning procedure actions.

2. Gather supplies needed: disposable gloves, emesis basin, two towels, commercially prepared swabs, lubricant for lips, plastic bag. If commercial swabs are not available, obtain tongue depressors, gauze sponges, a disposable cup, mouthwash, and water.

3. Cover the pillow with a towel. Use the second towel to cover the patient's chest.

4. Turn the patient's head to the side. Tip the head forward slightly so fluid and secretions will not run down the throat.

5. Place the emesis basin against the patient's chin.

6. Gently open the mouth.

7. Dip the pre-moistened applicators into water, mouthwash, or the solution used by the facility. Press against the side of the cup to remove extra water. Limit the amount of fluid used if the patient is unable to spit or swallow.

8. If prepared applicators are not available, wrap a gauze sponge around a tongue depressor. Dip the depressor into a cup containing half water and half mouthwash solution. Press the applicator against the side of the cup to remove extra solution.

9. Wipe the gums, teeth, tongue, and inside of the mouth with applicators.

10. Discard the used applicators in the plastic bag.

11. Apply lubricant to the lips.

12. Perform your procedure completion actions.

Care of Dentures

■ **dentures:** *artificial teeth*

Dentures are made of a hard plastic material. Most are removable, although some are permanently attached inside the mouth. They are necessary for eating, retaining the shape of the face and jaw, and giving the patient a sense of well-being. Many people are sensitive about wearing dentures and will not allow others to see them without their teeth. Always provide privacy when caring for dentures. Dentures are very expensive and break easily if dropped, so handle them with care.

General Guidelines for Denture Care

■ Always wear gloves when performing this procedure. Avoid contaminating environmental surfaces and clean supplies with your gloves.

■ Handle dentures very carefully.

■ Let the patient remove the dentures from her mouth, if able.

■ Check the dentures for cracks, chips, or loose teeth.

■ Store dentures in a marked denture cup. Some dentures are stored dry. Others are stored in water. Follow the directions for the type of dentures you are caring for. If in doubt, store dentures in clean, cool water.

PROCEDURE

 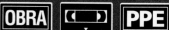

32 DENTURE CARE

1. Perform your beginning procedure actions.

2. Gather supplies needed: disposable gloves, emesis basin, denture cup, denture brush or toothbrush, denture paste or powder, towel, tissues, a disposable cup, paper towels, mouthwash, and water. If you will be removing the dentures, obtain a gauze sponge to place under your gloved hand. The gauze gives you a firm grip on the dentures to avoid slipping.

3. Drape the towel across the patient's chest.

4. Line the emesis basin with paper towels.

5. Ask the patient to remove the dentures, if able, and place them in the emesis basin.

6. Offer the patient a tissue to wipe her mouth after removing the dentures.

7. If the patient is unable to remove the dentures, remove them by grasping the center of the upper denture with your thumb and index finger. Gently move the denture up and down to break the seal. Gently pull the denture out of the mouth and place it in the emesis basin.

8. To remove a lower denture, gently grasp it with your thumb and index finger. Turn it to the side slightly and gently lift it from the mouth. Place it in the emesis basin.

9. Raise the side rail.

10. Line the bottom of the sink with paper towels and fill the sink half full of water so the dentures do not break if they drop (Figure 9-2).

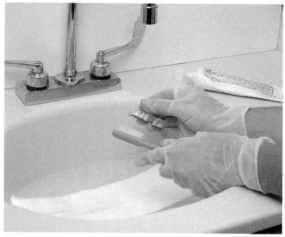

Figure 9-2 Fill the sink half full of water and line it with paper towels.

11. Wet the toothbrush and apply the denture paste or powder.

12. Hold the dentures securely and brush all surfaces.

13. Rinse the dentures well under running water. Place them in the denture cup.

14. Return to the bedside and lower the side rail.

15. Let the patient brush her gums and tongue, then clean and rinse her mouth with a solution of equal parts water and mouthwash before replacing the dentures.

16. Hold the emesis basin under the chin and allow the patient to spit out the solution.

17. Hand the patient the denture cup and ask her to insert the dentures, if able.

18. If the patient is unable to insert the dentures, grasp the middle front of the upper denture firmly with your thumb and index finger. Raise the upper lip with your other hand and slide the denture into the mouth. Place both index fingers in the mouth on each side of the upper denture and press firmly to ensure that the denture is in place.

19. Grasp the middle front of the lower denture securely with your thumb and index finger. With your other hand, pull the lower lip down and slide the denture into the mouth. Place both index fingers in the mouth on each side of the denture and press firmly to ensure that it is in place.

20. Raise the side rail.

21. Remove the towel and discard according to facility policy.

22. Rinse and dry the denture cup and return it, with your other supplies, to the top drawer of the bedside stand. If the patient does not want the dentures in her mouth, store them in the cup in the bedside stand. Some dentures are stored dry, but most should be kept moist. Ask the patient how the dentures should be stored. If in doubt, fill the cup with clean, cool water, and place the dentures in it. Cover the cup and place it in the bedside stand.

23. Perform your procedure completion actions.

■■■ BATHING THE PATIENT

Bathing is done to eliminate odor, stimulate circulation, provide mild exercise, and refresh and relax the patient. Washing removes secretions, excretions, dirt, and oil that are harmful to the skin. Bath time is also a good time for you to communicate with patients and make observations of their skin and overall appearance.

Types of Baths

■ **complete bath:** *washing the entire body of a patient*

■ **partial bath:** *washing the face, hands, underarms, back, and genital area*

Many types of baths are given in health care facilities. A complete bath is given when it is necessary to wash the entire body. Some facilities give all patients a partial bath at bedtime. The partial bath may be given as often as necessary to meet the patient's needs. Follow your facility policy for washing the hair. Some facilities do not consider a shampoo part of the bathing procedure, and may require a doctor's order to wash the hair.

Many patients can take a tub, shower, or whirlpool bath. Some facilities require a doctor's order for certain types of baths, so follow your facility policy. Many facilities have special shower chairs for the patient to sit in while taking a shower. Refer to the care plan for information about the type of bath and any special needs.

■ **bed bath:** *the bathing procedure used for a patient who is unable to get out of bed*

Patients who are either too weak or ill to receive a tub bath or shower are given a bed bath. The patient who receives a complete bed bath probably will be unable to assist you. If the doctor has written an order for complete bed rest, the patient must be given a bed bath. The care provider cleans the patient's entire body, one part at a time, while the patient remains in bed.

General Guidelines for Assisting with Bathing and Personal Care

- Consult the care plan for information about the type of bath to be given, special information, patient's self-care ability, routines, use of adaptive devices or other equipment, patient needs, and general care. Your care should be consistent with the care plan goals.
- Gloves are worn for part of the bathing procedure. You will have to change your gloves and wash your hands several times during a complete bath to apply the principles of standard precautions.
- Moving the patient to the side of the bed near you may be helpful if you are bathing the patient in bed. Follow the guidelines in Procedure 13.
- Provide privacy by closing the door, window curtain, and privacy curtain.
- Many personal care procedures involve exposing the patient, so be sure the room is warm and comfortable.
- Before beginning a procedure, organize your work. Anticipate what you will need and gather supplies in advance.
- Keep the patient's body covered with a bath blanket for modesty and warmth. Expose only the part of the body on which you are working.
- Bathe only one part of the body at a time, keeping the rest of the patient covered.

continues

General Guidelines for Assisting with Bathing and Personal Care, *continued*

- Offer the patient choices. Personal care should be given according to the patient's preference, considering medical needs. Consider culture, religion, and social and familial practices, as well as individual preference.
- If you find a technique that improves patient self-esteem or independence, share this information with other members of the interdisciplinary team.
- Change the water if it cools off or becomes soapy or dirty.
- Soap can be irritating and drying to the skin. Be sure it is rinsed completely off.
- When not using the soap, keep it in the soap dish, not in the wash basin.
- A bottle of lotion can be placed in the bath water at the beginning of the bath to warm it. After the bath it can be used on the patient's hands, arms, and back.
- After the bath, dry the skin well. Pay special attention to skin folds and creases. Drying helps prevent infection and skin breakdown.
- Follow your facility policy for use of powder. If permitted, use sparingly. Too much powder is not good for the skin.
- Apply deodorant after the bath, unless the patient objects.
- Upon completion of the bathing procedure, dress the patient in appropriate clothing, if permitted. If the patient must wear a hospital gown or other nightwear, cover the body as much as possible.
- Clothing should be appropriate for the patient's age and sex. Consider the season and color-coordinate the clothes as much as possible.
- Unless they interfere with medical treatment, assist the patient to put on undergarments, if preferred.
- If the patient will be getting out of bed, put nonslip footwear on his feet.

General Safety Guidelines for Personal Care Procedures

- Test the temperature of the bath water with a thermometer. As a rule, water that is 105°F is comfortable for bathing.
- If you will be transporting the patient in the hallway to a tub or shower room, be sure that the patient's body is covered.
- Use a transfer belt over clothing to move the patient.
- Use safety belts on tub lifts and shower chairs.
- Make certain that bath mats are secure.
- Help patients in and out of the tub and shower.   *continues*

> ## General Safety Guidelines
> ### for Personal Care Procedures, *continued*
>
> - Some facilities require you to stay with patients in the tub or shower. Follow your facility policy.
> - If the patient becomes weak or dizzy in the tub or shower, stay in the room and pull the emergency call signal. Begin to drain the water from the tub.

> ## General Infection Control Guidelines for Personal Care Procedures
>
> - Apply the principles of standard precautions and wear gloves and other personal protective equipment when indicated.
>   - Use of gloves is not necessary or desirable for the entire procedure. Use them only when contact with blood, body fluids (except sweat), secretions, excretions, mucous membranes, or nonintact skin is likely.
>   - If you are wearing gloves, remove them, wash your hands, and reapply new gloves *immediately before* contact with mucous membranes or nonintact skin. Mucous membranes are found in the eyes, nose, mouth, and **genital areas.**
>   - Avoid contaminating equipment or items in the room and environment with gloves used for patient care.
> - Wash from the cleanest area to the dirtiest.
> - Change the water, washcloth, and your gloves after washing a contaminated or dirty area.
> - Disinfect the tub, shower chair, or whirlpool according to facility policy before and after each use.
> - Follow your facility infection control policies for handling clean and soiled linen. Soiled linen or towels should not be left on the tub room floor.

■ **genital area:** *the area of the body where the external reproductive organs are located*

■ **axilla:** *the area under the arm; the armpit*

PROCEDURE

33 GIVING A BED BATH

1. Perform your beginning procedure actions.

2. Gather supplies needed: basin, bath thermometer, soap, washcloth, two towels, clean gown or clothing, bath blanket, lotion, comb or brush, disposable gloves, plastic laundry bag or hamper.

3. Place clean equipment on the overbed table. Follow your facility policy for covering the overbed table with a barrier.

4. Check the temperature of the room. Make sure that it is not too cold.

continues

PROCEDURE **33** *continued*

5. Offer the patient the bedpan or urinal before beginning the procedure. If you will be assisting, apply the principles of standard precautions.

6. Remove the bedspread and blanket. Fold and place them on the chair.

7. Place the bath blanket over the top sheet. Ask the patient to hold the blanket in place. Remove the sheet by pulling it down from underneath the blanket. Avoid exposing the patient. Place the soiled sheet in the hamper or dispose of it according to facility policy.

8. Remove the gown and dispose of it according to facility policy.

9. Raise the side rail.

10. Fill the basin with warm (105-degree) water. Check the temperature with a thermometer.

11. Return to the bedside and lower the side rail.

12. Place a towel across the patient's chest.

13. Allow the patient to wash her own face, if possible. If the patient is not able, you will wash the face. Check for the patient's preference regarding soap. Some people do not use soap on the face.

14. Apply disposable gloves to wash the eyes.

15. Make a mitten by folding the washcloth around your hand (Figure 9-3).

16. Wash the eyelids from the inner corner to the outer corner, using plain water without soap.

17. Dry the washed area.

18. Rinse the washcloth.

19. Remove the gloves and discard according to facility policy.

20. Wash the remainder of the face, neck, and ears.

21. Place a towel lengthwise under the patient's arm farthest from you.

22. Hold the arm up. Wash the arm from the shoulder to the wrist and fingertips, using long, firm, circular strokes (Figure 9-4).

23. Rinse and dry the arm.

24. Wash, rinse, and dry the axilla.

25. Repeat for other arm.

26. If possible, place the patient's hands in water. Wash, rinse, and dry hands, fingers, and nails. Clean under the nails with an orange stick, if permitted.

27. Place the towel across the chest. Pull the bath blanket down to the abdomen.

28. Fold the towel to expose half the chest.

29. Wash, rinse, and dry the chest. In the female patient, dry well under the breast. Repeat for the other side of the chest.

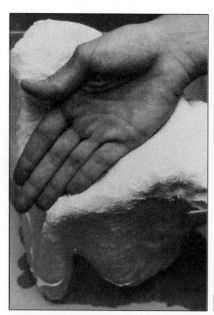
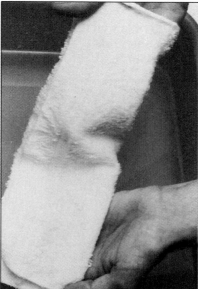
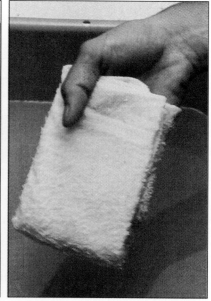

Figure 9-3 Make a mitten with a washcloth to avoid dragging the edges over the patient's skin.

continues

PROCEDURE **33** *continued*

30. Cover the chest with the towel.

31. Pull the bath blanket down to expose the abdomen.

32. Wash, rinse, and dry the abdomen.

33. Cover the patient with the bath blanket.

34. Remove the towel from under the blanket.

35. Uncover the leg farthest from you. Place the towel lengthwise under the leg. Bend the knee and place the foot on the bed, if able.

36. Wash, rinse, and dry the leg from the groin area to the toes (Figure 9-5).

37. Repeat for the other leg.

38. If the patient is able, place the basin on the towel and place feet in the basin one at a time.

39. Wash, rinse, and dry the feet. Wash, rinse, and dry well between the toes. Check the appearance of the toes and skin between the toes for redness, cracking, or irritation.

40. Cover the legs with the bath blanket.

41. Raise the side rail.

42. Empty the basin, rinse, and refill with clean (105-degree) water.

43. Return to the bedside and lower the side rail.

44. Assist the patient to turn with her back toward you.

45. Place the towel lengthwise on the sheet against the patient's back.

46. Wash, rinse, and dry the back and outer buttocks. Observe for signs of redness, irritation, or skin breakdown.

47. Put lotion on back (see Procedure 39).

48. Remove the towel and assist the patient to turn on her back.

49. Ask the patient if she would like to wash her genital area. If she is unable, apply disposable gloves.

50. Wash, rinse, and dry the genital area from the front to the rectal area (see Procedure 36).

51. Place the soiled linen in a hamper or plastic bag, according to facility policy.

52. Remove gloves and dispose of them according to facility policy.

53. Apply deodorant, if desired, and put a clean gown on the patient.

54. Raise the side rail.

55. Wash your hands.

56. Return to the bedside and put the side rail down.

57. Comb the hair and assist with other grooming aspects.

58. Replace bed linens, if indicated, or straighten the bed.

59. Perform your procedure completion actions.

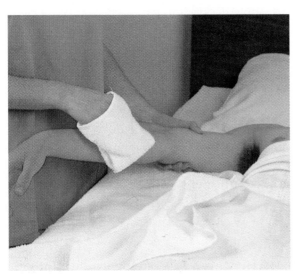

Figure 9-4 Place a bath towel under the arm, then wash, rinse, and dry.

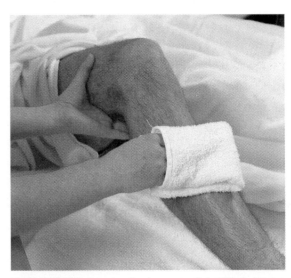

Figure 9-5 Expose only the part of the body you are washing.

PROCEDURE   OBRA   PPE

34   GIVING A PARTIAL BATH

1. Perform your beginning procedure actions.

2. Gather supplies needed: basin, soap, washcloth, two towels, clean gown or clothing, bath blanket, lotion, comb or brush, hamper or plastic laundry bag for soiled linen, and disposable gloves.

3. Place the equipment on the overbed table. Follow your facility policy for covering the overbed table with a barrier.

4. Offer the patient the bedpan or urinal. Apply the principles of standard precautions if you will be assisting with this procedure.

5. Remove the bedspread and blanket. Fold and place them on the chair.

6. Place the bath blanket over the top sheet. Ask the patient to hold the blanket in place. Remove the sheet by pulling it down from underneath the blanket. Avoid exposing the patient. Place the soiled sheet in the hamper or dispose of it according to facility policy.

7. Remove the gown and dispose of it according to facility policy.

8. Raise the side rail.

9. Fill the basin with warm (105-degree) water. Check the temperature with a thermometer.

10. Return to the bedside and lower the side rail.

11. Place a towel across the patient's chest.

12. Allow the patient to wash her own face, if possible. If the patient is not able, you will wash the face. Check for the patient's preference regarding soap.

13. Apply disposable gloves to wash the eyes.

14. Make a mitten by folding the washcloth around your hand.

15. Wash the eyelids from the inner corner to the outer corner, using plain water without soap.

16. Dry the washed area.

17. Rinse the washcloth.

18. Remove the gloves and discard according to facility policy.

19. Wash the remainder of the face, neck, and ears.

20. Place the towel under the hand farthest from you.

21. Wash, rinse, and dry the hand.

22. Repeat for the other hand.

23. Place the towel under the axilla.

24. Wash, rinse, and dry the axilla.

25. Repeat on the opposite side.

26. Assist the patient to turn with her back toward you.

27. Place the towel lengthwise on the sheet against the patient's back.

28. Wash, rinse, and dry the back and outer buttocks. Observe for signs of redness, irritation, or skin breakdown.

29. Put lotion on back (see Procedure 39).

30. Remove the towel and assist the patient to turn on her back.

31. Use gloves to wash the genital area. Wash from the front of the genital area to the rectal area (see Procedure 36).

32. Place the soiled linen in a hamper or plastic bag, according to facility policy.

33. Remove gloves and dispose of them according to facility policy.

34. Apply deodorant, if desired, and put a clean gown on the patient.

35. Raise the side rail.

36. Wash your hands.

37. Return to the bedside and put the side rail down.

38. Comb the hair and assist with other grooming requests.

39. Replace bed linens, if indicated, or straighten the bed.

40. Perform your procedure completion actions.

Perineal Care

■ **perineal care (peri care):** *washing the genital and anal areas of the body*

Perineal care is also called **peri care.** This procedure involves washing the genital area. In the female, the genital area includes the urinary opening, the vaginal area, and the rectum. In the male, the penis, scrotum, and rectum are included. Peri care must be given frequently when patients are incontinent. Urine and stool are very irritating and will promote skin breakdown.

PROCEDURE

35 ASSISTING THE PATIENT WITH A TUB OR SHOWER BATH

1. Perform your beginning procedure actions.

2. Check to see if the tub or shower room is available. Disinfect the tub or shower chair according to facility policy. Adjust the temperature in the room if necessary. Place a bath mat on the floor of the tub or shower and a disposable or cloth mat in front of the tub.

3. Gather supplies needed: disposable gloves, plastic laundry bag or hamper, washcloth, two or three towels, bath blanket, bath thermometer, soap, lotion, and personal grooming supplies.

4. Go to the patient's room and assist with toileting, if necessary. Apply the principles of standard precautions if you will be assisting with this procedure.

5. Assist the patient to the tub or shower room.

6. Regulate the water temperature. Always turn the cold water on first and off last. Check the water temperature with a thermometer. It should be comfortably warm, about 105 degrees.

7. If the patient is taking a tub bath, fill the tub half full of water.

8. Assist the patient to undress, if necessary. Give the patient a towel to place in front of the waist and lower abdomen.

9. Assist the patient to transfer to the tub or shower chair. If the patient is being transferred to a chair with a footrest, push the footrest back during the transfer, then pull it out to support the patient's feet.

10. Wash the back.

11. Allow the patient to complete the bath. If unable, you will wash and rinse the patient. Apply the principles of standard precautions if contact with blood, body fluids, secretions, excretions, mucous membranes, or nonintact skin is likely. You may have to change your gloves several times during this procedure to avoid cross-contamination.

12. Upon completion of the bathing procedure, assist the patient out of the tub or shower. Wrap with a bath blanket for modesty and warmth.

13. Pat the patient dry, or allow the patient to dry independently.

14. Apply lotion to the back, and other areas if the patient desires.

15. Return to the patient's room and assist with dressing and other personal care needs.

16. Perform your procedure completion actions.

17. After the patient is safe and comfortable, return to the tub or shower room. Discard the linen according to facility policy. Wear gloves when removing wet linen. Clean and disinfect the tub or shower chair.

General Guidelines for Giving Peri Care

- Always wear gloves during this procedure. Take care not to contaminate clean supplies and environmental surfaces with your gloves.
- Be kind and sensitive. Most people are very uncomfortable having someone else clean their genital area.
- Protect the patient's modesty and privacy by exposing only the part of the body on which you are working.
- Use warm, soapy water. Wash the cleanest area first. In the female, this means you will wash from front to back. In the male, begin at the end of the penis and move down toward the body, under the scrotum, then back to the rectum. Do not rub

continues

General Guidelines for Giving Peri Care, *continued*

■ **perineum:** *the area between the anus and vagina in the female; the area between the anus and scrotum in the male*

back and forth. Rinse the soap off well and dry thoroughly. Some facilities use special products for peri care. Follow your facility policy.

■ If the perineum is heavily soiled with excretions, remove them with tissues or disposable wipes. Place in bedpan for removal. After the heavy soiling is removed, discard your gloves. Wash your hands and reapply clean gloves before continuing the procedure.

■ If the patient has a catheter, wash it gently to remove urine, stool, mucus, or dried secretions. Catheter care is described in Chapter 11.

■ When washing the catheter, begin at the urinary meatus and wash downward three inches on the catheter. Do not rub back and forth.

■ Usually the patient care technician is expected to give perineal care to patients of both sexes.

■ **coccyx:** *the bone at the base of the spine*

PROCEDURE

36 FEMALE PERINEAL CARE

1. Perform your beginning procedure actions.
2. Gather supplies needed: basin, soap, washcloth, towels, clean gown or clothing, bath blanket, bed protector, hamper or plastic laundry bag, and disposable gloves.
3. Place the equipment on the overbed table. Follow your facility policy for covering the overbed table with a barrier.
4. Offer the patient the bedpan or urinal. Apply the principles of standard precautions if you will be assisting with this procedure.
5. Remove the bedspread and blanket. Fold and place them on the chair.
6. Place the bath blanket over the top sheet. Ask the patient to hold the blanket in place. Remove the sheet by pulling it down from underneath the blanket. Avoid exposing the patient. Place the soiled sheet in the hamper or dispose of it according to facility policy.
7. Remove the gown and dispose of it according to facility policy.
8. If the linen is wet or soiled, remove and dispose of it according to facility policy. Be sure the patient is lying on a clean, dry, surface.

9. Assist the patient to raise the hips. Place a bed protector under the buttocks. Remove the soiled bed protector, if present. Wear gloves if you will be handling a wet or soiled bed protector.
10. Raise the side rail.
11. Fill the basin with warm (105-degree) water. Check the temperature with a thermometer.
12. Return to the bedside and lower the side rail.
13. Position the bath blanket so the area between the legs is exposed.
14. Assist the patient to separate and bend the knees, placing the feet on the bed, if able.
15. Put on disposable gloves.
16. Make a mitten by folding the washcloth around your hand.
17. Apply soap to the washcloth. Avoid using too much soap, as it can be irritating to the skin.
18. Separate the labia with one hand.
19. With the other hand, wash the far side of the labia, using a single downward stroke from top to bottom (Figure 9-6).

continues

P R O C E D U R E **36** *continued*

20. Rinse the washcloth.

21. Wash the near side of the labia, using a single downward stroke from top to bottom.

22. Rinse the washcloth.

23. Wash the center of the labia, using a single downward stroke from top to bottom.

24. Rinse the area from top to bottom with the washcloth. Avoid rubbing back and forth.

25. Gently pat the area dry with a towel. Avoid rubbing back and forth.

26. Assist the patient to turn on the side away from you. Flex the upper leg forward, if possible.

27. Wet washcloth and make a mitt. Apply soap.

28. Expose the anal area.

20. Wash the area gently, wiping from the perineum to the coccyx (Figure 9-7).

30. Rinse the washcloth, then rinse the area well.

31. Gently pat the area dry with a towel. Avoid rubbing back and forth.

32. Assist the patient to return to her back.

33. Remove and dispose of the bed protector according to facility policy.

34. Place the soiled linen in a hamper or plastic bag, according to facility policy.

35. Remove one glove and raise the side rail with the ungloved hand. Dispose of both gloves according to facility policy.

36. Wash your hands.

37. Return to the bedside and lower the side rail.

38. Replace the top covers and remove the bath blanket.

39. Help the patient into a clean gown or other clothing of choice.

40. Perform your procedure completion actions.

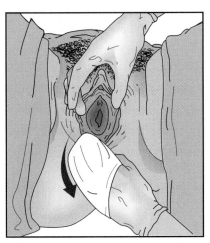

Figure 9-6 Spread the labia and wash using a single downward stroke.

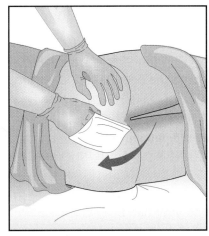

Figure 9-7 Wipe upward from the perineum to the coccyx.

P R O C E D U R E

37 MALE PERINEAL CARE

1. Perform your beginning procedure actions.

2. Gather supplies needed: basin, soap, washcloth, towels, clean gown or clothing, bath blanket, bed protector, hamper or plastic laundry bag, and disposable gloves.

3. Place the equipment on the overbed table. Follow your facility policy for covering the overbed table with a barrier.

continues

PROCEDURE **37** *continued*

4. Offer the patient the bedpan or urinal. Apply the principles of standard precautions if you will be assisting with this procedure.

5. Remove the bedspread and blanket. Fold and place them on the chair.

6. Place the bath blanket over the top sheet. Ask the patient to hold the blanket in place. Remove the sheet by pulling it down from underneath the blanket. Avoid exposing the patient. Place the soiled sheet in a hamper or dispose of it according to facility policy.

7. Remove the gown and dispose of it according to facility policy.

8. If the linen is wet or soiled, remove and dispose of it according to facility policy. Be sure the patient is lying on a clean, dry, surface.

9. Assist the patient to raise the hips. Place a bed protector under the buttocks. Remove the soiled bed protector, if present. Wear gloves if you will be handling a wet or soiled bed protector.

10. Raise the side rail.

11. Fill the basin with warm (105-degree) water. Check the temperature with a thermometer.

12. Return to the bedside and lower the side rail.

13. Position the bath blanket so the area between the legs is exposed.

14. Assist the patient to separate and bend the knees, placing the feet on the bed, if able.

15. Put on disposable gloves.

16. Make a mitten by folding the washcloth around your hand.

17. Apply soap to the washcloth. Avoid using too much soap, as it can be irritating to the skin.

18. With one hand, grasp the penis gently and wash. Begin washing at the urinary meatus and wash the penis in a circular motion toward the base of the penis (Figure 9-8).

19. If the patient is not circumcised, pull the foreskin back and wash it (Figure 9-9). Rinse the penis, dry gently, and replace the retracted foreskin.

20. Wash the scrotum, then gently lift it and wash the perineum.

21. Rinse the washcloth.

22. Make a mitten and rinse the entire area.

23. Gently dry the area with a towel.

24. Assist the patient to turn on the side away from you. Flex the upper leg forward, if possible.

25. Wet washcloth and make a mitt. Apply soap.

26. Expose the anal area.

27. Wash the area, wiping from the perineum to the coccyx.

28. Rinse the washcloth, then rinse the area well.

29. Gently pat the area dry with a towel.

30. Assist the patient to return to his back.

31. Remove and dispose of the bed protector according to facility policy.

32. Place the soiled linen in a hamper or plastic bag, according to facility policy.

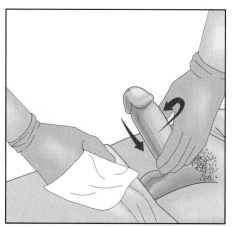

Figure 9-8 Wash from the tip of the penis down to the scrotum.

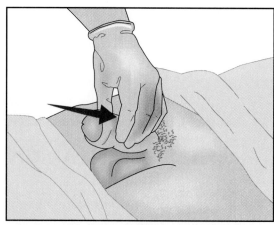

Figure 9-9 Retract the foreskin, wash, rinse, and pat dry. Replace the foreskin after washing.

continues

PROCEDURE **37** *continued*

33. Remove one glove and raise the side rail with the ungloved hand. Dispose of both gloves according to facility policy.
34. Wash your hands.
35. Return to the bedside and lower the side rail.
36. Replace the top covers and remove the bath blanket.
37. Help the patient into a clean gown or other clothing of choice.
38. Perform your procedure completion actions.

Shampooing the Patient's Hair. Follow your facility policy for washing the patient's hair. Some facilities require a doctor's order for this procedure. If permitted, the hair can be washed in the tub or shower. For patients on complete bed rest, this procedure must be done in bed. Some facilities use dry chemical shampoos that are brushed out. No-rinse shampoos are also available for patients in bed.

PROCEDURE

38 SHAMPOOING THE PATIENT'S HAIR IN BED

1. Perform your beginning procedure actions.
2. Gather supplies needed: chair, shampoo, basin of water (105 degrees), pitcher of water (110 degrees), bath thermometer, large (empty) basin, shampoo tray, water trough, plastic sheet, two bed protectors, three or four bath towels, washcloth, bath blanket, paper cup, cotton balls.
3. Place the chair next to the head of the bed with the back of the chair touching the mattress. Place a towel on the seat of the chair.
4. Place the empty basin on the chair.
5. Put cotton in the patient's ears.
6. Move the patient to the side of the bed (see Procedure 13).
7. Raise the patient's shoulders and move the pillow down so the head is extended. Cover the pillow with a bed protector. Place a second bed protector at the head of the bed.
8. Cover the patient with a bath blanket and remove the upper bedding without exposing the patient.
9. Place the shampoo tray under the patient's head (Figure 9-10). If a tray is not available, roll the plastic sheet inward at the top and both sides to make a trough. Place the end of the plastic sheet in the basin on the chair.

10. Fold the washcloth in thirds and use it to cover the patient's eyes.
11. Gently brush the patient's hair to remove any tangles.

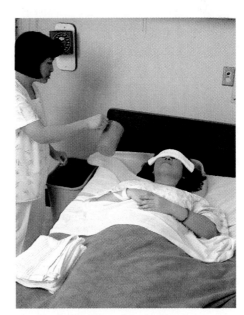

Figure 9-10 Place the shampoo tray under the patient's head with the trough over the washbasin next to the bed.

continues

PROCEDURE **38** *continued*

12. Fill the paper cup with water from the basin. (The pitcher of water is used to refill the cup with warm water.) Pour the cup of water over the patient's head and repeat until hair is thoroughly wet.

13. Place a small amount of shampoo in your hand. Apply the shampoo to the head and massage in with the fingertips of both hands. Avoid massaging with the fingernails.

14. Rinse the soap from the hair by pouring water from the cup. Repeat until all of the shampoo is removed from the hair.

15. Dry the patient's face, forehead, and ears. Remove the cotton balls.

16. Wrap the patient's head with a towel.

17. Remove the equipment from the bed. Remove the bed protector and replace the pillow under the patient's head. Cover the pillow with a towel or another bed protector.

18. Change the patient's gown, if necessary, and towel dry the hair.

19. Comb and blow dry the hair.

20. Cover the patient with the top linen and remove the bath blanket.

21. Perform your procedure completion actions.

■■■ APPLYING LOTION TO THE PATIENT'S SKIN

Massaging the patient's skin is comforting and refreshing. Massage can stimulate circulation and helps prevent skin breakdown. Refer to the care plan to see if massage is indicated. Each facility has a house lotion used for massaging patients' skin. Always massage the skin in smooth, light strokes. Do not massage red areas that may be Stage I pressure sores. Massaging these areas causes tissue destruction. Avoid massaging the legs, because it can cause complications related to blood clots. If the patient uses lotion on the legs, pat it on.

PROCEDURE OBRA

39 GIVING A BACKRUB

1. Perform your beginning procedure actions.

2. Gather supplies needed: basin of water (105 degrees), soap, washcloth, towel, hamper or plastic laundry bag for soiled linen, and disposable gloves if contact with nonintact skin, excretions, or any moist body fluid is likely.

3. Place the equipment on the overbed table. Follow your facility policy for covering the overbed table with a barrier.

4. Assist the patient to turn on the side away from you. Expose the back and upper buttocks.

5. Place the bottle of lotion in the basin of water to warm it.

6. Wash, rinse, and dry the back.

7. Apply a small amount of lotion to one hand.

8. Warm the lotion by rubbing it between your hands, if necessary.

9. Apply lotion to the back.

10. Rub the back with both hands, using gentle, firm strokes in a circular motion. Massage from buttocks to shoulders:

    a. Begin at the base of the spine and rub up the center of the back with long, soothing strokes (Figure 9-11A).

    b. Move your hands in a circular motion as you massage down from the shoulders to the buttocks (Figure 9-11B).

    c. Repeat this procedure for three to five minutes.

11. Wipe off excess lotion.

continues

PROCEDURE **39** *continued*

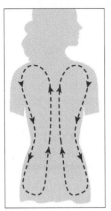

Figure 9-11A Beginning at the base of the spine, rub up and around, using long, soothing strokes.

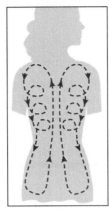

Figure 9-11B Rub in a circular motion from the shoulders down to the buttocks.

12. Close and retie the gown, or change the gown if necessary.
13. Straighten and tighten the bottom sheet and draw sheet.
14. Assist the patient to a comfortable position.
15. Perform your procedure completion actions.

GROOMING THE PATIENT

Proper grooming is important for the patient's self-esteem. Grooming includes combing hair, shaving, doing nail care, and applying makeup.

Shaving the Male Patient. Most men shave daily as part of the morning routine. If the patient can shave himself, provide the equipment and supplies and allow him to do it. If the patient is weak or unable, you will shave him. Check the care plan before shaving patients. Some patients may not be shaved because of their medical condition or medications they are taking.

Shaving may be done with an electric razor or a disposable razor. The patient may have brought the electric razor to the health care facility with him. If an electric razor is not available, a disposable safety razor is used. If you are using a

General Guidelines for Assisting Patients with Grooming

- Allow the patient to determine the routine. Respect the patient's preferences and choices.
- Encourage self-care. Assist by setting up supplies and providing equipment.
- Provide privacy.
- Dress and groom the patient appropriately for age, sex, and season, within the limitations of the patient's condition.
- Keep clean grooming items separate from soiled supplies.
- Clean all grooming items after using them.
- Discard disposable razors in a puncture-resistant sharps container.

PROCEDURE

OBRA

40 COMBING THE HAIR

1. Perform your beginning procedure actions.
2. Gather supplies needed: towel, comb, and brush.
3. Cover the pillow with a towel, or place the towel over the patient's shoulders if she is sitting in a chair.
4. Section the hair with one hand. Begin at the scalp and work toward the end of the hair (Figure 9-12).

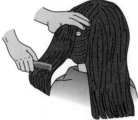

Figure 9-12 Section and support the hair. Comb downward, beginning at the ends to remove tangles.

5. Brush the hair well.
6. If the patient is in bed, assist her to turn away from you so that you can brush the back of her hair.
7. If the hair is tangled, separate it with the comb. Start with a small section of hair. Beginning at the end, comb downward. Hold the hair above where you are combing with your other hand so you do not pull on the patient's scalp. Continue working upward until you reach the scalp.
8. Style the hair attractively. If the patient has long hair, consider braiding it or putting it up. Coarse, tightly curled hair may require special treatment.
9. Remove the towel and discard according to facility policy.
10. Perform your procedure completion actions.

disposable razor, always wear gloves because of the high probability of contact with blood during this procedure.

Caring for the Patient's Hands, Feet, and Nails. Nails and feet require special attention to prevent injury and infection. In many agencies, only licensed per-

PROCEDURE

OBRA

41 SHAVING THE MALE PATIENT

1. Perform your beginning procedure actions.
2. Gather supplies needed: disposable gloves, washcloth, towel, electric or safety razor, shaving cream or preshave lotion, basin of water (105 degrees), mirror, aftershave lotion.
3. Place the equipment on the overbed table. Follow your facility policy for covering the overbed table with a barrier.
4. Provide privacy.
5. Drape a towel across the patient's chest.
6. Fill the washbasin with warm (105-degree) water and place it on the table.

7. Soften the beard by placing a warm, moist washcloth over it for two to three minutes.
8. Moisten the face with water and apply shaving cream.
9. Put on disposable gloves.
10. Hold the skin taut in front of the ear (Figure 9-13).
11. Starting at the sideburns, move the razor down over the cheeks to the chin, using short, even strokes. Continue until the entire cheek is shaved. Rinse the razor between strokes.
12. Repeat with other cheek.

continues

PROCEDURE **41** *continued*

13. Ask the patient to tighten the upper lip. Shave from the nose to the upper lip in short, downward strokes.

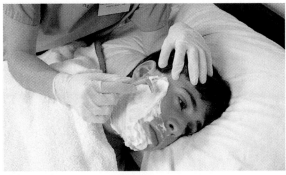

Figure 9-13 Hold the skin in front of the ear and shave downward in short, smooth strokes.

14. Ask the patient to tighten the chin. Shave the chin in downward strokes.
15. Assist the patient to tip his head back.
16. Apply shaving cream to the neck.
17. Hold the skin taut under the chin and shave the neck area in short, smooth, upward strokes.
18. Wash and dry the face and neck.
19. Apply aftershave lotion if the patient desires.
20. Remove the basin, empty and dry it, and return it to its storage place.
21. If you accidently nick the patient, report this to the supervisor.
22. Perform your procedure completion actions.

sonnel are allowed to cut fingernails, although the patient care technician is expected to clean them. As a rule, the patient care technician is not allowed to cut toenails, but is responsible for keeping the feet clean and dry.

The patient's feet require special care. Poor blood circulation to the feet is common, particularly in the elderly and persons with diabetes. Ingrown toenails cause breaks in the skin, which can lead to infection. The skin on the feet heals slowly if injured. Protecting the feet from injury is important. Know and follow your facility policy for foot and toenail care. Report to the supervisor if the nails need to be cut or if other abnormalities are noted.

General Guidelines for Providing Hand, Foot, and Nail Care

■ Know and follow your facility policy on who is allowed to clip and clean nails.

■ Cleaning and trimming nails is easier immediately after they are soaked or bathed.

■ Avoid the use of nail files and other sharp objects for cleaning nails. An orange stick is a disposable, pointed, wooden stick that can be safely used.

■ If your facility allows you to clip fingernails, use clippers, not scissors.

■ When trimming nails, be very careful not to accidentally clip or damage the skin surrounding the nail.

■ If you observe any abnormalities, such as redness, cracking, or signs of infection by the finger or toenails, report this finding to the supervisor.

continues

General Guidelines for Providing Hand, Foot, and Nail Care, *continued*

■ Fingernails are clipped straight across, then rounded at the edges with an emery board (Figure 9-14A).

■ Push the cuticles back with a washcloth or the dull end of the orange stick (Figure 9-14B).

■ Lotion may be applied to the hands or feet if the skin is dry. Do not apply lotion between the toes, as this may promote fungal growth.

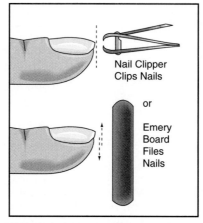

Nail Clipper
Clips Nails

or

Emery
Board
Files
Nails

Figure 9-14A Cut the nails straight across, then round the corners with the emery board.

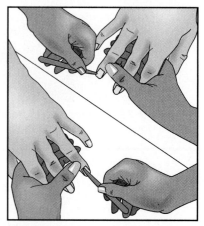

Figure 9-14B Gently push the cuticle back with the blunt end of the orange stick.

PROCEDURE

42 HAND AND FINGERNAIL CARE

1. Perform your beginning procedure actions.

2. Gather supplies needed: Disposable gloves if contact with moist body fluid or nonintact skin is likely, soap, towel, bed protector, basin of water (105 degrees), lotion, nail clippers, orange stick, emery board.

3. Place the equipment on the overbed table. Follow your facility policy for covering the overbed table with a barrier.

4. Position the overbed table in front of the patient and adjust the height. Cover the table with the bed protector.

5. Fill the washbasin with warm (105-degree) water and place it on the table.

6. Instruct the patient to place her hands in the water. A soft brush can be used to clean under the nails when the hands are soaking.

7. Soak the hands for 10 minutes. Placing a towel over the patient's hands and the basin will keep the water warm. Add more warm water if necessary.

8. Ask the patient to wash his or her hands. Gently push the cuticles back.

9. Lift the patient's hands out of the water and dry them with the towel.

10. Clip the nails if permitted by facility policy. The nail clippings will fall on the bed protector to be discarded later.

11. Round the edges of the nail with the emery board. Apply fingernail polish if requested by the patient.

12. Rub the hands with lotion.

continues

PROCEDURE **42** *continued*

13. Remove the basin, empty and dry it, and return it to its storage place.

14. Remove the bed protector containing the nail clippings and discard according to facility policy.

15. Perform your procedure completion actions.

■ SUPPORT HOSIERY

Support hosiery is used for patients with circulation problems. It is also used during and after surgery to prevent blood clots, edema, and other complications. The hose apply pressure to the legs, which increases the blood flow. The stockings are made of stretchable elastic and fit tightly. Support stockings may be knee length or cover the entire leg. They are called anti-embolism stockings, but are often referred to by the brand name, such as TED® Hose.

■ *anti-embolism stockings:*
elastic hosiery used on some patients to relieve edema and prevent blood clots

General Guidelines for Applying Anti-Embolism Stockings

■ Consult the care plan for wearing guidelines. The care plan will specify when the stockings should be put on and removed.

■ It is best to apply the stockings before the patient gets out of bed in the morning. Elevate the legs before applying the hosiery to reduce swelling and make hosiery easier to apply.

■ Anti-embolism stockings come in several sizes. The patient is measured with a tape measure to find the correct size. The hose must fit well to be effective.

■ The stockings must be applied smoothly with no wrinkles.

■ A light application of powder on the feet and legs will make the hosiery easier to apply.

■ Placing a plastic sandwich bag over the foot allows the hosiery to slide on easily. After the hose are applied, remove the bag through the opening in the toe area.

PROCEDURE

43 APPLYING ANTI-EMBOLISM STOCKINGS

1. Perform your beginning procedure actions.

2. Obtain hosiery in the correct size.

3. Expose one leg.

4. Hold the stocking with both hands at the top and roll or gather toward the toe end.

5. Apply the stocking over the toes and over the leg by rolling it upward (Figure 9-15).

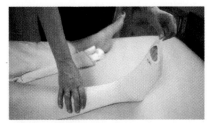

Figure 9-15 Pull the stocking evenly up the foot and leg.

continues

PROCEDURE **43** *continued*

6. Check the fit to be sure the stocking is even and there are no wrinkles.

7. Expose the other leg.

8. Repeat the procedure.

9. Perform your procedure completion actions.

■■■ PROSTHESIS CARE

A prosthesis is an artificial device used to replace a body part. Many types of prostheses are used. Some patients have an artificial eye or breast. Others have artificial arms, hands, legs, or feet. The prosthesis helps the patient function as normally as possible. Remember, the prosthesis is part of the patient's body and should be treated with care.

■■■ DRESSING AND UNDRESSING THE PATIENT

Patients in some health care agencies can be up and dressed each day. Self-esteem is improved when the patient is dressed and well groomed. It also affects other people's perception about the patient's health. Dressing and undressing are done several times a day. We remove night clothing and dress in day wear. At bedtime, we remove clothing and put on night wear. Sometimes in health care, more frequent changes of clothing are necessary due to tests, procedures, medical treatments, and accidental soiling of clothes. Some patients cannot dress and undress themselves. Others may need limited assistance. Patients with paralysis have special dressing needs.

■ *stump sock:* *a stocking that is placed over an amputated extremity before the prosthesis is applied*

General Guidelines for Caring for a Patient with a Prosthesis

■ Always check the care plan for special instructions regarding applying, removing, and caring for the prosthesis.

■ The prosthesis and the skin under the prosthesis must be kept clean and dry.

■ Check the skin under the prosthesis. Notify your supervisor of redness, irritation, dark spots, open areas, or blisters.

■ Follow the directions on the care plan for covering the extremity under the prosthesis. A **stump sock** is usually worn under artificial limbs.

■ Report to the supervisor if you think the prosthesis needs repair. Do not attempt to fix it yourself.

■ An artificial eye is usually cared for by the supervisor or an advanced care provider. If you will be caring for patients with artificial eyes, make sure you are properly trained. Follow your agency policy. Handle the eye carefully. The eye socket and the artificial eye must be cleaned as indicated on the care plan. Apply the principles of standard precautions when inserting, removing, and cleaning the eye.

General Guidelines for Dressing and Undressing Patients

- Provide privacy and avoid exposing the patient.
- Wear gloves and apply the principles of standard precautions if you anticipate contact with blood, body fluids (except sweat), secretions, excretions, mucous membranes, or nonintact skin.
- Check the care plan for special instructions and use of adaptive equipment.
- Encourage the patient to do as much self-care as possible.
- Allow the patient a choice of clothing, if possible.
- If the patient has one paralyzed or weak side, remove the clothing from the strong side first. Put clothing on the weak side first. Always support the weak or paralyzed extremity.
- It is easier to dress patients who can assist if they are standing or sitting.
- It is easier to dress a dependent patient in bed.
- Patients who are dressed in street clothes should wear proper undergarments.
- When dressing patients with catheters or tubes, treat them as part of the person's body. Avoid pulling on them or obstructing them. Do not disconnect them. Consult the supervisor for assistance.
- Gather sleeves and pant legs before putting them on the patient.

PROCEDURE

44 ASSISTING THE PATIENT WITH DRESSING

1. Perform your beginning procedure actions.
2. Gather needed supplies: bath blanket, clothing, deodorant, disposable gloves.
3. If the patient has a weak or paralyzed arm, work from the strong side.
4. Cover the patient with the bath blanket and remove the upper linens without exposing the patient.
5. For pants:
   a. Put one foot at a time into underwear. Slide them up over the feet and ankles.
   b. Gather the leg of the pants on the weak side. Slide the pant leg over the foot and ankle. Repeat with the strong leg.
   c. Slide the pants and underwear up the patient's legs.

   d. Ask the patient to raise the hips and buttocks while you pull underwear and pants into position.
   e. If the patient is unable to assist, roll onto the strong side. Pull the underwear and pants up on the weak side (Figure 9-16). Turn the patient to the weak side and finish pulling the clothing up. Fasten at the waist, if necessary.
6. Apply deodorant before putting on a shirt or sweater.
7. To put on garments that go over the arms or head:
   a. Stretch the neck as widely as possible and pull it over the patient's head (Figure 9-17).

continues

PROCEDURE   44   continued

b. Put your hand into the sleeve of the garment on the patient's weaker side. Grasp the patient's weak hand. Slide the sleeve off your wrist and pull patient's hand and wrist through the sleeve.

c. Pull the sleeve up and adjust it at the shoulder.

d. Lift the patient's arms and shoulders. Adjust the garment in the back.

e. Ask the patient to put the strong arm into the other sleeve. If unable, repeat step 7b.

f. Lift the patient's arms and shoulders, or roll the patient to the side. Pull down and adjust the garment in back.

8. To put on a shirt or blouse that opens in front:

a. Put your hand into the sleeve of the garment on the patient's weaker side. Roll the sleeve over your wrist. Grasp the patient's weak hand. Slide the sleeve off your wrist and over the patient's hand and wrist.

b. Pull the garment up the arm and adjust it at the shoulder.

c. Lift the patient's head and shoulders and pull the garment around the back. If you cannot lift the patient, roll him toward you and tuck the garment under him. Turn the patient away from you and pull the garment out. Then return the patient to the supine position.

d. Ask the patient to put the strong arm into the other sleeve. If unable, repeat step 8a.

e. Pull the garment up the arm and adjust it at the shoulder.

f. Fasten the garment in the front.

9. Reverse the procedure for undressing the patient.

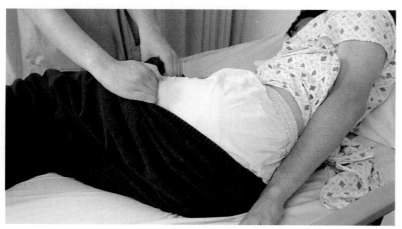

Figure 9-16 Roll the patient onto the strong side and adjust the pants and underwear on the weak side.

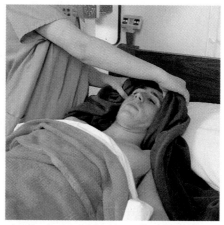

Figure 9-17 Position the neck of the shirt over the back of the patient's head, then stretch it to pull it over the face.

KEY POINTS IN CHAPTER

▬ *Good personal hygiene is essential to proper health.*

▬ *Activities of daily living are the things people do every day to meet their health and hygienic needs.*

▬ *The patient care technician assists patients to meet health and hygienic needs when they are unable to take care of these needs independently.*

▬ *Oral hygiene is the cleaning of the patient's mouth, teeth, gums, and tongue. Special oral hygiene is given frequently to patients who are unconscious, NPO, or receiving tube feeding or oxygen.*

▬ *Dentures are artificial teeth that require special care and handling.*

KEY POINTS IN CHAPTER

- *Bathing cleanses the skin, stimulates circulation, provides exercise, and refreshes and relaxes the patient.*
- *Bath time is an excellent time to make observations of the patient's skin and body.*
- *Bath water temperature is checked with a thermometer. A comfortable temperature for bathing is 105 degrees.*
- *When bathing patients, wash from clean to dirty areas.*
- *The bed bath is given to patients on complete bed rest and involves cleaning the patient's entire body.*
- *A partial bath involves washing the patient's face, hands, underarms, back, and genital area.*
- *When giving perineal care to a female, wash from front to back. Avoid rubbing back and forth.*
- *When giving perineal care to a male, wash from the tip of the penis to the rectum.*
- *Massaging the patient's back is comforting, refreshing, and stimulating to circulation. Giving a backrub helps prevent skin breakdown.*
- *In most agencies, the patient care technician does not cut finger and toenails.*
- *Anti-embolism hose increase blood flow to the legs and prevent blood clots, edema, and other complications.*
- *A prosthesis is used to replace a missing body part.*
- *The patient's self-esteem is enhanced when she is dressed and well groomed.*

REVIEW QUIZ

Multiple Choice Questions

1. Hygienic habits:
   a. develop over a person's lifetime.
   b. may be influenced by culture and religion.
   c. are a private matter for most people.
   d. all of the above.

2. ADLs are:
   a. all daily living.
   b. activities of daily living.
   c. all done lovingly.
   d. activities during life.

3. Incontinence is:
   a. loss of bowel or bladder control.
   b. difficulty breathing.
   c. inability to move or feel a body part.
   d. not a medical condition.

4. Always brush the patient's teeth:
   a. back and forth.
   b. in a circular motion.
   c. up and down.
   d. with the brush vertical to the teeth.

5. You are assigned to give Mr. Lee a partial bath. You know this means to wash the:
   a. face, abdomen, legs, underarms, and feet.
   b. face, hands, underarms, back, and perineum.
   c. face, arms, hands, perineum, and legs.
   d. face, underarms, perineum, and feet.

6. When bathing patients, always wash:
   a. vigorously in a circular motion.
   b. from the dirtiest area to the cleanest.
   c. from clean to dirty.
   d. the weakest side first.

7. The temperature of bath water should be:
   a. 85 degrees.
   b. 95 degrees.
   c. 105 degrees.
   d. 115 degrees.

8. Which of the following is *not* true about wearing gloves during the bathing procedure?
   a. Gloves are worn for the entire procedure.
   b. Gloves are changed immediately before contact with nonintact skin.
   c. Gloves are changed immediately before performing perineal care.
   d. Gloves should be changed if they become heavily soiled.

9. When assisting the female patient with perineal care, wash:
   a. from back to front.
   b. in a back-and-forth motion.
   c. in a circular motion.
   d. from front to back.

10. You are assigned to bathe Mrs. Lloyd. You notice that her toenails are long and dirty. You should:
    a. clean and cut the nails.
    b. clean the nails and consult the supervisor.
    c. do nothing about it, as you are not allowed to care for nails.
    d. clean the nails and file them with an emery board.

True/False Questions

11. ___ Massage Stage I pressure sores well with lotion.

12. ___ Shave a man's face using downward strokes.

13. ___ Assist the patient to sit in a chair before applying anti-embolism stockings.

14. ___ Always dress and undress the paralyzed arm first.

15. ___ A prosthesis is an artificial body part.

16. ___ HS care is given to prepare the patient for bed at night.

17. ___ Always wear gloves when giving oral care.

18. ___ It is not necessary to wear gloves when shaving patients.

19. ___ Always brush dentures while they are in the patient's mouth.

20. ___ Wear gloves when washing the patient's eyes.

Nutrition and Hydration

After reading this chapter, you will be able to:

Spell and define key terms.

Describe how proper nutrition influences health.

List the six categories in the food pyramid and give the number of daily servings from each.

List five common categories of diets served in health care facilities.

Describe how the PCT helps patients meet their nutritional needs.

List three alternative methods of feeding.

Identify the normal daily fluid requirement for adults.

Demonstrate accurate measurement of intake and output.

List the general rules for passing fresh water.

■■■ **NUTRITION**

Good nutrition is essential for good health. The PCT must maintain good health to be effective in the job. Patients need good nutrition to restore their health and promote healing. The body will not heal if it is not adequately nourished. Six **nutrients** are essential for good health:

- Water
- Vitamins
- Minerals
- Carbohydrates
- Proteins
- Fats

Vitamins are organic compounds found in foods that perform vital functions and regulate processes in the body. Each vitamin has a specific function. Absence of vitamins causes disease. **Minerals** are an essential part of all cells. They contribute to the formation of the bones, teeth, and nails, and help rebuild body tissues. **Carbohydrates** provide fuel and energy for the body. Sources of carbohydrates are fruits, vegetables, and grain products. **Proteins** are the fundamental structural element of all cells. Sometimes called "nature's building blocks," they are essential for growth, healing, and good health. Sources of protein are meat, fish, eggs, and milk products. **Fats** are used as a source of energy and heat.

■■■ **FOOD GUIDE PYRAMID**

The U.S. Department of Agriculture (USDA) is a governmental agency that studies nutrition and makes recommendations. The USDA has grouped foods into six categories. They recommend that everyone eat a certain number of servings

■ **nutrients:** *chemical substances in food that are necessary for life*

■ **vitamins:** *organic substances in food that are necessary for normal body function*
■ **minerals:** *inorganic compounds in food used to build body tissues*
■ **carbohydrates:** *foods that produce heat and energy in the body*
■ **protein:** *a nutrient in food that builds and repairs tissues*
■ **fats:** *food products, such as butter and oil, that are used for heat and energy production in the body*

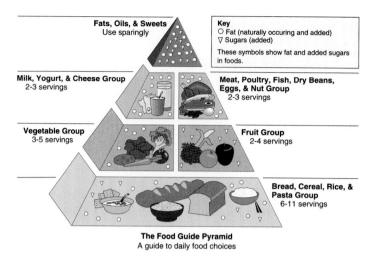

Figure 10-1 The USDA Food Guide Pyramid. (Courtesy U.S. Department of Agriculture)

■ **food pyramid:** *a U.S. Department of Agriculture diagram that provides a guide to a well-balanced diet*

from each category every day. The food pyramid (Figure 10-1) was developed to provide an easy-to-understand picture of daily nutritional requirements. The categories and USDA recommended servings are:

■ Bread, rice, cereal, and pasta group—6 to 11 servings a day

■ Fruit group—2 to 4 servings a day

■ Vegetable group—3 to 5 servings a day

■ Milk, yogurt, and cheese group—2 to 3 servings a day

■ Meat, poultry, fish, dry beans, eggs, and nuts group—2 to 3 servings a day

■ Fats, oils, and sweets—use sparingly

Eating according to the recommendations on the food pyramid will provide a well-balanced diet. Table 10-1 lists sample portion sizes from each category.

Table 10-1 Serving Sizes for Each Food Group

Food Group	1 serving from this group is:
Bread, cereal, rice, and pasta	1 slice of bread 1 tortilla ½ cup cooked rice, pasta, or cereal 1 ounce ready-to-eat cereal ½ hamburger bun, bagel, or English muffin 3–4 plain crackers 1 pancake (4-inch diameter) ½ large croissant ½ medium doughnut or danish 1/16 cake 2 medium cookies 1/12 of an 8″ pie
Vegetable group	½ cup chopped raw or cooked vegetables 1 cup raw, leafy vegetables ¾ cup vegetable juice ½ cup scalloped potatoes ½ cup potato salad 10 french fries

continues

Table 10-1, *continued*	
Food Group	**1 serving from this group is:**
Fruit group	1 piece fruit or melon wedge ¾ cup fruit juice ½ cup chopped, cooked, or canned fruit ¼ cup dried fruit
Milk, yogurt, and cheese group	1 cup milk or yogurt 1½ ounces cheese (natural) 2 ounces cheese (processed) 1½ cups ice cream or ice milk 1 cup frozen yogurt
Meat, poultry, dry beans, eggs, and nuts group	2½ to 3 ounces cooked lean beef, pork, lamb, veal, poultry, or fish (a portion the size of a deck of cards)
	½ cup cooked beans, 1 egg, 2 tablespoons peanut butter, or ⅓ cup of nuts equal one ounce of meat
Fats, oils, sweets	Use sparingly

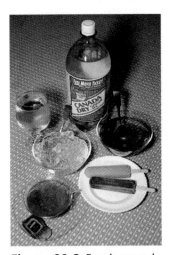

Figure 10-2 Foods served on a clear liquid diet

■ **regular diet:** *a normal diet based on the six food groups in the food pyramid*

■ **clear liquid diet:** *a diet high in water and carbohydrates, with little nutritive value*

■ HEALTH CARE FACILITY DIETS

Physicians write diet orders for their patients based on the patients' individual medical needs. Food served in the health care facility is prepared by the dietary department. A licensed dietitian writes the menus to be sure that diets are well balanced. The dietitian writes special menus for people with certain diseases to assure that the nutrients provided meet the patient's needs.

Many types of diets are served in health care facilities. Each facility has a listing of the types of diets served. Many facilities post the menu each day. Some health care facilities allow the patients to select what they want to eat. The common categories for diets served in health care facilities are:

■ Regular or general diet

■ Liquid diets

■ Soft or bland diets

■ Mechanically altered diets

■ Therapeutic diets

Regular Diets

The **regular diet** is a normal, unrestricted diet, served to patients with no restrictions on types of food. It is well balanced, with a wide variety of foods from the food pyramid groups.

Liquid Diets

Liquid diets are served to patients after surgery and before some tests. They are also used for patients who have nausea, vomiting, or diarrhea. They are not nutritionally complete and should be used only for a short time. The two main types of liquid diets are:

■ **Clear liquid diet** (Figure 10-2), which consists of liquids that you can see through. It includes broth, tea, soup, gelatin, and strained fruit juices. Clear soda pop and ginger ale may also be served with this diet.

■ **full liquid diet:** *a diet, used for patients with digestive disorders, that includes clear and milk-based liquids*

■ **soft (bland) diet:** *a diet containing foods that are low in residue, with limited or no seasoning*

■ **Full liquid diet**, which consists of all clear liquids plus milk-based liquids. It includes cream soups, milk, ice cream, eggnog, and yogurt.

Soft Diets

Soft or bland diets are served to patients who have certain conditions of the digestive system or those who cannot eat spiced or seasoned food. Food served on this diet includes soups, white meat and fish, cream cheese and cottage cheese, breads, crackers, and milk products.

Mechanically Altered Diets

■ **mechanically altered diet:** *a diet that is changed in texture to meet the needs of patients with chewing, swallowing, or digestive problems*

■ **pureed diet:** *a diet blenderized to a smooth consistency*

■ **mechanical soft diet:** *a diet that is finely ground or chopped for patients with chewing or swallowing problems*

Mechanically altered diets are served to patients who have chewing, swallowing, or digestive disorders. Any kind of diet can be blenderized to alter the mechanical consistency of the food. The two main types of mechanically altered diets are:

■ Pureed diet (Figure 10-3), which is blended with liquid so the food is smooth, without large particles. It is the consistency of baby food, but should not appear runny or watery. If a plastic spoon is placed upright in a pureed food, it should remain upright without falling over.

■ Mechanical soft diet (Figure 10-4), which includes some foods, such as bread, that are not blended. Hard-to-chew items, such as meats, are ground until they are finely chopped. The food is not reduced to liquid in this diet.

Therapeutic Diets

■ **therapeutic diet:** *a special or modified diet prepared to treat a patient's individual nutritional needs*

Therapeutic diets are served to treat certain medical diseases or conditions. The licensed dietitian plans these diets very carefully to meet the patient's treatment needs. Regular food is used, but preparation of the food may be different from that of a regular diet. For example, certain foods on a regular diet are prepared with salt. A patient on a salt-restricted diet would have the same food item prepared without salt. Each therapeutic diet has special requirements, and some foods may be restricted on certain diets. The following sections describe common types of therapeutic diets.

■ **diabetic diet:** *a diet calculated by the dietitian to meet the needs of a patient with diabetes mellitus; the diet limits free sugar and some other foods*

■ **calorie:** *a unit of energy-producing potential equal to the amount of heat that is contained in food and released upon use by the body*

■ **diabetes:** *a chronic disease caused by a disorder of carbohydrate metabolism*

Diabetic Diet. The diabetic diet serves normal foods, but without sources of free sugar. Some diabetic diets limit calories. Others restrict forms of concentrated sweets, such as sugar packets, fruits canned in sugar, cakes, pies, ice cream, and sweetened desserts. This type of diet is served to patients with diabetes mellitus. The recommended distribution of calories in a diabetic diet is 60% carbohydrate, 20–30% protein, and 20–30% fat.

Meal intake is very important for the diabetic patient. Meals and snacks must be served in a timely manner to maintain the patient's blood sugar levels. Diabetics receive medication to control their diabetes based on their food intake. If intake is inadequate, or meals are missed or delayed, serious complications may result. If a diabetic patient does not eat, report this information to your supervisor. You will usually be instructed to offer the patient another food of similar nutritive value to replace the uneaten items.

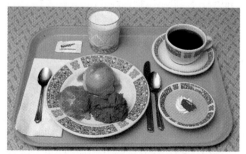

Figure 10-3 This pureed food is well blended but not watery.

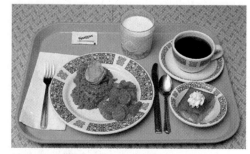

Figure 10-4 The mechanical soft diet serves foods that are easy to chew.

calorie-controlled diet: a diet that restricts the total number of calories served to the patient; usually served to overweight patients

sodium-restricted diet: a diet prepared with no or limited sodium

Calorie-Controlled Diets. Calorie-controlled diets are usually served to patients who are overweight. These diets are nutritionally complete, but the portions are usually smaller than those in a regular diet. Like the diabetic diet, sugar and forms of concentrated sweets are avoided on this type of diet.

Sodium-Restricted Diets. The sodium-restricted diet is served to patients with heart or kidney disease. The doctor may order a diet prepared completely without sodium (salt), or the patient may be allowed sodium in a limited amount. In this diet, salt packets are not served on trays. Some agencies use salt substitutes if the doctor agrees. Foods that are usually low in sodium are fresh fruits, vegetables, and some cereals. Some foods have a high sodium content and should be avoided. Some examples are:

- Potato chips and similar snacks
- Lunch meats and processed meats, ham, and bacon
- Certain soft drinks
- Pickles and olives
- Many canned foods

low-fat diet: a diet that is low in fat for patients with heart, blood vessel, liver, and/or gallbladder disease

low-cholesterol diet: a diet that is low in fat and cholesterol for patients with heart, blood vessel, liver, and/or gallbladder disease

Low-Fat/Low-Cholesterol Diets. Low-fat and low-cholesterol diets are served to patients with heart, blood vessel, liver, and gallbladder disease. Sources of fat are limited or avoided in food preparation, and fats such as butter are limited or restricted. This diet includes lean meats that are baked or broiled, fruits and vegetables, and low-fat dairy products.

Other Types of Diets. Patients have many unique needs, and sometimes other types of diets are necessary. Some diets restrict sources of fiber. Others may serve a high or low amount of protein. Some are high in calories. High-calorie diets are commonly served to burn patients or those who need extra nutrition for healing. Some patients are on special diets because of religious prohibitions on certain foods. Table 10-2 lists the special dietary requirements of many cultural and religious groups in the United States.

Table 10-2 Cultural and Religious Dietary Requirements

Religion/Group	Food Requirements and Prohibitions
Adventist, Seventh Day	Alcohol, coffee, and tea are prohibited. A vegetarian diet is encouraged.
American Indian	In some tribes, sharing food is customary. Explain to visitors that they should not share the patient's food in the health care facility. After prayer and certain ceremonies, berries, corn, and dried meat are consumed. These foods may be provided by family members or other members of the tribe.
Buddhist	Buddhists do not eat meat.
Catholic	Some patients do not eat meat on Fridays and other holy days.
Christian Scientist	Alcohol is prohibited. Some abstain from coffee and tea.
Hindu	Most Hindus are vegetarians. A light meal is eaten for breakfast, a heavy meal for lunch, and a light meal for supper. Dietary customs state that the right hand is used for eating and the left hand for toileting and personal hygiene.
Islamic	Alcohol, pork, and some shellfish are not allowed. *continues*

Table 10-2, *continued*	
Religion/Group	**Food Requirements and Prohibitions**
Jewish	Milk and meat are not eaten together. Predatory fowl, shellfish, and pork are not allowed. Fish with fins and scales are permitted. Other types of fish are not allowed. Some Jewish patients request kosher food, which requires very special preparation.
Mormon	Alcohol, coffee, and tea are not allowed.

■ **supplemental feedings:** *nourishments given to the patient in addition to meals to meet special nutritional needs*

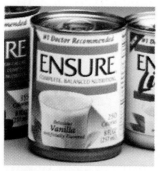

Figure 10-5 Prepared oral nutritional supplements provide good nutrition. (Photo used with permission of Ross Products Division, Abbott Laboratories, Columbus, Ohio)

Supplemental Feedings

Supplemental feedings are served to many patients. Sometimes common foods or beverages, such as milkshakes, ice cream, or juices, are served as supplements. Some facilities offer canned beverages such as Ensure® (Figure 10-5). Supplemental feedings are always served between meals. If they are served too close to meal time, the patient may not be hungry and will not eat. Diabetic patients are often given medication to control their diabetes. If supplements are served to a diabetic, the total calorie value of the supplement is included in the diet, because diabetic medication is calculated based on calorie count. It is important that supplements be given as ordered to maintain a proper balance between the food and medication.

■■■ ASSISTING PATIENTS WITH NUTRITION

Illness and certain medications can affect the patient's appetite. When preparing patients for meals, making the environment and the food as pleasant as possible is important.

Preparing Patients for Meals

Before meal time, prepare patients for meals so that when meals arrive they can be served quickly. This maintains proper temperature. Food can be a source of infection if the temperature is not maintained. Hot foods should be served hot and cold foods served cold.

Follow your facility policy for preparing the nursing unit for meals. Some facilities require removal of laundry hampers and housekeeping carts from hallways before tray carts arrive. Bring a clothing protector (Figure 10-6) to the room if needed by patient. Do not call a clothing protector a bib. "Bib" is a demeaning term to many adults.

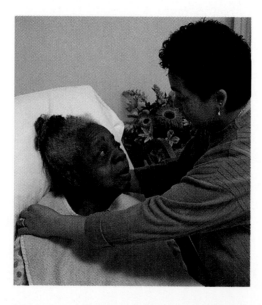

Figure 10-6 An adult clothing protector

General Guidelines for Preparing Patients for Meals

■ Make the environment as pleasant as possible. Remove bedpans, urinals, and other objectionable items. Eliminate odors.

■ Assist the patient with toileting and elimination needs. Provide incontinent care, if necessary. Apply the principles of standard precautions if you are assisting with these procedures.

■ Assist the patient to wash hands.

■ Be sure the patient has dentures, glasses, and hearing aid, if used.

■ If the patient will be eating in bed, elevate the head of the bed. Assist the patient to sit in a chair, if allowed.

■ Monitor the patient's position and distance from the food and make necessary adjustments.

■ Clear the top of the overbed table to receive the tray. Wipe the table top with a damp paper towel or according to facility policy.

■ Apply a clothing protector, if used by the patient.

When assisting patients to sit at dining tables or to use an overbed table, position is very important. The patient should sit upright with feet supported. Monitor the patient's distance from the table. Does the patient have to stretch and reach to eat? Monitor the height of the table. Some short patients may be sitting too low. Some adjustments in the type of table used, table height, or type of chair may be necessary to make eating easier. If the patient has to work to eat, she may not eat as well. It is usually easier to seat the patient in a straight-backed chair than it is to use a wheelchair. A straight-backed chair usually has lower armrests (or no armrests), making it easier to get close to the table. Chairs that are used in health care facilities are usually the correct height for the table. If an overbed table is used to serve the patient a meal, adjust the height and distance from the arms when you serve the tray.

Serving Meals. In most health care facilities, food is served on trays that are delivered to the nursing units in carts. Each tray is labeled with the patient's name, room number, and type of diet. After all trays are passed, check on patients while they are eating. If food is not being eaten, offer a substitute. Offer to replace or reheat food that has become cold.

General Guidelines for Serving Meals

■ Wash your hands.

■ Check the tray card for the patient's name and room number.

■ Check the food on the tray to see if it should be served on the patient's diet. If you think a food item is not appropriate, consult your supervisor.

■ Take the tray to the patient's room, identify the patient, and place the tray on the overbed table.

■ Prepare the tray, if necessary, by opening milk cartons, cutting meat, buttering bread, and putting condiments on food.

■ Provide adaptive eating devices, if used.

■ Feed the patient, if necessary.

General Guidelines for Feeding Patients

- Sit at or below the patient's eye level, if possible. This is less intimidating than standing over the patient. It also prevents the patient from choking, which could be caused if she must bend her head back to look up at you.
- Check the food temperature before feeding. Place a drop of hot food on the inside of your wrist to be sure it is not too hot.
- Tell the patient what is on the tray. Ask what the patient would like to eat first.
- Sometimes patients cannot handle utensils, but are able to eat their own finger foods, such as bread, crackers, or cookies. Encourage patients to do this.
- Offer liquids at intervals. Using a straw will make it easier for the patient to drink.
- Make pleasant conversation while feeding. Avoid making conversation if the patient has difficulty swallowing. Responding to conversation may cause accidental choking.
- Avoid rushing the patient.
- Be emotionally sensitive to the patient's needs. Focus on the patient when feeding. Avoid having conversations with others in the room.

PROCEDURE

 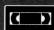

45 FEEDING THE DEPENDENT PATIENT

1. Perform your beginning procedure actions.
2. Place the tray on the overbed table and sit at or below the patient's eye level.
3. Inform the patient what is on the tray and ask what she would like to eat first.
4. Fill the fork or spoon half full (Figure 10-7). If the patient has had a stroke, place food in the unaffected side of the mouth.
5. Alternate liquids and solids.
6. Wipe the patient's mouth as often as necessary.
7. Remove the tray when the patient is finished.
8. Wash the patient's hands and face, if necessary.
9. Assist the patient with oral hygiene and toileting after meals.
10. Record the patient's appetite and fluid intake according to facility policy.
11. Perform your procedure completion actions.

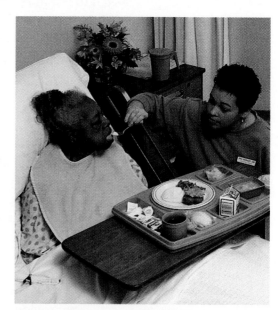

Figure 10-7 Sit at eye level with the patient and feed half a teaspoon of food each time.

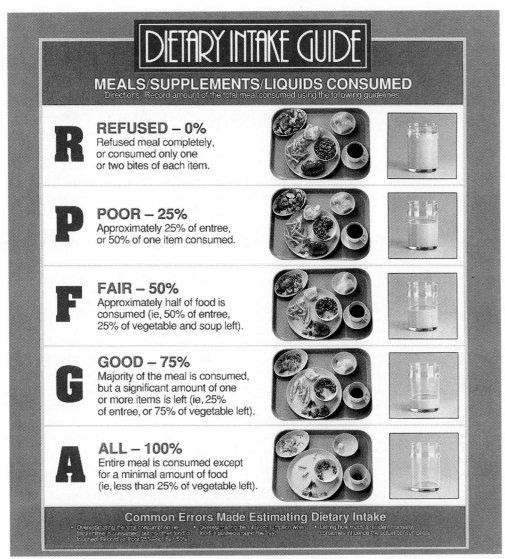

Figure 10-8 These simple guidelines describe how to estimate the patient's meal intake. (Photo used with permission of Ross Products Division, Abbott Laboratories, Columbus, Ohio)

Feeding the Patient

Some patients are not able to eat by themselves and must be fed. The patient may feel embarrassed and childish. Be sensitive to the patient's feelings.

After Meals

After meals, pick up trays and return them to the tray cart. Wipe spilled food off overbed tables, if necessary. Facilities record how much patients have eaten in different ways. Some write "good," "fair," or "poor." Other facilities use fractions or record the percentage of the diet consumed (Figure 10-8). Know and follow your facility policy. Record the amount of liquid taken if the patient is on intake and output. Before leaving the room, return the bed to a position of comfort and assist the patient to wash hands and meet other hygienic needs. Make sure that there is no food on the face or clothing. Wait until all uneaten trays have been passed before returning used food trays to the cart.

▪▪▪ ALTERNATIVE METHODS OF FEEDING

Sometimes patients cannot eat solid food and are fed by other methods. The patient care technician does not administer these feedings, but must have a basic understanding of how to care for patients being fed by alternative methods.

■ *nasogastric tube: a tube inserted into the nose and threaded through the esophagus into the stomach; can be used for feeding or medical procedures*

Tube Feeding

Feeding tubes are used for patients who have certain medical problems or are unable to swallow. A nasogastric tube is inserted through the nose and threaded through the esophagus to the stomach. A gastrostomy tube is surgically inserted through the abdominal wall into the stomach. The patient is fed liquid formula through the tube. The most common method of feeding is through a pump (Figure 10-9) that delivers the feeding at a slow rate over a long period of time. Several other methods of tube feeding may also be used.

Keeping the head of the bed elevated at least 45 degrees while the tube feeding is running is important. The head should remain elevated for 30 to 60 minutes, or according to facility policy, after the feeding is completed. If the alarm on the pump sounds, notify the supervisor. If you observe the patient coughing, choking, or vomiting, stay in the room and call for immediate assistance. Notify the supervisor if the feeding solution is not flowing through the tubing, or if the solution bag is low or empty.

Patients receiving tube feedings require frequent mouth care. Consult the care plan for specific instructions. When moving patients in bed, know the location of the tube at all times and avoid pulling on it. Serious complications can result if a tube is dislodged. The skin around the feeding tube must be kept clean. Sometimes the skin around a gastrostomy tube is covered with gauze. If the patient has a nasogastric tube, it may be pinned to the gown or clothing to prevent pulling.

Some patients with nasogastric tubes are being suctioned through the tube because of bleeding or other conditions. These patients will be kept NPO. You may be required to empty and clean the suction container. The stomach contents are a body fluid, so apply the principles of standard precautions during this procedure.

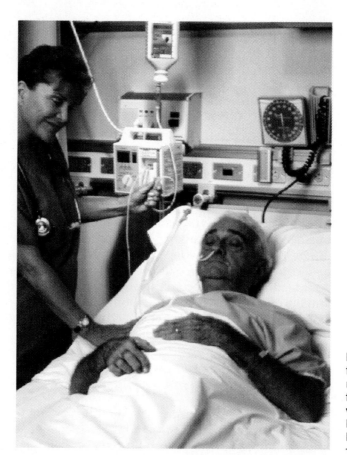

Figure 10-9 The tube feeding pump delivers a measured amount of tube feeding solution. (Photo used with permission of Ross Products Division, Abbott Laboratories, Columbus, Ohio)

Intravenous Feedings

■ *intravenous feeding (IV):* *administering sterile liquid and nutrients into a vein with a needle*

Intravenous feedings (IVs) are used for many purposes. Sometimes they are used to give the patient extra fluids or medications. The intravenous solution is attached to a needle or plastic cannula in a vein in the arm, leg, neck, or chest. Some IVs run by gravity (Figure 10-10); others are administered with a pump. For some patients, the intravenous feeding provides the only source of nutrition. Intravenous solutions are not nutritionally complete, so this will be used for only a short time.

Patients receiving intravenous feedings may also receive meal trays. Consult the care plan for instructions regarding meal trays.

Hyperalimentation

■ *hyperalimentation or total parenteral nutrition (TPN):* *a method of feeding a patient total nutrition intravenously, allowing the gastrointestinal system to rest*
■ *peripherally inserted central catheter (PICC):* *an intravenous line inserted in the arm and threaded through the venous system to the superior vena cava; used for long-term intravenous therapy and TPN*

Hyperalimentation may also be called **total parenteral nutrition (TPN)**. This intravenous feeding provides total nutrition. It is inserted into the subclavian vein in the chest or a special intravenous catheter in the arm called a **peripherally inserted central catheter (PICC)**. TPN bypasses the organs of the digestive system entirely, allowing them to rest and heal. The supervisor will care for the

■ *infusion site:* *the site where the intravenous needle is inserted into the body*

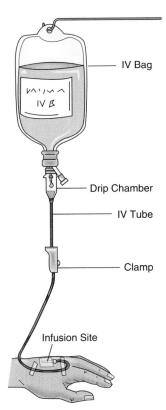

Figure 10-10 An intravenous infusion

General Guidelines for Caring for Patients with Intravenous Feedings

■ Make sure that the solution is flowing. Check the drip rate, if this is your facility policy and you have been trained in this procedure. The patient care technician is responsible only for monitoring the flow. Never try to adjust the rate of flow of the solution.
■ Handle the **infusion site** carefully.
■ Do not adjust the clamps on the tubing.
■ Avoid pulling on the tubing when moving the patient.
■ Keep the intravenous solution above the needle insertion site.
■ Avoid taking a blood pressure in the arm with an intravenous infusion.
■ Never disconnect the tubing. If the tubing or needle accidentally separates, put firm pressure on the needle insertion site with a gloved hand and call for the supervisor immediately.
■ Avoid kinks and obstructions in the tubing.
Report these observations to the supervisor:
■ An alarm sounds on an intravenous pump
■ Blood backing up into the intravenous tubing
■ Redness, swelling, or complaints of pain at the needle insertion site
■ Wetness or moisture at the insertion site or where the tubing connects to the intravenous catheter
■ An intravenous solution bag or bottle is empty or low (the container should never run dry)
■ The solution is not dripping, seems to be dripping too fast, or the drip chamber is completely full
■ The needle becomes dislodged
■ The tubing pulls apart from the needle
■ The solution appears to be leaking

IV Bag
Drip Chamber
IV Tube
Clamp
Infusion Site

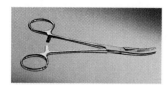

Figure 10-11 A Kelly is used to clamp the subclavian line close to the patient's body if it accidentally breaks. (Courtesy of Medline Industries, Inc.)

■ **Kelly:** *a special clamp used to close tubes quickly*

■ **dehydration:** *a serious condition resulting from inadequate water in the body*
■ **lethargy:** *abnormal drowsiness or sleepiness*

■ **intake and output (I & O):** *an estimated measurement of all the liquid the patient takes in and all the fluid he or she loses in a 24-hour period*

■ **force fluids:** *an order to encourage the patient to drink as much liquid as possible*

■ **fluid restriction:** *limiting the total amount of fluid the patient can have in a 24-hour period*

insertion site. Be sure the tubing is not obstructed or kinked. Be very careful to avoid dislodging the tubing when moving or caring for the patient. Many health care facilities keep a special clamp, called a Kelly (Figure 10-11), at the bedside of patients with intravenous lines in the subclavian vein. Serious complications occur if the tubing breaks or becomes dislodged. The Kelly clamp is used to clamp the tubing close to the patient's body if the line breaks or is accidentally pulled loose. It should be readily available at all times. Avoid storing it in a drawer or removing it from the room.

◼◼◼◼ FLUID INTAKE

An adequate intake of water and other fluids is essential to life. Two-thirds of the body is water. The body uses complex mechanisms to balance the fluid we take in with the fluid eliminated. In sickness and disease, ensuring that the patient drinks enough fluid is important. Fluid eliminated from the body may also be monitored, as described in Chapter 11.

We normally take in two to three quarts of liquid each day. Most of this is in the form of liquid beverages and water. Some fruits and vegetables also provide water. Dehydration occurs if patients do not take in adequate fluids. Dehydration is a serious condition resulting from inadequate fluid in the body. Signs of dehydration are mental confusion, lethargy, weakness, dry mucous membranes, rapid pulse, and low blood pressure. Dry skin that "tents" when you pinch it gently is also a sign of dehydration. This is called *poor skin turgor* and indicates lack of fluid in the subcutaneous tissues.

Because most patients are asleep during the night, most of the liquid taken in should be consumed during the day and the evening. We often measure how much liquid the patient takes in and the amount of urine and other drainage the patient excretes each day. This is called intake and output (I & O). Regardless of whether a patient is on intake and output, taking in enough liquid each day is still important. Offer patients liquids each time you are in the room. Pay particular attention to confused and dependent patients who may not be able to drink without your help.

Measuring and Recording Fluid Intake

Fluid intake is all liquid that the patient takes into the body. This includes everything the patient drinks and all fluid given in intravenous feedings and tube feedings. The supervisor is responsible for keeping track of fluid intake given through tubes, but the patient care technician is responsible for monitoring oral intake.

When monitoring intake and output, certain food items are also considered liquids, and should be recorded. These are things that would become liquid if allowed to stand at room temperature, such as ice cream, sherbet, gelatin, pudding, custard, and popsicles.

Force Fluids. Patients who require extra fluid often have an order to force fluids. This does not mean that you physically force the patient to drink. Rather, you will offer fluids frequently and encourage patients to drink throughout your shift. Finding out what beverages the patient likes may be helpful. Provide them, if allowed. Offer the patient a drink every time you are in the room and write down the amount the patient drinks each time. This will be totaled and recorded at the end of your shift.

Fluid Restrictions. Sometimes patients with heart or kidney disease, or other medical problems, are put on fluid restrictions. The total liquid allowed in a 24-hour period is calculated carefully. Usually the total is divided by three shifts, and the care plan lists how much fluid each shift may give the patient. The largest quantity is usually given by the day shift, because two meals are served on this shift. The night shift may have only a very small amount of fluid to give, because the patient is usually asleep during the night.

Water glass = 6 oz = 180 cc
Styrofoam cup = 6 oz = 180 cc
Juice glass (small) = 4 oz = 120 cc
Juice glass (large) = 8 oz = 240 cc
Full water pitcher (1 qt) =
    32 oz = 960 cc
Coffee or tea pot = 10 oz = 300 cc
Coffee cup = 5 oz = 150 cc
Milk carton = 8 oz = 240 cc
Soup bowl (small) = 6 oz = 180 cc
Soup bowl (large) = 10 oz = 300 cc
Gelatin = 4 oz = 120 cc
Ice cream cup = 4 oz = 120 cc
Creamer = 1 oz = 30 cc

Abbreviations
oz = ounce = 30 cc
pt = pint = 16 oz = 480/500 cc
qt = quart = 32 oz = 960/1000 cc
gal = gallon = 128 oz = 3840/4000 cc

Patients may not finish all fluids furnished to them. Estimate how much fluid has actually been taken and record the amount. For instance, the patient is given 8 ounces of milk but drinks only 4 ounces. Therefore, record intake of 120 cc.

Figure 10-12 Average container amounts

■ **milliliter (mL):** *a metric unit of measure used in health care facilities; 30 mL equals one ounce. One milliliter is the same as one cubic centimeter*
■ **cubic centimeter (cc):** *a metric unit of measure used in health care facilities; 30 cc equals one ounce*

■ **strict I & O:** *an accurate measurement of all the liquid the patient takes in and loses in a 24-hour period.*

Measuring Fluid Intake. The metric system is used to measure fluid intake and output. Fluid intake is measured in **milliliters** (mL) or **cubic centimeters** (cc). These two measurements are equivalent. Your facility will have a chart that gives the number of cubic centimeters in commonly used containers, such as the cups, dishes, and water pitcher (Figure 10-12). You must understand how to convert the commonly used measurements of ounces, pints, quarts, and gallons into metric measurements. Table 10-3 lists the common U.S. measurements for liquids and their metric equivalents.

When calculating how much liquid a patient drank, you must first know how much liquid the container holds when full. You will estimate how much the patient drank, then subtract it from the total. For example, a water glass holds 240 cc. The patient drinks half a glass, or 120 cc. 240 cc minus 120 cc equals 120 cc. You will record 120 cc under the intake column of the I & O record.

Usually an estimation of the amount of fluid the patient drinks is adequate. When we measure intake and output, our figures are close estimates. However, sometimes the doctor will order **strict I & O**. This means that the fluid must be measured exactly. Using the same example, the water glass holds 240 cc. The patient drinks approximately half a glass. You will pour the remaining water into a measuring device to see how much is left (Figure 10-13). After you do this, you find that 118 cc remains in the glass. 240 cc minus 118 cc equals 122 cc. You will record 122 cc on the I & O record. This method of measuring intake and output is more accurate, but as you can see, the figures are very close to the estimated amount in the first example.

Table 10-3

Common U.S. Measurement	Metric Equivalent	Common U.S. Measurement	Metric Equivalent
1 teaspoon	5 cc	1 quart	1,000 cc (or 1 liter)
1 ounce	30 cc	½ gallon	2,000 cc
½ pint	250 cc	1 gallon	4,000 cc
1 pint	500 cc		

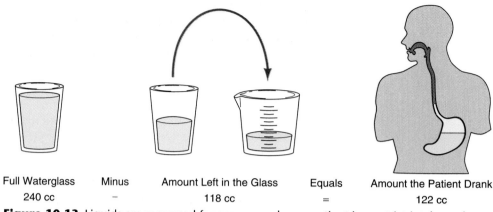

Full Waterglass	Minus	Amount Left in the Glass	Equals	Amount the Patient Drank
240 cc	−	118 cc	=	122 cc

Figure 10-13 Liquids are measured for accuracy when a patient is on strict intake and output.

You will be assigned to add the total intake at the end of your shift. Remember that most people drink 2,000 to 3,000 cc every 24 hours (Figure 10-14). If the patient's total intake for your shift seems inadequate, consult the supervisor. Your facility may have guidelines for you to follow. For example, a facility may require you to report to the supervisor if the patient takes in less than 1,200 cc on the day shift and 1,000 cc on the second shift. Consult your facility policy and procedure manual or supervisor.

▬ PASSING DRINKING WATER

The patient care technician is usually assigned to pass drinking water to patients every four to eight hours. Consult the care plan to see if the patient is allowed

Intake Section of Intake and Output Form

Time	Oral Kind	Oral Amount	Tube Feeding	Intravenous	Other
0700	Coffee	120 CC			
	Juice	100 CC			
	Milk	240 CC			
1000	Water	180 CC			
1200	Soup	120 CC			
	Juice	100 CC			
	Coffee	120 CC			
	Milk	240 CC			
8 Hour Total		1220 CC			
1500	Water	90 CC			
1800	Soup	200 CC			
	Milk	240 CC			
2000	Ensure	240 CC			
2210	Water	200 CC			
8 Hour Total		970 CC			
2300	Juice	120 CC			
8 Hour Total		120 CC			
24 Hour Total		2310 CC			

Worksheet

Oral Intake

1220 cc

970 cc

120 cc

Total 2310 cc

Figure 10-14 The oral intake is on the left side of the form. The type of fluid, time, and amount are recorded. The intake is totalled every 8 hours and cumulated every 24 hours.

to have ice. In certain medical conditions, beverages are served without ice. Also check to see if patients are NPO. Most facilities remove the cup and water pitcher from the room while a patient is NPO. The method of passing drinking water and the type of ice dispenser will vary with your facility. However, certain common rules for passing water apply in all facilities.

General Guidelines for Providing Fresh Drinking Water

■ Wash your hands before beginning this procedure. If your hands become contaminated, or if you assist a patient, wash your hands again before continuing. Your hands remain clean if you are touching only clean items.

■ Follow facility policy and good infection control practices.

■ Avoid contaminating the ice scoop, ice machine, or supply of clean ice with your hands, a cup, pitcher, or ice scoop. Avoid touching the ice scoop against the pitcher when you are filling it with ice.

■ Do not pour water from a cup back into a water pitcher.

■ Avoid filling a pitcher or cup directly over the clean ice supply. Ice from the scoop will hit the outside of the container and fall back into the clean ice supply, causing contamination. Fill the pitcher over a plastic bag, sink, or other container.

■ Avoid mixing the pitchers and cups if there is more than one patient in the room. Pitchers that are reused should be labeled with the patient's name. Return the correct pitcher to each patient.

KEY POINTS IN CHAPTER

― *Water, vitamins, minerals, carbohydrates, fats, and proteins are essential for good health.*

― *The USDA food pyramid recommends a specific number of servings from each of the six food groups each day.*

― *FIve common categories of diets are served in health care facilities.*

― *Therapeutic diets are planned by a licensed dietitian to meet a patient's specific medical needs.*

― *The patient care technician is responsible for preparing patients for meals, serving trays, feeding patients, and removing trays after patients have eaten.*

― *Tube feeding, intravenous feeding, and hyperalimentation are alternative methods of feeding patients with special needs.*

― *Adults need 2,000 cc to 3,000 cc of liquid each day for their bodies to function properly.*

― *Measuring fluid intake and output is an important responsibility of the patient care technician.*

― *The patient care technician applies principles of medical asepsis when passing fresh drinking water to patients.*

REVIEW QUIZ

Multiple Choice Questions

1. How many nutrients are essential for good health?
   a. Two
   b. Three
   c. Five
   d. Six

2. The type of food called "nature's building blocks" is:
   a. minerals.
   b. proteins.
   c. carbohydrates.
   d. vitamins.

3. According to the USDA food pyramid, how many servings of fruit should you have each day?
   a. 2 to 4
   b. 3 to 5
   c. 1 or 2
   d. 6 to 11

4. According to the USDA food pyramid, how many servings of bread, rice, cereal, or pasta should you have each day?
   a. 2 to 4
   b. 3 to 5
   c. 1 or 2
   d. 6 to 11

5. You are assigned to serve a full liquid diet to Mr. Johnson. Which of the following would you expect to find on his tray?
   a. Vegetable soup
   b. Pureed fish
   c. Yogurt
   d. Peach cobbler

6. Therapeutic diets:
   a. are planned by the dietitian for patients with special medical needs.
   b. are rarely used in the health care facility.
   c. have no effect on patients with heart disease or diabetes.
   d. are always limited in sugar.

7. Foods that are high in sodium include:
   a. fresh fruit.
   b. fresh vegetables.
   c. bread and whole grains.
   d. lunch meat and ham.

8. Guidelines for passing trays to patients include:
   a. handwashing and identifying the patient.
   b. preparing the tray and providing adaptive devices.
   c. checking the food on the tray to see if it is allowed.
   d. all of the above.

9. If you think a food is too hot to feed to a dependent patient, you should:
   a. return the food to the tray cart uneaten.
   b. blow on the food to cool it.
   c. leave the food until it cools.
   d. put the food in the refrigerator.

10. When feeding a patient with a paralyzed side, direct the food:
    a. to the unaffected side of the mouth.
    b. to the affected side of the mouth.
    c. in the center of the mouth.
    d. to the back of the throat.

11. Alternative methods of feeding include:
    a. therapeutic diets.
    b. TPN.
    c. mechanically altered diets.
    d. all of the above.

12. When a patient is receiving a tube feeding, the head of the bed should be:
    a. flat.
    b. elevated 20 degrees.
    c. elevated 45 degrees.
    d. tilted back.

13. When caring for a patient with an intravenous feeding, notify the supervisor if:
    a. blood backs up in the tubing.
    b. the insertion site is swollen.
    c. the container is almost empty.
    d. all of the above.

14. The normal daily fluid requirement for adults is:
    a. 100 to 1,000 cc.
    b. 500 to 2,000 cc.
    c. 2,000 to 3,000 cc.
    d. 3,500 to 4,000 cc.

15. A condition that results from inadequate fluid in the body is:
    a. hydration.
    b. dehydration.
    c. mechanical alteration.
    d. none of the above.

16. Lethargy is:
    a. hyperactivity.
    b. abnormal thirst.
    c. abnormal drowsiness.
    d. an indication of overhydration.

17. The metric equivalent for 1 quart is:
    a. 100 cc.
    b. 250 cc.
    c. 500 cc.
    d. 1,000 cc.

18. 30 cc is equivalent to:
    a. 1 teaspoon.
    b. 1 ounce.
    c. 1 cup.
    d. 1 quart.

19. 8 ounces is equivalent to:
    a. 24 cc.
    b. 80 cc.
    c. 240 cc.
    d. 800 cc.

20. 500 cc is equivalent to:
    a. 1 pint.
    b. 1 quart.
    c. 1 gallon.
    d. none of the above.

Elimination

After reading this chapter, you will be able to:

Spell and define key terms.

Describe the purpose of the urinary system.

Identify the common problems with urinary elimination associated with aging, trauma, and disease.

List the PCT's responsibilities in assisting patients with urinary elimination.

Describe the purpose of the urinary catheter.

Demonstrate the ability to perform catheter care, empty the drainage bag, and apply an external catheter.

Describe accurate measurement of urinary output.

State the purpose of collecting urine and stool specimens and demonstrate the procedures.

Identify the common problems with bowel elimination and list the PCT's responsibilities in assisting patients with bowel elimination.

Demonstrate administering a cleansing enema and retention enema and giving colostomy care.

■ **kidneys:** *the organs that filter waste and remove it from the bloodstream*
■ **ureters:** *two hollow tubes leading from the kidneys to the bladder*
■ **bladder:** *a hollow muscle that stores urine until it is eliminated from the body*
■ **urethra:** *the hollow tube leading from the bladder to the outside of the body*
■ **urination (voiding, micturition):** *the act of passing liquid waste to the outside of the body*
■ **urinary meatus:** *the external opening to the urethra where urine leaves the body*
■ **labia majora:** *two large, hair-covered structures on the external female genitalia*
■ **labia minora:** *two small, liplike structures inside the labia majora on the external female genitalia*
■ **penis:** *the external male organ used for sex and elimination*

THE URINARY SYSTEM

The urinary system (Figure 11-1) removes waste products and regulates water in the body. The urinary system consists of the kidneys, ureters, bladder, and urethra. The kidneys filter waste products from the blood and form urine. The urine leaves the kidneys through the ureters and travels to the bladder, where it is stored until it is eliminated from the body. When urine is eliminated, it leaves the bladder through the urethra and passes to the outside of the body. Several medical terms are used to describe the elimination of urine from the body: urination, voiding, and micturition. Most people feel the urge to urinate when the bladder contains 250 cc.

External Organs

The external organs associated with elimination in the female are the urinary meatus, labia majora, and labia minora (Figure 11-2A). The external organs in the male are the penis, urinary meatus, and foreskin (Figure 11-2B).

Normal Elimination

You have learned that the normal fluid intake for most adults is 2,000 to 3,000 cc per day. The average adult eliminates about 1,500 cc of urine a day from the bladder. The remaining liquid is eliminated from the body as sweat, moisture in respiratory secretions, and liquid in bowel elimination. Many factors influence urine production. Some factors, such as disease, ingestion of salt, and certain medications, reduce urine production and cause the body to retain fluid. Coffee, tea, alcoholic beverages, and some medications increase urine production.

■ *foreskin:* *the loose tissue*
at the tip of the penis

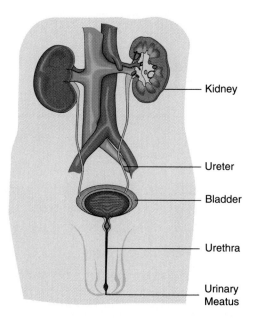

Figure 11-1 The urinary system

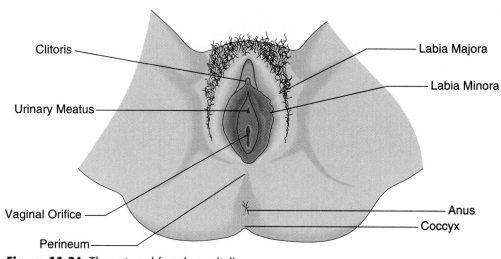

Figure 11-2A The external female genitalia

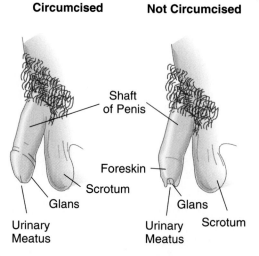

Figure 11-2B The external male genitalia

■■■ COMMON PROBLEMS RELATED TO THE URINARY SYSTEM

Aging, medications, and many different diseases can all cause problems with elimination. Elimination is very private for most people, and even a change in routine can cause embarrassment. This is particularly true if someone else must assist with this very personal body function. Physical changes in elimination can have a major impact on the patient's self-esteem. Protecting the patient's feelings when assisting with urinary elimination procedures is important. The PCT must be sensitive, understanding, and professional.

Incontinence is a medical problem. Health care workers often use underpads, incontinent pads, and briefs to contain urine, prevent skin breakdown, and avoid embarrassment to the patient. Select your words carefully—do not call these medical aids *diapers* or use other words that can be demeaning. Appropriate terms include *adult brief, garment protector,* and *clothing protector.* Your facility may have specific names for the products you will be using.

Changes in Urinary Function Associated with Aging and Disease

The aging process affects the urinary system. The kidneys do not filter the blood as efficiently as they did previously, so less urine is produced. Muscle tone decreases with aging and some diseases. The bladder is a muscle. Although the bladder is still able to hold urine, the capacity of the bladder is reduced and it cannot hold as much as it once did. A common myth is that incontinence is a normal part of aging. This is not true. Incontinence usually indicates a physical problem. It can also occur in mentally confused patients because they cannot express the need to use the bathroom. However, if they are taken to the bathroom and seated on the toilet, they will frequently urinate.

■ **prostate:** *a gland surrounding the urethra in the male patient*
■ **urinary retention:** *inability to empty the bladder completely*

Elderly men often develop prostate problems. The prostate gland surrounds the urethra just below the bladder and secretes fluid in semen (Figure 11-3). As men age, the prostate gland enlarges and applies pressure to the urethra. This causes problems with frequent dribbling of urine, urinary retention, or inability

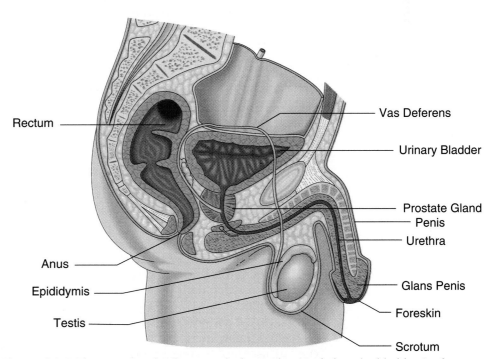

Rectum

Vas Deferens

Urinary Bladder

Prostate Gland
Penis
Urethra

Anus

Epididymis

Testis

Glans Penis

Foreskin

Scrotum

Figure 11-3 The prostate gland surrounds the urethra just below the bladder. It often enlarges with age and compresses the urethra, making urination difficult.

to urinate at all. Because men are used to urinating while standing, assisting the male patient to stand will help him empty his bladder more efficiently.

Many diseases also affect the urinary system. In heart disease, the blood is not circulated through the body efficiently, so less urine is produced. Edema often results. High blood pressure causes severe kidney damage over time. Other conditions, such as strokes, trauma, and neurological diseases, affect sensation and may make the patient unable to feel the urge to urinate when the bladder is full. Some patients do not feel the need to urinate until the bladder is very full, and then the need is immediate. If they have to wait, accidents will result.

Urinary Incontinence

Incontinence—the inability to control the passage of urine from the bladder—can be temporary or permanent. In addition to the problems listed earlier, other common causes of incontinence are disease, trauma, surgery, infection, stress, anxiety, tumors, mental confusion, loss of muscle control, and constipation. Inability to communicate the need to use the bathroom, or physical inability to get to the bathroom, also contribute to incontinence. When caring for patients who are incontinent, provide perineal care after each incontinent episode, following the guidelines in Procedures 36 and 37. Some facilities used premixed sprays for this purpose. Some are rinsed off with water; others are no-rinse solutions. Follow the directions for the type of product you are using, but apply the principles of peri care when you perform the procedure. Notify the nurse of any signs of skin redness, irritation, or breakdown.

Types of Incontinence.   Some patients have a condition called stress incontinence. This is a common problem in women, caused by weak muscles, having multiple children, and aging. In stress incontinence, the bladder leaks urine when the pelvic muscles are strained in activities such as laughing, coughing, sneezing, and lifting.

Urge incontinence is often caused by infection. Other causes include tumors, neurological problems, reproductive problems, and constipation. Patients with this condition have little warning of the need to use the toilet. When they feel the urge, the need is immediate. If the urine begins to escape, the patient may be unable to control it and the bladder will empty involuntarily.

Functional incontinence occurs when the patient is physically unable to get to the toilet on time, or is disoriented and unable to find the bathroom. It is easily treated by anticipating patient needs in advance, answering call signals immediately, and meeting patients' needs responsively. If the patient is in a restraint, she will be unable to get to the bathroom without your help. Anticipate the need and offer to take the patient routinely.

Mixed incontinence is a combination of urge and stress incontinence. Overflow incontinence occurs when the bladder is very full. When it can hold no more, urine leaks out to ease the pressure. Reflex incontinence is loss of urine that occurs without awareness in patients who are paralyzed or have other neurological problems.

Mentally Confused Patients.   Patients who are mentally confused present a particular challenge to the care provider. Most are able to urinate if they are taken to the toilet. Some patients who are mentally confused have behavior problems caused by the discomfort of needing to use the toilet. They are not able to express themselves verbally, so they yell, scream, hit, or cry. After they have eliminated the urine, the behavior problems cease. Some confused patients become restless and will pull at or remove their clothing. Anticipate the need for toileting and take confused patients to the bathroom every two hours, unless contraindicated. Managing incontinence requires planning and effort on your part. However, preventing accidents makes your work easier. A wet bed is a warm, moist, dark environment that presents an ideal breeding ground for bacteria. The risk of skin and bladder infections is increased by incontinence. Preventing incontinence also prevents skin breakdown, discomfort, and other complications for the patient.

■ **constipation:** *difficult passage of hard, dry stool from the lower bowel*

■ **stress incontinence:** *inability to control the passage of urine due to muscular weakness*

■ **urge incontinence:** *inability to control the passage of urine when the need to urinate is very strong and sudden, preventing the patient from getting to the toilet on time*

■ **functional incontinence:** *inability to control the passage of urine due to physical inability to get to the toilet*

■ **mixed incontinence:** *a combination of urge and stress incontinence*

■ **overflow incontinence:** *the escape of urine that occurs when the bladder is very full and can hold no more urine*

■ **reflex incontinence:** *a loss of urine that occurs without awareness in patients who are paralyzed or have other neurologic problems*

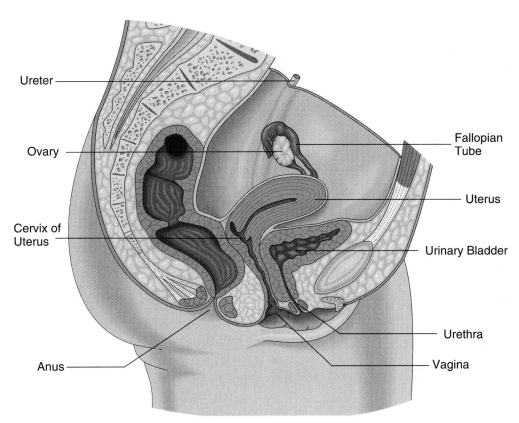

Figure 11-4 Bacteria enter the female urethra and easily make their way to the bladder, causing infection.

Urinary Tract Infections. Urinary tract infections (UTI) are common in women. The urethra in the female is 2½ to 3 inches long (Figure 11-4). Because the urethra is so short, bacteria can easily enter the urethra and travel to the bladder. This is why following the correct procedure for perineal care is so important. The urethra in the male patient is 6 to 8 inches long. Bacteria can travel through the male urethra, but because of the length, the problem is less common than it is in women.

Urine is normally amber or straw-colored, and clear. There is no mucus or sediment. It has a faint odor. A urinary tract infection may cause an unusual color, odor, blood, mucus, or pus in the urine. If you think the urine appears abnormal, save it for the supervisor to observe. Pain in the flank, or the area of the back immediately above the waist, may indicate an infection. Other signs and symptoms include voiding frequently in small amounts, incontinence, burning or pain on urination, feeling an urgent need to void, and getting up frequently at night to urinate. If you observe any of these signs in a patient, notify the supervisor. If a patient who normally has bladder control begins to have episodes of incontinence, this is also an important observation. If the patient has not voided at all on your shift, this could indicate a problem. Notify the supervisor of these findings as well.

■ *flank:* the area of the back immediately above the waist where the kidneys are located

ROLE OF THE PCT IN ASSISTING PATIENTS WITH URINARY ELIMINATION

The patient care technician has a very important responsibility in assisting patients with elimination. Always apply the principles of standard precautions when assisting patients with elimination. Avoid contaminating environmental surfaces with your gloves. Wear a gown, eye protection, and face mask if splashing is likely.

General Guidelines for Assisting Patients with Urinary Elimination

■ Provide adequate fluid intake. Many patients drink less because they believe they will urinate less. The opposite is true. If the patient does not drink enough fluids, the bladder capacity will shrink, and the patient will void more frequently.

■ Answer call signals promptly. Take patients to the bathroom, or provide a **bedpan**, **urinal**, or bedside commode, if necessary.

■ Assist patients to assume an upright position for urination. Emptying the bladder in the supine position is difficult.

■ Provide privacy by closing the door, privacy curtain, and window curtain. Cover the patient with a bath blanket when using the bedpan or commode, even if alone in the room. Leave the patient alone if doing so is safe. Return immediately when the patient signals. If the patient is unable to safely be left alone, remain nearby.

■ Never restrain a patient on the toilet or commode.

■ Allow the patient adequate time to empty the bladder. Leave toilet paper and the call signal nearby.

■ If the patient has difficulty urinating, try running a slow, steady stream of water so the patient can hear it. Placing the patient's hands in warm water, offering the patient a drink of water, or pouring warm water over the genital area may also be helpful.

■ After the patient has voided, give perineal care if needed, or if this is your facility policy.

■ Bedpans and urinals should always be covered when they are removed from the bedside. Some agencies use covers designed for this purpose. Others use disposable underpads. Wear gloves when handling the bedpan or urinal. Avoid contaminating side rails, door knobs, and faucets with your gloves. Wearing a glove on one hand is a good method of preventing environmental contamination. If removing a glove is not possible, use a paper towel under your gloved hand to avoid touching environmental surfaces.

■ Before discarding the specimen, check to see if a urine specimen is needed, or if the patient's urinary output must be measured.

■ Follow your facility policy for discarding urine and disinfecting the bedpan or urinal after each use.

■ Assist the patient to wash hands after emptying the bladder.

■ **bedpan:** *a device used for elimination in bed*
■ **urinal:** *a container used for urinary elimination by the male patient*

Assisting Patients with the Bedpan, Urinal, and Bedside Commode

Patients who are confined to bed must use a bedpan or urinal for elimination. The most common bedpans are regular bedpans and fracture pans (Figure 11-5A). Adjusting to using a bedpan in bed may be difficult for patients. The urinal (Figure 11-5B) is a plastic or metal container, with a handle, that the male patient uses for urination. It is usually marked on the side with measurements in cubic centimeters. Male patients use a bedpan for bowel movements.

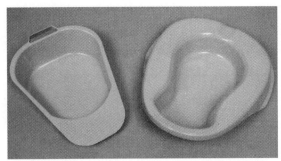

Figure 11-5A The bedpan on the left is a fracture, or orthopedic, bedpan. The bedpan on the right is a regular bedpan.

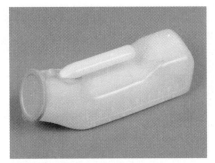

Figure 11-5B The male urinal is covered to avoid contamination.

PROCEDURE

OBRA 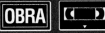 PPE

46 ASSISTING THE PATIENT WITH A BEDPAN

1. Perform your beginning procedure actions.

2. Gather supplies needed: disposable gloves, bedpan, bedpan cover, two bed protectors, toilet tissue, basin of water, soap, washcloth, towel.

3. Cover the top linen with a bath blanket and remove the upper linen without exposing the patient, or fold the upper linen down to expose the buttocks.

4. Ask the patient to flex knees, resting weight on the heels, and lift the buttocks off the bed, if able.

5. Help the patient to raise buttocks by putting one hand under the small of the back and gently lifting while the patient pushes with the feet. With the other hand, insert the bed protector under the buttocks.

6. If the patient is unable to lift the buttocks:

   a. Assist the patient to turn on the side, with his back facing you.

   b. Place the bed protector on the bed.

   c. Place the bedpan flat against the buttocks (Figure 11-6).

   d. Assist the patient to roll back, while holding the bedpan in place.

7. Cover the patient with the top sheet or bath blanket.

8. Roll the head of the bed up for comfort.

9. Remove the disposable gloves.

10. Raise the side rail.

11. Dispose of gloves according to facility policy.

12. Wash your hands.

13. Give the patient the call signal and toilet tissue and leave the room.

14. Return immediately when the patient calls.

15. Put on disposable gloves.

16. Lower the side rail.

17. Remove the bedpan by asking the patient to raise his hips.

18. If the patient is unable to raise his hips, hold the bedpan securely while the patient rolls to the side with back toward you (Figure 11-7). Remove the bedpan. Cover the pan with a bedpan cover or disposable underpad, according to facility policy.

19. Place the bedpan on a bed protector on the chair in the room, or according to facility policy. It is usually not placed on the overbed table or bedside stand.

20. Remove one glove to avoid environmental contamination.

21. Fill the washbasin with water (105 degrees). Help the patient to clean the perineal area. If you will be assisting with the procedure, wear two gloves. Follow the guidelines in Procedure 36 or 37 for perineal care.

22. Remove one glove and raise the side rail with the ungloved hand.

continues

PROCEDURE **46** *continued*

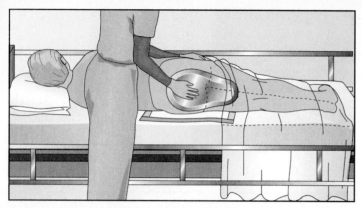

Figure 11-6 Hold the bedpan securely against the buttocks while the patient turns on his back.

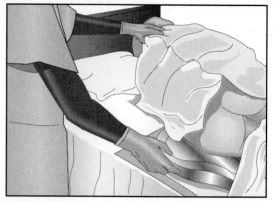

Figure 11-7 Hold the bedpan firmly against the bed when the patient turns to the side, to prevent spilling.

23. Take the covered bedpan to the bathroom. Empty and disinfect it according to facility policy. Use the ungloved hand to turn on faucets and flush the toilet. Store the bedpan in its proper location.

24. Assist the patient with handwashing.

25. Perform your procedure completion actions.

26. Report or record output. Note color, amount, or any abnormalities.

PROCEDURE OBRA [■] PPE

47 ASSISTING THE MALE PATIENT WITH THE URINAL

1. Perform your beginning procedure actions.

2. Gather supplies: disposable gloves, urinal with cover, a basin of water, soap, washcloth, towel.

3. Put on disposable gloves.

4. Lift the top covers and hand the patient the urinal. If the patient is unable to take the urinal, place it between the patient's legs and insert the penis into the opening.

5. Remove the disposable gloves and discard according to facility policy.

6. Raise the side rail.

7. Wash your hands.

8. Give the patient the call signal and leave the room.

9. Return immediately when called.

10. Fill the washbasin with water (105 degrees).

11. Put on one disposable glove.

12. Ask the patient to hand you the urinal. Remove it if he is unable, using the gloved hand.

13. Take the urinal to the bathroom, using the ungloved hand to open the door. Empty and disinfect the urinal according to facility policy. Store the urinal in its proper location.

14. Remove the glove and dispose of it according to facility policy.

15. Wash your hands.

16. Lower the side rail.

17. Help the patient to wash his hands.

18. Raise the side rail.

19. Perform your procedure completion actions.

20. Report or record output. Note color, amount, or any abnormalities.

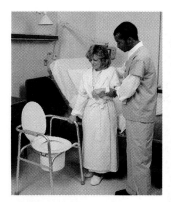

Figure 11-8 There are many different types of bedside commodes.

Assisting the Patient with the Bedside Commode. The bedside commode (Figure 11-8) is a raised seat placed over the regular toilet, or is used at the bedside with a bedpan or other container placed under the seat. It is used for patients who can get out of bed but are unable to walk to the bathroom. It positions the patient in a natural position for elimination and is used to increase patient independence. The bedside commode is more secure for some patients to sit on because it has sturdy arms that help with sitting, rising, and positioning. Some commodes have wheels. If this is the case, they should be locked securely at all times. Most commodes have a cover over the container used for elimination. However, the commode should be emptied each time it is used. The cover is used when transporting the container to the designated area for emptying and disinfecting.

The procedure for transferring a patient to the commode is the same as for transferring from bed to chair. Apply the principles of standard precautions when handling the container the patient uses for elimination.

URINARY CATHETERS

■ **catheter:** *a hollow tube used to drain secretions from the body*

A **catheter** is a hollow tube inserted into the bladder. Most are inserted through the urethra and held in place with a balloon inflated with sterile water (Figure 11-9). Sometimes the patient will complain of feeling the urge to urinate after the catheter is inserted. This is due to the pressure of the balloon on the internal sphincter of the urethra. The pressure feels the same as the sensation of urine pressing on the sphincter. If the patient complains of feeling the urge to void, notify the supervisor.

■ **suprapubic catheter:** *a hollow tube surgically inserted into the bladder through the abdomen*
■ **indwelling catheter:** *a hollow tube inserted into the bladder to remove urine; remains in the body for a period of time*
■ **condom (external) catheter:** *a catheter applied to the outside of the penis in incontinent males*
■ **intermittent:** *alternating or cyclic*

A **suprapubic catheter** is inserted surgically through the abdomen directly into the bladder. Sometimes such a catheter is called a "Foley," which is a common brand name for **indwelling catheters**. A **condom catheter** is an **external catheter** used in males. It is applied over the penis and attached to drainage tubing. An **intermittent** catheter is inserted into the bladder for emptying the bladder or obtaining a urine specimen. After the bladder is emptied, the catheter is removed.

Purpose of Catheters

Catheters are used for many reasons. Some catheters are intermittent, some are temporary, and others are used permanently. Catheter use is avoided whenever possible because it presents a very high risk of infection. Because the catheter provides a direct opening into the bladder, pathogens can make their way up the tubing and cause serious problems.

Catheters are never used for staff convenience. Many patients with neurological problems or trauma are catheterized, because the neurological condition has affected sensation and the patient cannot feel the urge to void. Some patients retain urine until the bladder is stretched beyond capacity. This is very painful. Catheters are used to empty the bladder in this case. Catheters are also used

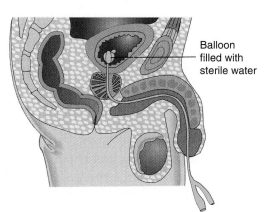

Balloon filled with sterile water

Figure 11-9 The catheter is inserted into the bladder. A balloon filled with sterile water holds it in place.

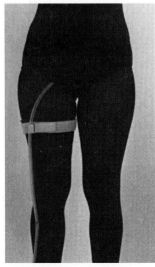

Figure 11-10 The catheter strap holds the catheter securely against the leg to prevent irritation and pulling. (Courtesy Skil-Care Corp.)

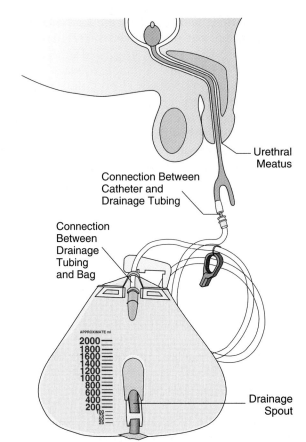

Figure 11-11 The closed drainage system

■ **sepsis:** *systemic poisoning of the body caused by bacteria; a serious infection*

■ **closed drainage system:** *a drainage bag and tubing connected to a catheter that is not opened*
■ **drainage bag:** *a bag connected to a catheter to collect urine*
■ **sterile:** *free from all microbes*
■ **leg drainage bag:** *a bag attached to a catheter to collect urine that is secured to the leg with an elastic or Velcro® strap*

after many surgical procedures. These catheters are used temporarily and are removed when the patient is able to use the toilet again. Patients with severe skin problems may also use catheters temporarily, allowing time for the skin to heal without the irritation of urine on the wound. Occasionally catheters are inserted into mentally confused patients to prevent incontinence. However, because of the high risk of infection, it is far better to toilet these patients routinely than to use a catheter. Sepsis may occur in patients who are elderly and those with weakened immune systems because of bladder infections.

Drainage Systems. Catheters must be ordered by a physician and inserted by licensed personnel and advanced care providers. They must always be secured to the patient's body with tape or a special strap (Figure 11-10). Securing the catheter prevents accidental pulling on the catheter during movement. Pulling can cause damage to the bladder and urethra and is very uncomfortable for the patient. After the catheter is inserted, it is connected to a closed drainage system (Figure 11-11) by a long tube that empties urine into a drainage bag. As long is the system is not opened, it remains sterile (free from pathogens). Each time the system is opened, the risk of infection increases.

Some facilities use leg drainage bags (Figure 11-12) on both indwelling catheters and condom catheters. These are used for ambulatory patients who are up and about during the day. The bag is attached to the leg with elastic straps or Velcro® bands. It holds a smaller amount of urine than a normal drainage bag and must be emptied more often. Use of the leg bag is avoided whenever possible, because it requires frequent manipulation and opening of the closed system and increases the chance of infection. Some facilities have policies and procedures for disinfecting and reusing them; others use a new bag each day. Patients who use a leg bag are connected to a normal catheter drainage bag when they return to bed. Follow your facility policy for use of the leg bag.

Sometimes other types of drainage systems are used to meet a patient's medical needs. These involve open systems and irrigation of sterile fluids into the

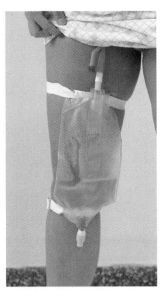

Figure 11-12 The leg bag must be emptied frequently.

bladder. Maintaining this type of system is also the responsibility of the licensed supervisor or advanced care provider.

Caring for a Catheter. The patient care technician is usually responsible for maintaining the closed drainage system. The tubing may be secured to the bed linen with a rubber band and safety pin. Maintaining the sterility of this system is an important responsibility. Apply the principles of standard precautions, and use the correct personal protective equipment when working with catheters.

You may be assigned to care for a patient who has recently had a catheter removed. Sometimes patients have difficulty urinating after the catheter is removed, or the bladder does not empty completely. After the catheter is removed, monitor the patient and record the time and amount of each voiding for the rest of your shift. If the patient has not voided by the end of your shift, notify the supervisor. This monitoring of the patient's urination will continue for at least 24 hours after removal of the catheter.

General Guidelines for Maintaining a Closed Drainage System

- Always wash your hands and apply gloves before handling the catheter and closed drainage system.
- The catheter, bag, and tubing are never disconnected unless sterile technique is used.
- When the patient is in bed, the closed drainage bag is attached to the frame of the bed, never the side rail (Figure 11-13).
- When the patient is in a chair or wheelchair, the closed drainage bag is attached to the frame of the chair between the wheels in the back.
- When the patient is ambulating, the tubing and drainage bag are carried below the level of the bladder.
- Many facilities use cloth catheter bags (Figure 11-14) for privacy. If this is the policy of your facility, the cloth bag is connected to the bed or chair frame, and the urinary drainage bag is placed into it.
- The urinary drainage bag must *never* touch the floor, as this contaminates the system.

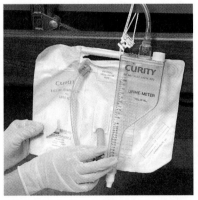

Figure 11-13 The drainage bag is attached to the bed frame above the floor.

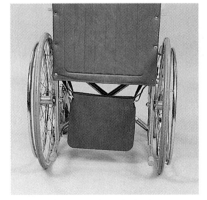

Figure 11-14 The cloth drainage bag provides privacy for the patient. (Courtesy Skil-Care Corp.)

continues

General Guidelines for Maintaining a Closed Drainage System, *continued*

- The urinary drainage bag and tubing must *never* be elevated above the level of the bladder. This causes a backflow of urine into the bladder, greatly increasing the risk of infection.
- Secure the catheter with tape or a strap. Some facilities secure the catheter to the leg in women and the abdomen in men. When securing the catheter to the leg, it is positioned on the top. Avoid placing the catheter under the leg, as it may be pinched and obstruct the flow of urine. Know and follow your facility policy.
- Attach the tubing to the bed with a rubber band and safety pin.
- Make sure the urine is draining freely through the system and there are no kinks or obstructions in the tubing.
- Never disconnect the tubing unless you are trained to do so.
- Use care when lifting, moving, and transferring patients with catheters, to avoid accidentally dislodging the catheter by pulling on the tubing.
- Monitor the level of urine in the drainage bag. Most people excrete about 50 to 80 cc of urine each hour. If the level of urine in the bag does not change, report this information to the supervisor.
- Notify the supervisor if the catheter is leaking, if no urine is present in the bag, or if the urine has an abnormal color, odor, or appearance.
- Notify the supervisor if redness, irritation, drainage, crusting, or open areas are present at the catheter insertion site.
- Notify the supervisor if the patient complains of pain, burning, or tenderness, or has other signs or symptoms of urinary tract infection.
- Most facilities routinely measure intake and output on patients using urinary catheters. Follow your facility policy.

Providing Catheter Care. The patient care technician is responsible for providing catheter care to most patients with catheters. Always apply the principles of standard precautions when caring for the catheter. Use **aseptic technique** when caring for the catheter or the drainage system. The perineum should be as clean as possible, so perform perineal care before caring for the catheter.

■ ***aseptic technique:*** *practices used that are free of all microbes*

Some facilities use specially packaged catheter care kits, but most use soap and water when providing perineal and catheter care. The supplies for performing this procedure will vary depending on which method you use, but the principles of care are the same.

Caring for the External Catheter. The risk of infection is not as great with an external catheter. However, the catheter must be cared for correctly because infection can occur. Other complications, such as irritation and circulatory problems, can also occur. The external catheter is applied over the penis. It is usually attached with an adhesive strip. The strip should always be applied in a spiral. If it completely encircles the penis, severe injury can result. The inside of some external catheters contains a self-adhesive film, making the adhesive

PROCEDURE

48 PROVIDING INDWELLING CATHETER CARE

1. Perform your beginning procedure actions.

2. Gather supplies needed: catheter care kit or basin, soap, two washcloths, towels, clean gown or clothing, bath blanket, bed protector, hamper or plastic laundry bag, and disposable gloves.

3. Place the equipment on the overbed table. Follow your facility policy for covering the overbed table with a barrier.

4. Perform perineal care, following the guidelines in Procedures 36 or 37.

5. Using a clean washcloth, wash the catheter for three inches from the insertion site into the body. Begin washing at the urinary meatus and wash downward. Avoid rubbing back and forth on the tubing.

6. Thoroughly rinse and dry the tubing.

7. Secure the tubing to the leg.

8. Perform your procedure completion actions.

strip on the outside unnecessary. About one inch of the catheter should extend beyond the tip of the penis and attach to the drainage tubing. Always apply the principles of standard precautions when caring for an external catheter.

General Guidelines for Caring for an External Catheter

- Provide perineal care, following the guidelines in Procedure 37, before applying the external catheter.
- Wear gloves and apply the principles of standard precautions when caring for an external catheter and drainage system.
- Dry the penis well before applying the catheter. Report redness, irritation, or signs of infection to the supervisor.
- Roll the tip of the condom catheter over the tip of the penis and up the shaft. Leave one inch of space at the end.
- Wrap the adhesive strip in a spiral.
- Attach the connecting tube of the catheter to the drainage tubing and urinary drainage bag.
- Change the catheter daily. Discard the external catheter and apply a new one each day, and more often if necessary. Never reuse a catheter after it has been removed.
- To change the catheter, remove the adhesive strip and roll the condom down over the tip of the penis. Discard it in the biohazardous waste container, according to facility policy.
- Observe the skin on the penis for redness, irritation, swelling, and open areas. If noted, report your observations to the supervisor before applying a new condom catheter.
- After the catheter has been removed, it is not reapplied until after perineal care has been done.

PROCEDURE

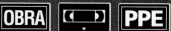

49 EMPTYING THE URINARY DRAINAGE BAG

1. Perform your beginning procedure actions.

2. Gather supplies needed: disposable gloves, mask and eye protection, if necessary, graduate pitcher, paper towel, alcohol sponge.

3. Place the paper towel on the floor and place the graduate pitcher on top of it (Figure 11-15A).

4. Remove the drainage spout from the bag and center it over the graduate. Avoid touching the tip of the drainage spout with your hands or the side of the graduate.

5. Open the clamp on the drainage spout and drain the urine into the graduate (Figure 11-15B).

6. After the urine has drained into the graduate, wipe the spout with the alcohol sponge, if this is your facility policy. Some facilities do not wipe the tip of the spout unless it has contacted your hands or the graduate.

7. Replace the drainage spout into the holder on the side of the catheter bag. Pick up the graduate and dispose of the paper towel.

8. Note the amount, color, and character of urine.

9. Discard urine and disinfect the graduate according to facility policy. Store the graduate in its proper location.

10. Perform your procedure completion actions.

11. Report or record output. Note color, amount, or any abnormalities.

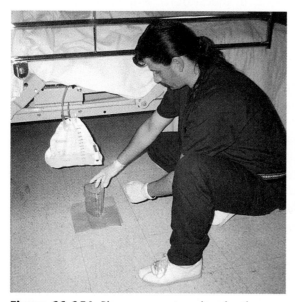

Figure 11-15A Place a paper towel under the graduate.

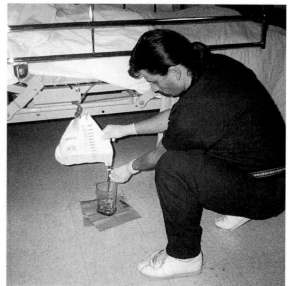

Figure 11-15B Center the drain spout over the graduate. If the drain spout contacts your fingers or the sides of the container, wipe it with an alcohol sponge.

Emptying the Urinary Drainage Bag. The patient care technician is responsible for emptying the urinary drainage bag at the end of the shift, and more often if the bag becomes full. The output is measured and recorded. Apply the principles of standard precautions when performing this procedure. All facilities require you to wear gloves. Some also require the use of a face mask and eye protection, because of the risk of splashing if the drainage bag is full. Know and follow your facility policy.

▬ MEASURING URINARY OUTPUT

You have learned that most people eliminate about 1,500 cc of urine each day, and the reasons for recording intake and output. If the patient is incontinent,

PROCEDURE

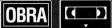

50 MEASURING URINARY OUTPUT

1. Perform your beginning procedure actions.

2. Gather supplies needed: graduate, intake and output worksheet, disposable gloves.

3. After the patient has voided, empty the urine into the graduate (Figure 11-16A). Measure the amount of urine in the container at eye level (Figure 11-16B).

4. Empty the graduate into the toilet, and rinse and disinfect the container.

5. Rinse and disinfect the bedpan, urinal, or commode container.

6. Remove your gloves and discard according to facility policy.

7. Wash your hands.

8. Perform your procedure completion actions.

9. Record the output on the intake and output worksheet, or according to facility policy.

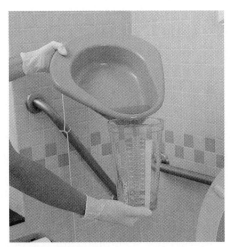

Figure 11-16A Carefully pour the urine into the graduate.

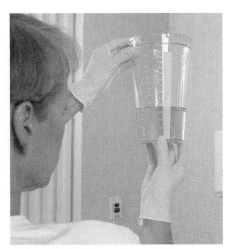

Figure 11-16B Record the amount of urine at eye level.

follow your facility procedure for recording fluid output. Some facilities count the number of episodes of incontinence. Others measure the size of the urine puddle or weigh the pad underpad. The dry weight of the pad is subtracted from the total weight, and an estimation of the amount of urine eliminated is made.

■ **graduate:** *a measuring device with markings on the side*

A **graduate** is a container used for measuring liquids in the health care facility. The graduate is marked on the side in ounces and cubic centimeters. Measuring the urine in a graduate is more accurate than using the markings on a catheter bag or estimating the output.

If you will be measuring urinary output, remind the patient not to drop toilet tissue into the container holding the urine. The toilet tissue is discarded into a plastic bag, or according to facility policy. Apply the principles of standard precautions when measuring urinary output.

■ **laboratory requisition:** *a document with identifying patient information that specifies the type of lab test to be performed on a specimen*

▬▬ COLLECTING A URINE SPECIMEN

The patient care technician is responsible for collecting routine urine specimens for analysis by the laboratory. The physician will use the information gathered by the lab to aid in diagnosis and treatment of the patient. A **laboratory requisition** is completed and sent to the lab with each specimen.

Urine is collected in a clean bedpan, urinal, or specimen collection container in the toilet. This container may be called a specimen collection "hat" or "nuns' hat." The specimen is poured into a closed urine specimen container with a lid. A routine urine specimen is collected using clean technique. The specimen does not have to be sterile, but must be free from outside contamination.

A **clean-catch**, or **midstream**, urine **specimen** is as sterile as possible. The cup in which the specimen is collected is sterile. Urine in the bladder is normally sterile. Precautions are taken when obtaining the specimen to avoid as much contamination as possible. The perineum is washed before obtaining the specimen to eliminate microbes on the skin. The patient starts to void into the toilet

■ *clean-catch (midstream) specimen: a urine sample collected from the middle of the urinary stream*

General Guidelines for Collecting a Urine Specimen

■ Apply the principles of standard precautions.

■ The lid to the specimen container is always placed top side down on the table, so the clean inner side faces up.

■ Avoid touching the inside of the container or lid with your hands.

■ The specimen container is always labeled with the patient's name and other identifying information. Follow your facility policy for labeling the container.

■ Ask the patient not to discard toilet tissue into the specimen. The toilet tissue is discarded into a plastic bag, or according to facility policy.

■ Pour the specimen into the specimen collection container. If you will be placing the container on a counter or other flat surface, place a paper towel under it.

■ After you have obtained the specimen, put the lid on the container and place it in a sealed **transport bag** labeled with a biohazardous waste label (Figure 11-17A).

■ If the urine specimen cannot be transported to the lab immediately, it can be stored in a designated refrigerator or cooler for lab specimens (Figure 11-17B).

■ *transport bag: a sealed plastic bag labeled with a biohazard emblem, used to contain laboratory specimens during transport*

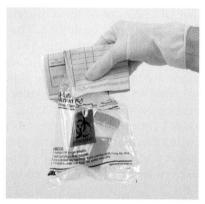

Figure 11-17A The specimen container is placed in a sealed, plastic transport bag with a biohazard label. The laboratory requisition is taken to the lab with the specimen.

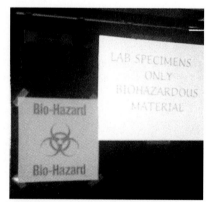

Figure 11-17B Lab specimens are stored in a specially marked refrigerator away from food and beverages.

PROCEDURE

51 COLLECTING A ROUTINE URINE SPECIMEN

1. Perform your beginning procedure actions.
2. Gather supplies needed: specimen collection container, label, transport bag, bedpan, urinal, commode, or specimen hat, disposable gloves.
3. Complete the label and put it on the container.
4. Ask the patient to urinate into the designated collection device. Instruct the patient not to place toilet tissue into the specimen. Provide a plastic bag for this purpose.
5. Provide privacy and make sure the call signal and toilet tissue are within reach.
6. Return immediately when the patient signals.
7. Open the specimen collection container and place the lid on the counter, with the top side down.
8. Apply gloves.
9. Take the container of urine to the toilet and raise the seat.
10. Measure the urine if the patient is on intake and output.
11. Hold the specimen collection container over the toilet. Pour the urine into the collection container. The container should be about three-quarters full. Discard the rest of the urine into the toilet.
12. Put the lid on the specimen container. Place the container on a paper towel on the counter.
13. Rinse and disinfect the bedpan or other container according to facility policy.
14. Remove one glove and place the specimen into the transport bag. Handle the transport bag with your ungloved hand.
15. Remove the other glove and discard according to facility policy. (Gloves can be discarded in the plastic bag with toilet tissue.)
16. Wash your hands.
17. Record output, if the patient is on intake and output.
18. Perform your procedure completion actions.
19. Take the specimen to the designated location.
20. Discard the plastic bag containing the waste in the biohazardous waste container.
21. Report that the specimen was collected and any abnormalities to the supervisor.

or other container and then stops the flow of urine partway through. The sterile specimen collection container is placed under the urethra and the patient voids into the container until an adequate amount of urine is obtained. The patient stops voiding again and then finishes the elimination in the toilet.

PROCEDURE

52 COLLECTING THE CLEAN-CATCH URINE SPECIMEN

1. Perform your beginning procedure actions.
2. Gather supplies needed: clean-catch specimen kit or other equipment used by your facility, sterile specimen cup, bedpan, urinal, or commode, transport bag, plastic bag for waste disposal, and disposable gloves.
3. Open the clean-catch specimen collection kit. Remove the specimen collection container. Apply disposable gloves.
4. Remove the towelettes or swabs from the collection kit.
5. Clean the penis or female perineal area with the swabs or towelettes, using the guidelines in Procedures 36 and 37. Use each swab or towelette once, then discard in a plastic bag. Do not place the used swabs near the clean kit. Discard in plastic bag after use.

continues

PROCEDURE **52** *continued*

6. In a female patient, keep the labia separated until the specimen has been collected. In an uncircumcised male patient, keep the foreskin retracted until the specimen is collected.

7. Explain the procedure to the patient and ask her to begin urinating into the toilet or other container. Ask the patient to stop the stream. Hold the collection cup under the patient without touching the patient's body and collect the specimen. Ask the patient to stop urinating, and remove the container. Instruct the patient to finish urinating in the toilet. Assist the patient to use toilet tissue, if necessary.

8. Put the lid on the specimen container. Place it on a paper towel on the counter.

9. Remove gloves and discard according to facility policy.

10. Wash your hands.

11. Assist the patient to wash hands, and return to bed, if necessary.

12. Wash your hands and apply clean gloves.

13. Rinse and disinfect the bedpan or other container, if used, according to facility policy.

14. Remove one glove and place the specimen into the transport bag. Handle the transport bag with your ungloved hand.

15. Remove the other glove and discard according to facility policy.

16. Wash your hands.

17. Record output, if the patient is on intake and output.

18. Perform your procedure completion actions.

19. Take the specimen to the designated location.

20. Discard the plastic bag containing the waste in the biohazardous waste container.

21. Report that the specimen was collected and any abnormalities to the supervisor.

THE GASTROINTESTINAL SYSTEM

■ **peristalsis:** *muscular contractions of the digestive tract that move food and waste products through the intestines*

Excretion of wastes from the gastrointestinal system (Figure 11-18) is called bowel elimination. A process called **peristalsis** moves the food from the upper end of the gastrointestinal system to the lower end. Peristalsis is caused by the contraction and relaxation of the muscles in the intestines. As the muscles contract, the food is propelled downward in the system. Food and fluids are taken in orally and partially digested by the stomach. They are mixed with digestive juices, then move from the stomach to the small intestine where nutrients are absorbed and more digestion takes place. The food mass passes to the large intestine where extra water is absorbed. After the liquid is absorbed, the food mass is called **feces**. The feces move from the large intestine to the rectum, where they are stored until excreted through the **anus**. Additional water is absorbed from the stool in the rectum. The material excreted may be called feces, **fecal material**, **stool**, or **bowel movement**. The process of eliminating the waste from the anus is called **defecation**.

■ **feces (fecal material, stool, bowel movement):** *solid waste eliminated from the digestive system*
■ **anus:** *the outlet of the colon to the outside of the body*
■ **defecation:** *elimination of solid waste from the lower bowel*

Bowel Elimination

The frequency of bowel movements varies with the individual. Some people have more than one bowel movement a day. Others have a bowel movement every two or three days. Fecal material is usually brown, but the color can be affected by certain foods, medications, and diseases. The bowel movement is normally soft and formed. If it passes through the colon too quickly, the stool is loose and watery. This is called **diarrhea**. If it passes through too slowly, the fecal material becomes hard, dry, or sticky and pasty in consistency. This is called *constipation*. Some foods and medications can cause constipation and diarrhea. **Flatus** is intestinal gas. As foods move through the gastrointestinal tract by peristalsis, gas is formed. When the gas is expelled from the body, it is called "passing flatus" or *flatulence*. If the gas is not passed, it accumulates in the abdomen. The abdomen will enlarge and appear bloated. This is called **abdominal distention** and is an important observation to report to the nurse.

■ **diarrhea:** *passage of loose, watery, liquid stools*
■ **flatus:** *gas expelled from the digestive tract*
■ **abdominal distention:** *enlargement of the abdomen due to excess gas, fecal matter, or urinary retention*

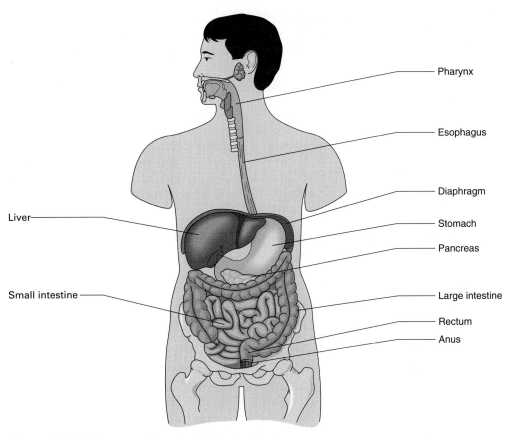

Figure 11-18 The gastrointestinal (digestive) system

Observations to Make When Assisting Patients with Bowel Elimination. You must observe the color, odor, character, and consistency of the patient's bowel movement before discarding it. Notify the supervisor if it has an unusual color, odor, amount, or if there is blood, mucus, or parasites in the stool. If you think a stool is abnormal, save the specimen for the supervisor to assess.

▇▇▇▇ COMMON PROBLEMS RELATED TO THE GASTROINTESTINAL SYSTEM

The most common problems in the gastrointestinal system are related to constipation, diarrhea, and excessive flatulence. Other problems are caused by cancer, diseases, and trauma.

Constipation and Fecal Impaction

■ *fecal impaction: a large, hard, dry mass of stool that the patient is unable to pass*

Report problems with constipation to the supervisor. If the patient has not had a bowel movement in more than three days, or if the patient strains or passes hard, marble-like stools, this is an indication of constipation. Fecal impaction is the most serious form of constipation, caused by retention of stool in the rectum. Water is absorbed in the rectum, causing the fecal mass to become hard and dry. The patient may be unable to pass it. The patient may complain of abdominal or rectal pain, nausea, or lack of appetite. Sometimes fecal impaction will cause mental confusion and fever. Other signs and symptoms of fecal impaction are passing excessive flatus, bloating, frequent urination, inability to empty the bladder, or leaking around the catheter. Patients may complain of feeling the need to have a bowel movement, but being unable to do so. Eventually, liquid stool begins to seep from the rectum. This is easily mistaken for diarrhea. It occurs because liquid feces pass through the colon to the rectum, but are obstructed by the hard fecal mass. The rectum becomes so full that the fluid escapes around the impaction and is eliminated from the body. Fecal impaction is a very serious condition that is usually treated by manual removal of the mass by the licensed supervisor or advanced care provider. Laxatives and enemas are also used to treat fecal impaction. The best thing to do is observe the patient's bowel elimination carefully and prevent fecal impaction from occurring.

Diarrhea

Diarrhea occurs when peristalsis in the stomach is very rapid. This is caused by certain foods, medications, infections, and diseases. The need to defecate may be very urgent if the patient is having diarrhea. The patient may also complain of abdominal pain and cramping. Some patients may become incontinent because of the force with which the fecal material moves through the intestines.

Diarrhea can cause dehydration and other serious medical problems if undetected or untreated. Most health care facilities do not consider one loose stool to be diarrhea. Diarrhea is usually defined as three or more loose stools in a designated period of time. Remember to be objective in reporting your observations. When reporting loose stools to the supervisor, report the color, odor, consistency, character, amount, and frequency of stools. Also report any patient complaints of pain or other discomfort.

Changes in Function of the Gastrointestinal System Associated with Aging and Disease

Change in bowel function may be caused by aging, disease, surgery, diet, and medications. Lack of privacy may also affect the patient's ability to have a bowel movement. In aging, movement of the colon is decreased. Food absorption is slowed and fewer digestive juices are produced. Constipation is a common problem. Other factors that affect bowel function are:

- Bed rest
- Inactivity
- Inadequate exercise
- Inability to chew foods properly
- Loose or missing teeth
- Inadequate fluid intake
- Stress
- Change in environment
- Change in diet

A diet that does not contain enough fiber, fruits, or vegetables may cause constipation and other nutritional problems.

Bowel Incontinence. *Bowel incontinence* is involuntary passage of fecal material from the anus. It has many causes, including trauma, neurological diseases, inability to reach the toilet in time, and mental confusion. Fecal material is very irritating to the skin, so the patient must be cleansed well after each episode of incontinence. Skin exposed to fecal material will break down quickly. Bowel incontinence may lower the patient's self-esteem. Be professional, compassionate, and understanding when assisting patients with bowel elimination and incontinence.

ROLE OF THE PCT IN ASSISTING PATIENTS WITH BOWEL ELIMINATION

Assisting with bowel elimination is a very important responsibility. Always apply the principles of standard precautions when assisting patients with elimination. Avoid contaminating environmental surfaces with your gloves. Wear a gown, eye protection, and face mask if splashing is likely.

General Guidelines for Assisting Patients with Bowel Elimination

- Encourage the patient to consume an adequate amount of fluid. Maintaining fluid intake is as important for bowel elimination as it is for urinary elimination.
- Encourage the patient to eat a well-balanced diet.
- Allow adequate time for the patient to eat meals.
- Encourage the patient to chew food well. Cut food into small pieces if necessary. Report chewing problems to the supervisor for further assessment.
- If you observe that the patient has not eaten fiber foods, fruits, or vegetables, offer a substitute. The dietitian may have to visit the patient to discuss likes and dislikes and assure that the patient will eat the foods served.
- Encourage exercise and activity as allowed and as tolerated.
- Assist the patient with toileting at regular intervals and provide privacy.
- Help the patient into a sitting position, if allowed, for bowel elimination.
- If the patient is using a bedpan or commode, use a bath blanket to cover the patient for privacy and warmth.
- Leave the call signal and toilet tissue within the patient's reach and respond to the call signal immediately.
- Allow adequate time for defecation.
- Provide perineal care as needed, or according to facility policy. Feces are very irritating to the skin and promote skin breakdown and infection.
- Assist patients with cleaning the anal area (this may be called the rectal area by some health care providers).
- Assist patients with handwashing and other personal hygiene after bowel elimination.
- Monitor bowel elimination and report irregularities.
- Record bowel movements on the flow sheet or other designated location. If a patient is independent with bowel elimination, ask if she has had a bowel movement each day.
- Report to the supervisor: frequent stools, absence of stools, pain, cramping, excessive flatulence, abnormal color or consistency of stool, extremely small amounts of stool, hard, dry stool, or bloating and enlargement of the abdomen.
- Specific abnormalities in stools to report are presence of blood, pus, mucus, or parasites or black or other unusual color.

■■■ ENEMAS

■ *enema: introduction of fluid into the lower bowel*

An **enema** is the introduction of fluid into the body to cleanse the anus, rectum, and lower colon. Enemas are ordered by the physician and are used to relieve constipation and empty the colon before some tests and surgeries. Occasionally enemas are given to relieve excessive flatulence. The physician always specifies the type of enema to give and the solution to use. The patient care technician is responsible for administering enemas in many health care facilities. Always

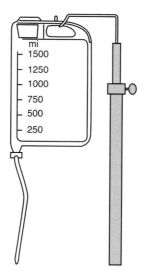

Figure 11-19 A disposable enema bag. Some facilities use a disposable plastic canister.

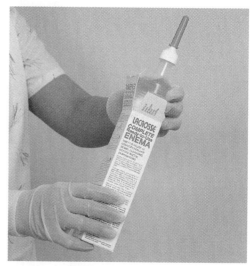

Figure 11-20 The commercially prepared enema is ready to administer. The tip of the container is pre-lubricated.

apply the principles of standard precautions when you are performing this procedure. Avoid contaminating environmental surfaces with your gloves.

A **cleansing enema** is used to soften and remove fecal material, cleanse the lower bowel, and stimulate peristalsis. A water-based solution is used in a cleansing enema. The cleansing enema is administered through a special enema bag or other container (Figure 11-19).

A **retention enema** may be given for constipation or fecal impaction. An oil-based solution is used in the retention enema. It usually comes in a small, commercially packaged container. The purpose of this enema is to soften hard stool and gently stimulate evacuation. It also lubricates the rectum, making it easier to pass the stool.

Commercially prepared enemas (Figure 11-20) are administered in small, premeasured containers. Commercially prepared enemas are available with either cleansing or retention enema solutions.

■ **cleansing enema:** introduction of fluid into the lower bowel to remove solid waste

■ **retention enema:** introduction of fluid into the lower bowel to soften, lubricate, and remove solid waste

■ **commercially prepared enema:** an enema solution pre-packaged in a small dispenser

General Guidelines for Enema Administration

- Administer an enema only upon the direction of a licensed nurse.
- Consult the care plan or licensed supervisor for the amount and type of solution to use and any special instructions.
- Provide privacy. Cover the patient with a bath blanket during the procedure.
- Check the temperature of a water-based solution with a bath thermometer. The solution temperature should be 105 degrees.
- Commercially prepared enemas can be administered at room temperature, or warmed by placing the container in a basin of warm water.
- Lubricate the tip of the enema tubing well with a water-based lubricant before inserting it into the rectum. Most disposable units are pre-lubricated. However, if the tip appears dry, apply additional lubricant before inserting it into the rectum.

continues

General Guidelines for Enema Administration, *continued*

- Insert the enema tube gently into the rectum. The tube should be inserted two to four inches. If you meet resistance, do not force the tube. Remove it and consult the supervisor.
- An enema in a bag should be raised 12 to 16 inches above the rectum. Follow your facility policy.
- Administer the enema solution slowly. Instruct the patient to inhale and breathe in slowly through the nose and exhale through the mouth. If the patient complains of pain, stop the solution briefly before proceeding. If the patient complains of severe, persistent pain, stop the solution and notify the supervisor.
- Hold the enema tubing in place with your gloved hand when administering the solution.
- Instruct the patient to retain the enema solution for the designated time.
- Ensure that the bathroom, bedside commode, or bedpan is readily available.
- The patient should be assisted to a sitting position on the bedpan, commode, or toilet, if possible, to expel the enema.
- Leave the patient alone to expel the enema solution, if doing so is safe. Place the call signal and toilet tissue within reach.
- Respond promptly when the patient signals.
- After the patient expels the enema, save the results for the supervisor to observe before discarding.
- Assist the patient to cleanse the perineal area and wash hands after the enema has been expelled.

■ **Sims' position:** *a side-lying position in which the patient is placed on the left side with the right leg flexed and bent; used for rectal examinations and treatments*

Sims' position (Figure 11-21) is commonly used for giving enemas, rectal examinations, and other rectal treatments. This position promotes evacuation of the bowel. To assist a patient into Sims' position, turn her onto the left side. Position the shoulder, arm, and hip for comfort. Bend the right leg at the knee and flex the leg forward slightly.

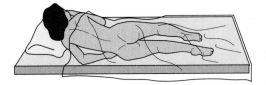

Figure 11-21 Sims' position is used for rectal treatments and examinations.

PROCEDURE

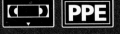

53 ADMINISTERING A CLEANSING ENEMA

1. Perform your beginning procedure actions.
2. Gather supplies needed: assembled enema kit, prescribed solution, water-soluble lubricant, bath blanket, bath thermometer, bed protector, bedpan, toilet tissue, washcloth, towel, washbasin, paper towel, plastic bag, and disposable gloves.
3. Close the clamp on the enema container.

continues

PROCEDURE 53 *continued*

4. Prepare the enema solution in the bathroom or utility room, according to facility policy. Fill the enema container with water in the specified amount. This usually varies from 500 to 1,500 cc, but more or less solution can be used. Check the water temperature with a bath thermometer.

5. If you are instructed to administer a soapsuds enema, empty the contents of the soap packet into the container *after* the water has been added. Squeeze and agitate the bag slightly to mix the solution.

6. Open the clamp on the tubing and allow the solution to flow through the tubing to the tip. This prevents the injection of air into the body. Close the clamp when the solution begins to flow through the tip.

7. Take the solution to the bedside. Squeeze some water-soluble lubricant onto a paper towel or gauze sponge.

8. Place the bed protector under the patient's buttocks. Cover the upper bedding with a bath blanket, then remove the linen from under the blanket without exposing the patient.

9. Assist the patient into Sims' position and ensure that he is comfortable.

10. Apply disposable gloves.

11. Expose the rectal area.

12. Remove the cap from the end of the tubing. Lubricate the tube if it is not pre-lubricated. If the tip appears dry, apply extra lubricant.

13. Separate the buttocks to expose the anal area.

14. Tell the patient you are going to insert the tube and ask him to take a deep breath, then exhale.

15. When the patient is exhaling, gently insert the enema tubing 2 to 4 inches.

16. Hold the solution 12 to 16 inches above the rectum, or according to facility policy.

17. Unclamp the tubing and allow the solution to flow into the rectum. Instruct the patient to retain the solution. Remind the patient to relax.

18. Allow the desired amount of solution to flow into the rectum. When the fluid level reaches the bottom of the bag, clamp the tubing to avoid injecting air into the rectum.

19. Remove the tubing and insert the tip into the enema administration container.

20. Instruct the patient to retain the solution for the designated amount of time.

21. Place the enema container in a plastic bag.

22. Remove your gloves and place them in the plastic bag.

23. Assist the patient to the bathroom or commode, or place the bedpan. Instruct the patient not to flush the toilet after expelling the enema.

24. Make sure the patient is safe, warm, and comfortable. Leave the call signal and toilet tissue within reach.

25. Wash your hands.

26. Leave the room if doing so is safe. Take the plastic bag containing the enema container and gloves and discard in the biohazardous waste container.

27. Return immediately when the patient signals.

28. Apply gloves and assist the patient with cleansing and perineal care.

29. Remove one glove to turn on the faucet, and assist the patient with handwashing.

30. Remove the bed protector with the gloved hand and discard according to facility policy.

31. Remove the other glove and discard according to facility policy.

32. Wash your hands.

33. Assist the patient back to bed, or position in bed for comfort and safety.

34. Observe results of the enema and save for the nurse, or discard according to facility policy.

35. Perform your procedure completion actions.

36. Observe and report to the supervisor:
    a. type of enema and amount of solution
    b. results of the enema, estimated amount of solution returned, amount and consistency of stool
    c. unusual observations (if noted, save the returns for the supervisor to assess)
    d. presence of blood, mucus, or parasites in stool
    e. response of patient to the procedure

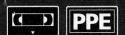

P R O C E D U R E

54 ADMINISTERING A COMMERCIALLY PREPARED ENEMA

1. Perform your beginning procedure actions.

2. Gather supplies needed: commercial enema, water-soluble lubricant, bath blanket, bed protector, bedpan, toilet tissue, washcloth, towel, washbasin, plastic bag, paper towel, and disposable gloves.

3. Warm the container of enema solution in a basin of warm water, if this is your facility policy. Dry the outside of the container.

4. Take the solution to the bedside.

5. Place the bed protector under the patient's buttocks. Cover the upper bedding with a bath blanket, then remove the linen from under the blanket without exposing the patient.

6. Assist the patient into Sims' position and ensure that she is comfortable.

7. Apply disposable gloves.

8. Expose the rectal area.

9. Remove the cap from the end of the container and lubricate the tip, if it is not pre-lubricated.

10. Separate the buttocks to expose the anal area.

11. Tell the patient you are going to insert the tip and ask her to take a deep breath, then exhale.

12. When the patient is exhaling, gently insert the tip of the container.

13. Gently squeeze and roll the container until the desired quantity of solution is administered. A small amount of solution will remain in the container. Avoid releasing pressure on the container, or the solution will return.

14. Instruct the patient to hold her breath, then gently remove the tip of the container.

15. Place the enema container in a plastic bag to avoid contamination.

16. Remove your gloves and place them in the plastic bag.

17. Assist the patient to the bathroom or commode, or place the bedpan. Instruct the patient not to flush the toilet after expelling the enema.

18. Make sure the patient is safe, warm, and comfortable. Leave the call signal and toilet tissue within reach.

19. Wash your hands.

20. Leave the room if doing so is safe. Take the plastic bag containing the enema container and gloves and discard in the biohazardous waste container.

21. Return immediately when the patient signals.

22. Apply gloves and assist the patient with cleansing and perineal care.

23. Remove one glove to turn on the faucet, and assist the patient with handwashing.

24. Remove the bed protector with the gloved hand and discard according to facility policy.

25. Remove the other glove and discard according to facility policy.

26. Wash your hands.

27. Assist the patient back to bed, or position in bed for comfort and safety.

28. Observe results of the enema and save for the nurse, or discard according to facility policy.

29. Perform your procedure completion actions.

30. Observe and report to the supervisor:
    a. type of enema and amount of solution
    b. results of the enema, estimated amount of solution returned, amount and consistency of stool
    c. unusual observations (if noted, save the returns for the supervisor to assess)
    d. presence of blood, mucus, or parasites in stool
    e. response of patient to the procedure

◼◼◼ COLLECTING A STOOL SPECIMEN

Stool specimens are collected and analyzed by the laboratory for the presence of blood, parasites, fat, bacteria, and other abnormalities. Analysis of the stool assists the physician with diagnosis and treatment of the patient. The patient is instructed to defecate in a specimen collection device, commode, or bedpan. The stool is then transferred into the specimen collection container and packaged

PROCEDURE [PPE]

55 COLLECTING A STOOL SPECIMEN

1. Perform your beginning procedure actions.

2. Gather needed supplies: bedpan and cover, commode, or specimen collection pan, specimen container with lid, transport bag, tongue blade, toilet tissue, plastic bag, and disposable gloves.

3. Complete the label and put it on the container.

4. Ask the patient to defecate into the designated collection device. Instruct her not to discard toilet tissue into the collection device. Provide a plastic bag for this purpose.

5. Provide privacy and make sure the call signal and toilet tissue are within reach.

6. Return immediately when the patient signals. Remove the stool specimen collection container and provide a clean container or bedpan for urination, if necessary. Allow the patient to urinate. Provide privacy.

7. Cover the specimen collection container and assist the patient with cleansing, returning to bed, or positioning.

8. Take the collection device to the bathroom or other designated location according to facility policy.

9. Open the specimen collection cup and place the lid on the counter, with the top side down.

10. Apply gloves.

11. Uncover the container. Use the tongue blade to remove the fecal material from the collection device and place it in the specimen container. About two tablespoons of stool are necessary. Taking a small sample from each part of the stool is best. Discard the tongue blade in the plastic bag.

12. Put the lid on the specimen container. Place it on a paper towel on the counter.

13. Rinse and disinfect the bedpan or other collection container according to facility policy.

14. Remove one glove and place the specimen into the transport bag. Handle the transport bag with your ungloved hand.

15. Remove the other glove and discard according to facility policy.

16. Wash your hands.

17. Perform your procedure completion actions.

18. Take the specimen to the designated location.

19. Discard the plastic bag containing the waste in the biohazardous waste container.

20. Report that the specimen was collected and any abnormalities to the supervisor.

according to facility policy prior to transport to the lab. The patient should be instructed not to urinate into the stool specimen. Follow the general guidelines for collecting a urine specimen when collecting a stool specimen. Apply the principles of standard precautions. Some stool specimens must be analyzed while warm, so they must be transported to the laboratory immediately. Check the care plan or with the supervisor for special directions for the type of specimen you are collecting.

▬▬▬ CARING FOR PATIENTS WITH OSTOMIES

■ **ostomy:** *a surgically created opening into the body*

■ **stoma:** *the opening of an ostomy to the outside of the body*

An ostomy is a surgically created opening into the body. There are many types of ostomies (Figure 11-22). Some are performed for bowel elimination. These are usually done because of cancer, bowel disease, and trauma. The opening to the outside of the body is called a stoma. An ostomy may be temporary or permanent. The location of the ostomy is determined by the part of the colon that is injured or diseased.

Colostomies

The colostomy is the most common type of ostomy. This ostomy is located between the colon and the abdomen. The intestines are brought to the outside of

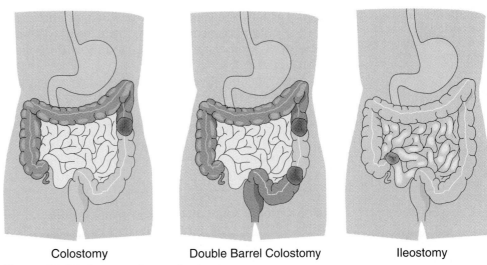

| Colostomy | Double Barrel Colostomy | Ileostomy |

Figure 11-22 Common types of ostomies

the body to create the stoma. A bag is attached to the stoma to collect fecal material. When the ostomy is first performed, the stool is loose and watery, but over time it becomes soft and formed. The amount of liquid in the stool is also determined by how much of the colon remains after surgery. If a large amount of

General Guidelines for Caring for an Ostomy

- Remove and apply the ostomy appliance gently to prevent irritation to the skin. It may help to apply gentle traction to the skin next to the appliance when you are removing the adhesive.
- Empty the reusable bag and wash it thoroughly with soap and water after each bowel movement. Secure the clamp at the bottom of the bag to prevent leaking. Discard and replace a disposable bag.
- Observe the skin around the stoma for redness, irritation, and skin breakdown, and report any problems to the supervisor.
- After the appliance has been removed, gently wipe the area surrounding the stoma with toilet tissue. Discard the tissue in the toilet or a plastic bag. If a plastic bag is used, discard it in the biohazardous waste container.
- Wash the skin around the stoma with mild soap when the appliance is removed. Rinse well and gently pat dry.
- Apply skin barriers, lubricants, or medicated creams to the area surrounding the stoma as stated on the care plan. Apply only a thin layer. Avoid caking the products on the skin.
- You may be required to cut an opening into the appliance before applying it to the skin. Cut the area about $\frac{1}{8}$ inch larger than the size of the stoma.
- When reapplying a new appliance, seal the entire area surrounding the stoma to prevent leaking.
- Observe the color, character, amount, and frequency of stools, and report abnormalities to the supervisor.

■ **appliance:** *a plastic collection device used to contain the excretions from an ostomy*

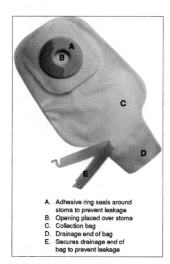

A. Adhesive ring seals around stoma to prevent leakage
B. Opening placed over stoma
C. Collection bag
D. Drainage end of bag
E. Secures drainage end of bag to prevent leakage

Figure 11-23 The colostomy appliance should be sealed tightly against the abdominal skin to prevent leaking.

colon is left, the colon will absorb water and the stools will be formed. If most of the colon has been removed, the body will be unable to absorb the water in the stool, so the stools in the ostomy will be more liquid. Flatus is also passed through the stoma.

Many people live successfully for years with an ostomy, but this type of surgery is very difficult for the patient to adjust to psychologically. Patients are often upset by this change in normal function. They worry about the appliance showing under their clothing. They also worry about offensive odors and sounds. The patient may have to adjust his or her diet to avoid gas-forming foods. Adjusting a dietary pattern established over a lifetime may be difficult. The patient with an ostomy requires you to be very professional, tactful, patient, and understanding.

The Ostomy Appliance. The ostomy **appliance** (Figure 11-23) is the container into which the contents of the bowel are emptied. It is fastened to the body with a belt or a self-adhesive seal around the bag. Remember that fecal material is very irritating to the skin. A new ostomy is sore and tender. The fecal material, particularly liquid stool, causes additional irritation. Even established ostomies become irritated from the combination of fecal material and adhesive on the skin. The care plan will guide you in caring for the ostomy. Report redness or skin irritation to the supervisor. Always apply the principles of standard precautions when caring for an ostomy appliance.

Odors from ostomies are a particular problem. Good personal hygiene is essential. The skin around the stoma is washed and dried well each time the bag is removed. A special skin barrier product may also be used. The used bag is discarded with biohazardous waste. Various deodorizing products may be placed inside the bag to reduce or eliminate odors.

KEY POINTS IN CHAPTER

- *The urinary system regulates water in the body; it also filters waste products from the blood and eliminates them from the body.*

- *The average adult eliminates 1,500 cc of urine from the body each day. Additional fluid is lost through respiration, perspiration, and bowel elimination.*

- *Incontinence is a medical problem.*

- *Urinary tract infections are more common in women than in men because the female urethra is shorter.*

- *Patients with catheters are at high risk of infection because the catheter provides an opening directly into the bladder.*

- *Maintaining sterility of the catheter by using aseptic technique is a very important responsibility.*

- *A graduate is used to accurately measure urinary output.*

- *Feces are a solid waste product eliminated through the digestive system.*

- *Constipation, fecal impaction, and diarrhea are common problems that the patient care technician will assist with.*

- *The patient's self-esteem is affected by problems with elimination, and the care provider must be professional, sensitive, and compassionate in meeting the patient's elimination needs.*

- *An enema is an injection of fluid into the rectum to cleanse the lower bowel.*

- *An ostomy is a surgically created opening into the body. Several different types of ostomies are used to treat disorders of bowel elimination.*

REVIEW QUIZ

Multiple Choice Questions

1. The urinary system:
   a. removes solid waste from the digestive tract.
   b. removes waste from the blood and regulates water in the body.
   c. recirculates waste products through the system.
   d. none of the above.

2. The average adult eliminates:
   a. 500 cc of urine per day.
   b. 1,000 cc of urine per day.
   c. 1,500 cc of urine per day.
   d. 4,500 cc of urine per day.

3. Which of the following affect urinary elimination?
   a. Beverages the patient consumes.
   b. Salt.
   c. Medications.
   d. All of the above.

4. Incontinence:
   a. occurs naturally in aging.
   b. is always a psychological problem.
   c. is a medical problem.
   d. none of the above.

5. Aging and disease may affect:
   a. bladder muscle tone.
   b. the kidneys' ability to filter efficiently.
   c. the prostate gland in the male.
   d. all of the above.

6. A common cause of urge incontinence is:
   a. infection.
   b. multiple childbirths.
   c. physical inability to get to the bathroom.
   d. all of the above.

7. Which of the following are signs or symptoms of urinary tract infection?
   a. Pain or burning on urination.
   b. Voiding frequently in small amounts.
   c. Presence of blood, pus, or mucus in urine.
   d. All of the above.

8. A container that the male patient uses for urination in bed is the:
   a. urinal.
   b. regular bedpan.
   c. fracture bedpan.
   d. indwelling catheter.

9. A catheter is used:
   a. for staff convenience.
   b. to drain urine from the bladder.
   c. to obstruct the bladder so urine cannot escape.
   d. all of the above.

10. The inside of the unopened closed drainage system is:
    a. clean.
    b. contaminated.
    c. septic.
    d. sterile.

11. When a patient is in bed, the catheter drainage bag should be positioned:
    a. above the level of the bladder.
    b. on the bed frame above the floor.
    c. on the side rail above the floor.
    d. on the floor.

12. When caring for a catheter, you should practice:
    a. standard precautions.
    b. good handwashing.
    c. medical asepsis.
    d. all of the above.

13. The catheter should always be:
    a. secured to the patient's body with tape or a strap.
    b. opened and cleaned twice a day.
    c. washed from bottom to top with alcohol.
    d. all of the above.

14. The tape or strap that secures the external catheter to the penis should be wrapped:
    a. in a circle.
    b. diagonally.
    c. in a spiral.
    d. none of the above.

15. Condom catheters should be disposed of in the:
    a. trash can in the patient's room.
    b. biohazardous waste container.
    c. puncture-resistant container.
    d. sanitary sewer.

16. You are assigned to measure urinary output on Mr. Davis, a patient with an indwelling catheter. To obtain an accurate measurement, you should:
    a. record the level of urine according to the markings on the catheter bag.
    b. empty the catheter bag into a bedpan.
    c. withdraw the urine with a syringe.
    d. empty the catheter bag into a graduate.

17. When preparing to collect a clean-catch urine specimen from a female patient, you should wipe the labia:
    a. from top to bottom.
    b. from bottom to top.
    c. back and forth.
    d. from side to side.

18. Water is absorbed from fecal material in the:
    a. stomach.
    b. small intestine.
    c. large intestine.
    d. liver.

19. The medical term for passing gas is:
    a. impaction.
    b. distention.
    c. flatulence.
    d. obstruction.

20. The most serious form of constipation is:
    a. flatulence.
    b. impaction.
    c. distention.
    d. diarrhea.

21. Which of the following affect normal bowel elimination?
    a. Immobility.
    b. Inadequate fluid intake.
    c. Change in diet.
    d. All of the above.

22. The enema tubing is inserted into the rectum:
    a. 1 to 2 inches.
    b. 2 to 4 inches.
    c. 4 to 6 inches.
    d. 6 to 8 inches.

23. The opening of a colostomy to the outside of the body is called the:
    a. rectum.
    b. insertion site.
    c. stoma.
    d. none of the above.

24. Fecal material is:
    a. very irritating to the skin.
    b. normally liquid.
    c. excreted through the urethra.
    d. all of the above.

25. The ostomy appliance is:
    a. an irrigating device.
    b. similar to a catheter.
    c. difficult to apply.
    d. a plastic bag.

BASIC PATIENT CARE SKILLS

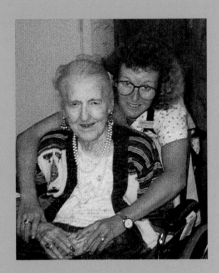
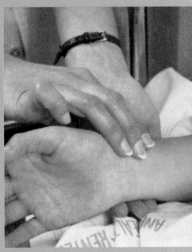
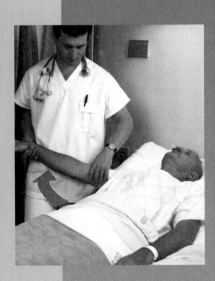

After reading this chapter, you will be able to:

Spell and define key terms.

Define restraints and list six reasons for using restraints.

Describe when and how restraints are used as enablers.

List the guidelines for using restraints.

List the complications of restraint use.

Demonstrate correct application of the vest, belt, and extremity restraints.

Define restraint alternative and describe when to use an alternative device.

RESTRAINTS

■ **restraint:** *a device attached or adjacent to the patient's body that the patient cannot remove easily; prevents access to the body*

Restraints are safety devices that serve many useful purposes. Reasons for using restraints include:

■ Prevention of injury and falls
■ To prevent the patient from injuring others
■ To prevent pulling on tubes, drains, wound coverings, or other forms of treatment
■ To prevent patients from accidentally injuring themselves
■ To help maintain position when the patient is in bed or a chair. Some patients are repositioned by staff only to change position quickly, often causing complications or skin problems. Use of a restraint helps maintain position in some situations.
■ To support the patient in good anatomical alignment to prevent discomfort and deformity.

Restraints are most commonly used to prevent falls and wandering and to protect patients from injury. They are also used for mentally confused and psychiatric patients because of behavior problems. These patients may be unaware of hazards in the environment and unknowingly jeopardize their own safety, as well as the safety of others.

Definition of Restraints

■ **physical restraint:** *physical, manual, or mechanical device attached or adjacent to the patient's body that the patient cannot remove easily; prevents access to the body*

■ **chemical restraint:** *a medication or drug used to alter behavior only for staff convenience and not required to treat a patient's medical symptoms*

Restraints are physical, manual, or mechanical devices attached or adjacent to the patient's body that the patient cannot remove easily. They are used to prevent injury to the patient and others and to allow medical treatment when the patient is confused and uncooperative. Restraints may not be used on alert patients who have refused specific treatments. Refusing treatment is the patient's right, and a restraint is not used to administer treatment that the alert patient does not want.

Restraints restrict freedom of movement and prevent normal access to one's body. **Physical restraints** are devices applied to the patient's body or chairs that prevent the patient from standing. For example, side rails are physical restraints. **Chemical restraints** are drugs used for discipline and staff convenience and not required to treat a patient's medical symptoms. Tranquilizers and mood-altering drugs are chemical restraints. In some patients these drugs have the opposite effect from that intended. Instead of calming the patient, they may worsen agitation. They also may cause the patient to be very lethargic. Side effects from long-term use of these drugs can be very serious. Licensed nurses and advanced care providers are responsible for medication administration. This chapter focuses on the use of physical restraints.

Enablers. Enablers are devices that allow patients to function at their highest possible level. For example, a patient in a wheelchair is unable to sit up straight to feed herself, so she is fed by staff. If a supportive device is applied to correct her posture and allow her to feed herself, the device is an enabler. Devices used as enablers are commonly called postural supports. Used correctly, postural supports can give patients a higher degree of independence and enable them to perform tasks they were previously unable to do. In this case, using the restraint improves the patient's self-esteem.

■ **enabler:** *a device that empowers patients and allows them to function independently*

■ **postural support:** *a device that maintains good body alignment and posture*

Using Restraints

Unfortunately, most restraints are not used as enablers. They are used to manage behavior problems and prevent falls. Several studies have shown that injuries related to falls are more severe in patients who were in restraints, compared with patients who were not restrained. Because patients tend to fight restraints, their behavior may be more exaggerated than it was before use of the restraint.

Before restraints are applied, the staff must assess the patient's capabilities and reasons for the restraint. If the reason for the patient's problem can be determined and corrected, restraint use may not be necessary. For example, if use of restraints is being considered to prevent the patient from falling, all risk factors associated with falls are assessed. If some risk factors can be eliminated, this reduces the risk of falls, and restraint use may not be necessary.

If a patient is a danger to himself or others, or requires emergency medical treatment, restraints may be appropriate. However, less restrictive alternatives to restraints must be considered first. Sometimes the environment can be modified to avoid restraint use. Many alternative devices are available to use instead of restraints. If a restraint is determined to be the best approach, it is applied. However, a continuous assessment of the factors necessitating use of the restraint is done, and the interdisciplinary team works to reduce or eliminate use of the restraint.

If the interdisciplinary team determines that restraints are needed, the least restrictive restraint required to keep the patient safe should be selected. The restraint should be used as infrequently as possible. Use of restraints requires careful assessment, care planning, and monitoring by members of the interdisciplinary team. Studies have proven that it actually takes more time to care for a patient in restraints than for one who is not. The physician must agree to the use of restraints and write an order before they can be used. The care plan will provide information about the type of restraint to use, when the restraint is to be applied, and other special information and instructions.

Factors to Assess and Risk Factors to Eliminate. The patient care technician makes a valuable contribution to the interdisciplinary team's assessment of the need for restraints. Because you have the most direct contact with the patient, you may be in the best position to know what works and does not work in managing the problem causing the need for the restraint. Other important information to consider is:

■ Does the patient see and hear well? Does the patient normally wear glasses? Is she wearing them now? Are they clean? Does the hearing aid work? Are the patient's ears plugged with wax? Sometimes behavior problems, balance problems, and other risk factors arise because the patient is out of touch with the environment.

■ Is the patient able to make her needs known? Sometimes unsafe behavior is caused by an unmet need.

■ Does noise or confusion in the environment cause the patient to become agitated? Eliminating the noise may stop the behavior.

■ Does the behavior occur during a certain time of day, during a certain activity, or with a specific care provider?

■ Does the patient seem uncomfortable? Physical pain, hunger, thirst, or need to use the bathroom can cause unsafe behavior.

■ Does the patient seem lonely or isolated? Bored? Boredom, loneliness, or looking for a misplaced item can cause unsafe behavior.

■ Does the patient try to get out of bed or chair without help? Is the patient steady on her feet? Does she normally use a cane or walker? Is she using it now? Is the call signal available, and does the patient know how to use it? Would the patient benefit from use of an alarm that sounds when she stands up? Would use of this device remind the patient to sit down, alert the staff, and eliminate the need for a restraint?

Complications of Restraints. Caution is needed in making the decision to use restraints, because many complications and side effects are associated with their use. (See Table 12-1.) Patients have been severely injured and died struggling to free themselves from restraints, so restraint use must be taken very seriously. If a patient is seriously injured as the result of restraint use, the Safe Medical Device Reporting Act requires that the injury be reported to the government for investigation. Accrediting and licensing organizations require health care facilities to reduce physical restraint use and track all restraint-related incidents.

Table 12-1 Complications of Restraints

Potential Physical Problems	Potential Psychosocial Problems
Decreased independence	Worsening of behavior problems
Pressure sores	Withdrawal, loss of social contact
Weakness	Depression
Decreased range of motion	Forgetfulness
Muscle wasting	Fear
Contractures (frozen, deformed joints)	Anger
Loss of ability to ambulate	Shame
Edema of ankles, lower legs, feet, fingers	Agitation
Decreased appetite, weight loss	Mental confusion
Dehydration	Combativeness
Acute mental confusion	Restlessness
Distended abdomen	Sense of abandonment
Urge to void frequently	Loss of self-esteem
Incontinence	Screaming, yelling, calling out
Urinary tract infection	
Constipation	
Fecal impaction	
Lethargy	
Shortness of breath	
Pneumonia	
Bruising, redness, cuts	
Falls	
Impaired circulation	
Blood clots	
Choking	
Death	

APPLYING RESTRAINTS

Despite the efforts of staff, restraints must sometimes be used. The law is clear regarding the use of restraints: it specifies that restraints must be applied according to manufacturers' directions. Each manufacturer determines the best way to apply its restraints. This information is sent to the government, which approves the application instructions. There are many restraint manufacturers, so you must become familiar with the directions for applying the types of restraints your facility uses. Consideration is also given to the size of the restraint. Each manufacturer lists weight and size guidelines for its restraints. Many restraints are color-coded so the size is known at a glance. An improperly fitted restraint is dangerous. Select the correct size to fit the patient.

Restraint straps are tied where the patient is unable to reach them. This is usually under the frame of the chair, or under the springs of a hospital bed. Many types of hospital beds are used in health care facilities. When applying a restraint in bed, fasten the straps to the moveable part of the bed frame, so if the bed is repositioned the restraint will move with the patient. Avoid tying restraints to the side rails. When applying restraints to a patient in a chair, the straps are usually inserted between the seat and the armrest. A common mistake is threading the straps through the armrest. This places the restraint straps around the abdomen and fails to keep the hips down. If the patient attempts to stand or slides forward, injury may result. Attention to manufacturer's directions for strap placement in the wheelchair is very important for preventing injuries.

Most restraints are tied in a slip knot. This allows for quick release in case of choking, fire, or other emergency.

After restraints have been applied, you must visually check the patient every 15 to 30 minutes, or according to your facility policy. The restraint must be completely released every 2 hours for 10 minutes. During this time, the patient should be repositioned, ambulated, taken to the bathroom, and exercised. The restraint may be reapplied after the 10-minute release.

General Guidelines for Using Restraints

- Each facility has policies and procedures for the use and application of restraints. Know and follow your facility policies.
- Restraints are never used for staff convenience. They are used for the safety of the patient and others.
- Restraints are applied only with a physician's order.
- The patient and family should clearly understand the purpose of the restraint. Emphasize safety; restraints are not used for punishment.
- The need for restraints is assessed by members of the interdisciplinary team, and alternatives are considered.
- The least restrictive type of restraint is used to keep the patient safe.
- The restraint is applied for as short a time as possible.
- Restraints are applied only according to manufacturers' directions.
- The proper size restraint must be used for the patient's weight and body size.
- Check the care plan for instructions on using restraints. The plan will specify the type of restraint to use, the reason for the restraint, when it should be applied, when it should be released, and any special information. *continues*

General Guidelines for Using Restraints, *continued*

- Check the restraint before using it. If it is worn, torn, cut, or frayed, discard it and obtain another restraint in good repair.
- Restraints used on the torso are always applied over clothing. They should not be applied directly against the skin. Extremity restraints are applied either over or under clothing on the arms and legs, but are padded to prevent restriction of circulation.
- The restraint straps should be smooth. Avoid twisting.
- When applying a restraint to a female patient, make sure the breasts are not under the strap.
- After a restraint is applied, check the fit to be sure it is not too loose or too tight.
- The skin under the restraint is closely monitored for signs of redness, irritation, or breakdown from the restraint.
- Check the skin above and below the restraint for signs of impaired circulation, such as abnormal color or swelling.
- If the patient is restrained in a chair, his feet must be supported to prevent pain and circulatory problems.
- Restraints are tied in slip knots or bows so the health care provider can release them quickly in an emergency.
- The patient should be positioned using good body mechanics and good posture while in a restraint. Props and supports may also be necessary to keep the patient in good alignment.
- Lock the brakes to a wheelchair before applying a restraint.
- When the patient is restrained in a chair, the hips should be kept back. The purpose of the restraint is to keep the hips down. Restraint straps applied to the waist area instead of the hips may be incorrectly applied. Check the manufacturer's recommendations. The restraint should be at a 45-degree angle to keep the hips back.
- Most restraints are tied under the chair, to the frame. Avoid tying them around the back of the chair, unless the manufacturer's directions clearly say to do so.
- When the patient is restrained in a wheelchair, the brakes should be locked when the chair is parked. The large part of the small front wheels of the chair should face forward. This changes the center of gravity of the chair and makes the chair more stable, preventing tipping.
- Facility policies vary, but overall the patient should be visually checked every 15 to 30 minutes while restrained.
- The patient should have the call signal, water, and other needed items within reach while restrained.
- The restraint is released every 2 hours for 10 full minutes. During this time the patient is repositioned, exercised, ambulated, and taken to the bathroom.
- Report any changes in behavior or side effects to the restraint.
- Restraint use must be recorded on the medical record. A flow sheet is commonly used for this purpose.

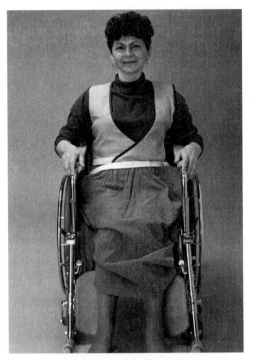

Figure 12-1 The properly applied vest restraint holds patients securely. The vest is always crossed in the front. (Courtesy of Skil-Care Corp.)

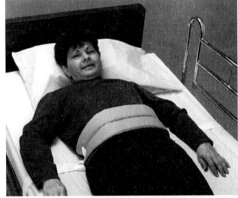

Figure 12-2 The belt restraint may be used in bed or chair. (Courtesy of Skil-Care Corp.)

■ *vest restraint:* a safety device applied to the patient's upper body to limit movement and prevent rising
■ *belt restraint:* a safety device that encircles the patient's waist and/or hips and serves as a reminder to prevent rising
■ *extremity restraint:* a safety device that encircles the arm or leg and prevents movement

Common Restraints

Although many types of restraints are available from different manufacturers, similar restraints are used in most health care facilities. The most common types are the vest restraint (Figure 12-1), belt restraint (Figure 12-2), and extremity restraints. They are all applied in a similar manner, regardless of the manufacturer.

Vest Restraints. The vest restraint is a very secure restraint used for patients at high risk of incident or injury. It is called a vest because it looks like a vest. The

---

PROCEDURE

56 APPLYING A VEST RESTRAINT

1. Perform your beginning procedure actions.

2. Get help from another care provider, if necessary.

3. Slip the patient's arms through the armholes of the vest.

4. Straighten the patient's clothing to be sure it is not wrinkled under the vest.

5. Pull the vest down and smooth it over the clothing.

6. Cross the vest in the front and thread the straps through the slots on the sides.

7. Thread the straps *between* the seat and the armrest or *between* the back of the seat and back of the chair, according to manufacturers' directions. If the patient is in bed, attach the straps to the moveable part of the bed frame.

8. Pull the straps securely and tie them in a slip knot under the chair or the moveable part of the bed frame, according to manufacturers' directions.

9. Insert three fingers under the restraint and check to be sure that it is not too tight.

10. Perform your procedure completion actions.

vest crosses over in the front. Other similar restraints are pulled over the head. These are called by different names, such as *jacket* or *poncho,* but the principles of application are the same for all three devices. Years ago, health care providers were taught to cross the vest restraint over the patient's back. This is no longer acceptable and should never be done. Crossing the vest in the back greatly increases the risk of choking. A properly fitted vest restraint, crossed in front according to manufacturers' directions, will safely and securely hold the patient.

The vest restraint is applied by placing the patient's arms through the sleeves, then crossing the vest over itself in the front. The straps thread through the vest on the side. The vest should be pulled down as low as possible on the patient's torso. The straps are drawn behind the patient and fastened to the bed or chair frame.

Belt Restraints. A belt restraint may also be called a *waist restraint* or a *soft tie.* It is a wide, padded strap that encircles the patient's waist and attaches to the chair at a 45-degree angle to keep the hips down. Belts may serve as a gentle reminder to prevent the patient from rising.

Extremity Restraints. Extremity restraints are used to hold the patient's arms and legs. They are usually used to prevent the patient from pulling at tubes or dressings, or to keep the patient still during a medical procedure. Many different restraints that encircle the arms and legs are available. Most are padded with sheepskin or foam, so additional padding is not necessary. If your agency uses unpadded restraints, wrap a washcloth or other padding around the extremity before applying the restraint, to prevent circulatory problems. Some facilities require handrolls to be placed in the patient's hands when wrist restraints are used. Commercial devices should be used. Use of rolled washcloths as handrolls should be avoided, because they promote squeezing and can cause deformities. The patient's skin must be kept clean and dry under the handroll. Use of handrolls is discussed in Chapter 15.

For patients who hit, scratch, or pull tubes even if restrained, several types of mitten restraints are available. The fingers are inserted into the mitten. The bottom is padded to maintain alignment, prevent pulling at tubes, and prevent injury. Mittens with mesh on top are common because you can see through them to check the patient's circulation.

When caring for patients in wrist restraints, remember that the restraint renders the patient helpless. You must feed the patient and offer fluids frequently. The call signal should be positioned close to the dominant hand. If the patient

PROCEDURE

57 APPLYING A BELT RESTRAINT

1. Perform your beginning procedure actions.

2. Get help from another care provider, if necessary.

3. If the patient is in a wheelchair, move his hips as far back as possible, position the footrests to support his feet, and lock the brakes.

4. Place the belt around the patient's waist. Cross the straps through the loops behind the patient.

5. After the straps are threaded through the loops, tighten the belt securely around the patient's waist.

6. Insert the straps between the seat and armrest, or between the seat and backrest, according to manufacturers' recommendations for the type of restraint you are using.

7. Bring the straps down and tie them to the kickspurs of the wheelchair, using a quick-release knot, according to manufacturers' directions.

8. Insert three fingers under the restraint and check to be sure that it is not too tight.

9. Perform your procedure completion actions.

PROCEDURE

58 APPLYING AN EXTREMITY RESTRAINT

1. Perform your beginning procedure actions.

2. Get help from another care provider, if necessary.

3. Position the patient's extremity in good alignment. The joints should be bent slighty in a state of **flexion**.

4. Pad the skin with a washcloth or other padding, if an unpadded restraint is used.

5. Insert handrolls into the hands, if this is your facility policy.

6. Encircle the extremity with the restraint, and loop it over itself according to manufacturers' directions.

7. Place two fingers under the restraint to check for tightness. Observe the toes or fingers **distal** to the restraint to be sure circulation is adequate.

8. Tie the ends of the restraint to the bed frame or springs, according to facility policy.

9. Check the patient's circulation and pulse in the restrained extremity every 15 minutes

10. Perform your procedure completion actions.

■ **flexion:** bending at a joint
■ **distal:** situated farthest away from the center of the patient's body

cannot push the call signal because of a mitten, an alternative type of signal should be provided, such as a manually operated bell.

Side Rails as Restraints. By definition, side rails are restraints. They can also be enablers that allow the patient to position and turn herself in bed. Side rails must always be up on the bed of patients who are restrained in vests, belts, or extremity restraints.

Acute care hospitals vary on the use of side rails as a restraint. Side rails are used more frequently in hospitals than in other settings because medications, anesthesia, and procedures in the hospital cause a high degree of risk to the patient for injury.

Facilities that hold a long-term care license, including hospital skilled units and some subacute centers, consider side rails to be a restraint. In fact, the OBRA legislation makes it clear that side rails are restraints. Studies have shown that injuries are often very serious if a resident attempts to climb over side rails and falls. Leaving the rails down in this case may be safer, or an alarm that sounds if the patient attempts to get up may be used. Facilities and commercial manufacturers have developed many excellent alternatives to the use of side rails. Many long-term care residents use them as enablers and may feel more secure if the rails are up. Know and follow your facility policy for use of side rails.

■■■ ALTERNATIVES TO RESTRAINTS

Ideally, alternatives to restraints will be used before the patient is placed in a more secure restraining device. However, the reverse may occur: the patient may be placed in a restraint until alternatives can be explored and obtained. Health care workers are not always aware of the wide variety of alternatives available. Some can be made from common items. Others are available from commercial manufacturers and are reasonably priced. If you know of a restraint alternative that you feel would be useful to a patient, inform the supervisor.

Types of Restraint Alternatives

The wheelchair lap tray (Figure 12-3), is a simple restraint alternative. The tray is attached to the back of the wheelchair with Velcro® straps. It can be used for patients to lean on and provide a surface to hold personal items and reading and writing supplies. A tray may enable the patient to feed himself by moving the

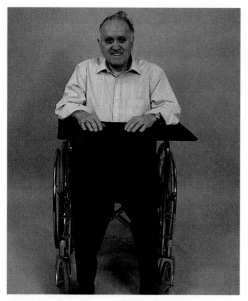

Figure 12-3 The wheelchair lap tray attaches to the wheelchair with Velcro® straps. It serves as a reminder for the patient to remain seated and is convenient for meals and activities. (Courtesy of Skil-Care Corp.)

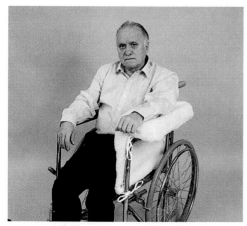

Figure 12-4 Lateral armrests are used for supporting patients who lean to the side. (Courtesy of Skil-Care Corp.)

food closer so he can reach it. The tray also reminds the patient not to leave the chair. If the patient does not have the physical or mental ability to remove the tray, it is considered a restraint. If the tray can be removed by the patient, it is a restraint alternative.

Lateral body supports (Figure 12-4) improve sitting posture. They are commonly used for patients who have paralysis on one side of the body. The foam support prevents leaning to the side and supports the patient's arm to prevent discomfort and swelling.

Lateral stabilizer armrest bolsters (Figure 12-5) are also used to correct leaning. These are commonly used for patients who have no paralysis, but have problems with motor control or balance.

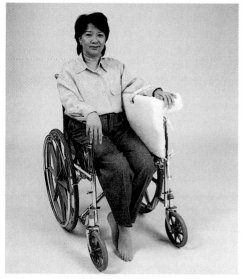

Figure 12-5 Lateral armrest bolsters assist patients with poor motor control to sit upright. (Courtesy of Skil-Care Corp.)

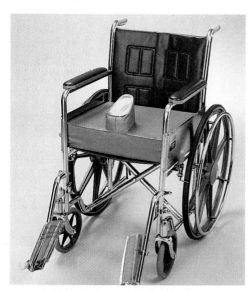

Figure 12-6 The slide guard wedge keeps the hips to the back of the chair and is useful for patients who slide forward. (Courtesy of Skil-Care Corp.)

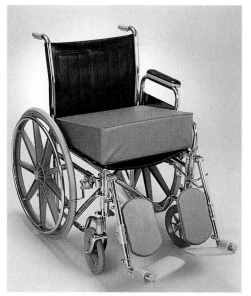

Figure 12-7 The wedge cushion prevents patients from sliding forward. The cushion makes it difficult for patients to stand up unassisted. (Courtesy of Skil-Care Corp.)

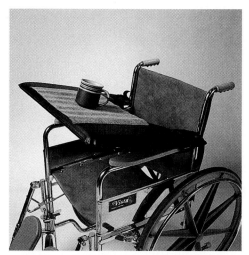

Figure 12-8 Nonslip matting has many uses. (Courtesy of Skil-Care Corp.)

The slide guard wedge (Figure 12-6), also called a *pommel cushion,* shifts the patient's weight to the back of the seat. The shape of the cushion and the pommel in the center prevent the patient from sliding. It is used for patients who slide forward on the seat of the chair.

The vinyl wedge cushion (Figure 12-7) is used for residents who slide forward in the chair. The cushion also makes it more difficult to stand up because the hips are lower than the knees when the wedge is in place.

Nonslip matting (Figure 12-8), sometimes called *gripper* or Dycem®, is a useful restraint alternative for many activities of daily living. It can be used as a placemat for patients who scoop their food away from their body. Using the matting prevents dishes from sliding away. The matting can be used alone on the seat of a wheelchair to prevent rising. It can also be placed under a wedge cushion for extra security. The matting comes on a roll so you can cut off a section of the correct size. It may be rinsed with water if it becomes soiled. Hang the matting to dry. The surface becomes slippery when wet, so do not use it until it is completely dry.

Supporting the feet when the patient is seated in a chair is very important. Dangling the legs is painful and may cause complications such as blood clots. The patient's legs may be too short to reach the floor or footrests of the chair. In this case, a footrest extender pad (Figure 12-9) may be helpful. The pad provides a firm base of support and makes it more difficult to tip the chair.

Bed control bolsters (Figure 12-10) are a good alternative to side rails. The bolsters can be used alone or in pairs. They protect the patient from rolling off the bed and act as a reminder not to get up. The bolsters are half the length of the bed. They can also be used as a support to maintain good body alignment. Patients who are restless also benefit from the use of bolsters because they prevent injury caused by striking the side rails.

Other Restraint Alternatives. Other restraint alternatives include:

■ Magnetic sensor bracelets (Figure 12-11) that set off alarms if the patient enters a dangerous area or tries to leave the premises. These work on the same principle as the magnetic detectors in stores that prevent shoplifting. They are applied to the dominant hand to make them difficult to remove.

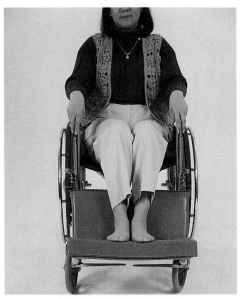

Figure 12-9 The patient's feet must be supported when sitting in a chair. The footrest extender is helpful to patients with short legs. (Courtesy of Skil-Care Corp.)

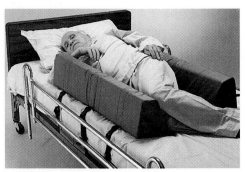

Figure 12-10 Bedrest bolsters remind the patient not to get up and protect the patient from falling out of bed in his sleep. (Courtesy of Skil-Care Corp.)

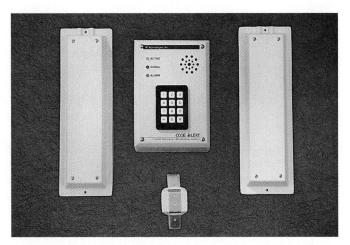

Figure 12-11 The magnetic sensor is attached to a bracelet on the patient's dominant hand. The control panel alerts staff if the patient tries to exit the facility. (© 1996, RF Technologies. Used by permission)

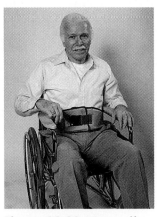

Figure 12-12 Many self-releasing seat belts are available. They remind the patient to call for help before getting up. (Courtesy of Skil-Care Corp.)

- Alarm cushions that sound an alarm when the patient leaves the chair or bed. Some facilities attach the signal cord to the patient's gown or clothing; if the patient rises, it pulls the call signal.
- Self-releasing seat belts (Figure 12-12), similar to lap belts used in a car. Some belts have buckles and some have Velcro® fasteners.
- "Lap buddies" or foam cushions placed on the lap.
- Chairs designed to make it more difficult for the resident to get up. Many chairs are available for patients with special positioning needs. Use caution, however. A common restraint alternative is a commercial reclining chair designed for health care facilities. Although some patients benefit from this device, it causes complications in others. Patients in this type of chair for prolonged periods develop weakness in the neck muscles and lose the ability to hold the head up. They are unable to feed themselves in the reclining position, so they are fed by staff. Eventually they lose the ability to feed themselves. Patients in reclining chairs look at the ceiling all day and may be out of touch with the environment because they cannot see it. If possible, use a headrest to position the head forward and promote eye contact.

REVIEW QUIZ

Multiple Choice Questions

1. Restraints are:
   a. safety devices.
   b. enablers.
   c. devices that restrict freedom of movement.
   d. all of the above.

2. An enabler is:
   a. a type of drug therapy.
   b. something that improves independent functioning.
   c. a mechanical device to manage behavior problems.
   d. a form of punishment.

3. Restraints may be used:
   a. if the care provider feels they are needed.
   b. to punish the patient.
   c. with a physician's order.
   d. for convenience when short of staff.

4. Modifying the environment involves:
   a. eliminating risk factors that contribute to the need for a restraint.
   b. assessing the patient for the proper size restraint.
   c. always restraining unsafe patients when out of bed.
   d. all of the above.

5. Which of the following will guide you in the type of restraint to use and when to apply it?
   a. The patient
   b. The care plan
   c. The family
   d. The progress notes

6. Which of the following are complications of restraints?
   a. Dehydration
   b. Incontinence
   c. Fecal impaction
   d. All of the above

7. Which of the following should be considered when evaluating the patient for use of restraints?
   a. Age
   b. Sex
   c. Ability to see and hear
   d. Paralysis and pain

8. Which of the following are considerations when selecting a restraint to put on a patient?
   a. Restraint size
   b. Condition of the restraint
   c. Correct type of restraint
   d. All of the above

9. Restraints should be released:
   a. every 15 to 30 minutes.
   b. every 2 hours.
   c. every 4 hours.
   d. every shift.

10. When the patient is restrained in a chair, the hips should be:
    a. as far forward as possible.
    b. flexed as much as possible.
    c. as far back as possible.
    d. extended as much as possible.

11. When applying a vest restraint to a patient:
    a. apply the restraint directly against the patient's skin.
    b. cross the vest in the front.
    c. thread the straps through the armrests of the chair.
    d. all of the above.

12. Restraint alternatives are:
    a. devices that hold patients very securely.
    b. devices to use instead of restraints.
    c. always postural supports.
    d. all of the above.

13 Measuring Vital Signs, Height, and Weight

OBJECTIVES:

After reading this chapter, you will be able to:

Spell and define key terms.

Define vital signs and explain why accurate measurements are important.

Accurately measure the patient's temperature, pulse, respirations, and blood pressure.

Identify abnormal vital signs.

Accurately record vital signs.

Accurately measure and record height and weight.

■ **temperature:**
measurement of heat within the body
■ **pulse:** *the expansion and contraction of an artery, which can be felt on the outside surface of the body*
■ **respiration:** *the act of breathing in and out*
■ **blood pressure:** *the force of blood on the walls of the arteries*

VITAL SIGNS

Vital signs are an indication of body function. Measurements of temperature, pulse, respiration (TPR), and blood pressure are called *vital* signs because they are measurements of the most important functions of the body. Temperature is a measurement of heat within your body. The pulse measures how fast your heart is beating. The blood pressure is a measurement of how hard your heart is working. Measuring respirations gives an indication of how fast you are breathing. Vital signs fall within certain normal ranges. Readings above or below these values may be symptoms of illness and disease. Measurement of vital signs gives the health care provider an indication of whether the patient's condition is improving, worsening, or staying the same. The physician depends on these readings to order diagnostic tests and make changes in the treatment regimen. Accurately measuring vital signs is a very important responsibility.

TEMPERATURE

■ **thermometer:**
instrument used to measure temperature

Temperature indicates how much heat is in the body, and is measured with a thermometer. In some conditions, such as infection, the temperature will be elevated. In other conditions, the temperature will be low. These are important findings. The body attempts to regulate temperature on its own. If you feel hot, your body will sweat and you will feel thirsty. If you feel cold, you will shiver to stimulate circulation and increase the temperature. Diseases, medications, and many other factors affect temperature within the body. Some changes in temperature require immediate attention from the licensed supervisor or physician.

Many different types of thermometers are used in health care facilities. Temperature is measured by different methods, depending on the needs of the patient. Your facility will teach you how to use the equipment, which recording scale to use, and how to document your findings.

The care provider must use good judgment in deciding which method to use for taking the temperature. You must evaluate the patient's condition and other safety factors and select a method that is safe for the patient and will give you the most accurate reading. Four common methods are used to measure body temperature:

■ **oral temperature:** the temperature taken by placing the thermometer in the mouth

■ **rectal temperature:** the temperature taken by inserting the thermometer into the anus

■ **axillary temperature:** the temperature taken in the armpit or groin

■ **aural (tympanic) temperature:** the temperature taken at the tympanic membrane inside the ear

■ **Fahrenheit scale:** a scale commonly used for measuring temperature

■ **Celsius (or centigrade) scale:** a scale for measuring temperature in which the boiling point is 100

■ Oral temperature is taken by inserting a thermometer in the mouth under the tongue. This is the most common method.

■ Rectal temperature is taken by inserting the thermometer into the anus. This method is commonly used in children and adults in whom you are unable to take the temperature orally.

■ Axillary temperature is taken by placing the thermometer under the arm or in the groin. This is the least accurate method and is used only when taking the temperature by other methods is not possible.

■ Aural, or tympanic temperature is taken in the ear. This method is controversial. It is an accurate, safe method of taking a temperature, and is quicker than the other methods. However, variations in equipment and technique can affect the accuracy of the reading. Some facilities previously used this method, but have now eliminated it because of these variations.

Temperature Values

Health care facilities use different methods of recording temperature. The Fahrenheit scale is used most often. An "F" written after the temperature value indicates a Fahrenheit reading. A "C" written after the value indicates the Celsius, or centigrade, scale. In the United States, we commonly use the Fahrenheit scale. The formulas used to convert temperature readings between the two scales are found in Table 13-1. Both scales are recorded in degrees. The symbol for degree is "°," so a properly recorded temperature would be written "98.6°F" or "37°C."

The normal temperature ranges for adults and children are listed in Tables 13-2 and 13-3. Memorize these values. If a patient's temperature falls outside the values, report this information to the supervisor immediately.

Table 13-1 Formulas for Converting Fahrenheit and Celsius Temperature Readings

	Celsius (C)	Fahrenheit (F)
Freezing	0°	32°
Body Temperature	37°	98.6°
Pasteurization	63°	145°
Boiling	100°	212°
Sterilizing (Autoclave)	121°	250°

Conversion Formulas

$$\text{F to C} \quad C = \frac{5}{9}(F - 32) \qquad\qquad \text{C to F} \quad F = \frac{9}{5}(C + 32)$$

For example: To convert a Celsius temperature of 100 to Fahrenheit, follow the procedure:

$$100 \times \frac{9}{5} = \frac{900}{5} = 180 + 32 = 212°F$$

For example: To convert a Fahrenheit temperature of 100 to Celsius, follow the procedure:

$$100 \times \frac{5}{9} = (212 - 32) = \frac{5}{9} \times 180 = 100°C$$

Table 13-2 Temperature Variations in the Same Person (Adult)

	Oral	Axillary	Rectal
Average Temperature	98.6°F	97.6°F	99.6°F
Range	97.6-99.6°F (36.5-37.5°C)	96.6-98.6°F (36-37°C)	98.6-100.6°F (37-38.1°C)

Documentation. Facilities have different methods of recording temperature. The information may be recorded on a flow sheet or graphic chart (Figure 13-1). Some facilities list the method by which the temperature was taken in parentheses next to the reading. For example, writing the letter "O" indicates an oral reading. If recording in this manner is your facility policy, you would record the oral temperature value listed previously as "98.6°F(O)." Common abbreviations for vital signs, height, and weight are listed in Table 13-4.

Gloves. Facility policies vary greatly regarding whether gloves are worn when care providers are measuring temperature. The principles of standard precautions should be followed at all times. Gloves are always worn when taking a rectal temperature, with either glass or electronic thermometers. Many agencies require gloves for the oral temperature procedure using a glass thermometer because of the possibility of contacting saliva, which is a body fluid, and the mucous membranes in the mouth. Use of gloves with an oral electronic thermometer is usually not necessary. Standard precautions do not require the use of gloves for contact with perspiration (sweat), so your agency may not require glove use for taking an axillary temperature. However, if you are using this method to take the temperature in the groin, gloves are worn. Wearing gloves when using a tympanic thermometer is not necessary. Know and follow your facility policy. Remember, there may be exceptions to the rule. Your agency may not require gloves for oral temperatures. However, if the patient has open lesions in or around the mouth, or is drooling excessively, use good judgment and apply gloves. The use of standard precautions requires you to be familiar with the principles and apply them as needed in procedures to protect yourself. In health care, there are so many variables that the rules must be flexible. Using the one-glove technique is convenient for taking temperatures. If your ungloved hands accidentally contact a body fluid or mucous membrane during this, or any, procedure, wash them immediately.

Types of Thermometers

Three basic types of thermometers are used in health care facilities. The patient care technician must be able to operate and read all three types. Although vari-

Table 13-3 Average Temperatures in Infants and Children. Temperature Control in Infants and Children is Less Stable.

Age	Temperature	Age	Temperature
3 months	99.4°F	3 years	99.0°F
6 months	99.5°F	5 years	98.6°F
1 year	99.7°F	9 years	98.0°F

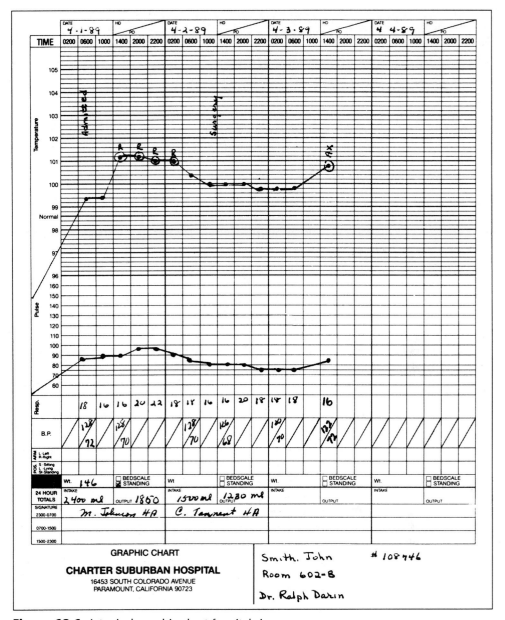

Figure 13-1 A typical graphic chart for vital signs

ations exist between thermometers and manufacturers, they all operate in basically the same way.

Glass Thermometers. Glass thermometers are thin, hollow tubes with a column of mercury inside that provides the temperature reading. Three types of glass thermometers are used: oral, security, and rectal. Figure 13-2 compares glass thermometers. As you can see, the size and shape of the bulbs are different. Oral thermometers may be marked with a blue dot on the end. Rectal thermometers are often marked with a red dot. Security thermometers are commonly used in health care facilities

Facilities using glass thermometers usually cover them with a plastic, disposable sheath (Figure 13-3). Although glass thermometers are normally disinfected after each use, the sheath provides further protection against pathogens. It also protects the patient by containing the glass and mercury if the thermometer is accidentally cracked or broken.

Table 13-4 Common Abbreviations for Vital Signs

Abbreviation	Vital Sign	Abbreviation	Vital Sign
V.S.	vital signs, vitals	F	Fahrenheit
TPR	temperature, pulse, and respiration	C	centigrade (or Celsius)
BP or B/P	blood pressure	°	degrees
(O) or (PO)	oral temperature	T	temperature
(R)	rectal temperature	P	pulse
(Ax) or (A)	axillary temperature	R	respiration
No abbreviation, (AU), (A), or (T), depending on facility policy	aural (tympanic) temperature	Ht.	height
		Wt.	weight
		mm Hg.	millimeters of mercury

Reading the Glass Thermometer. The glass thermometer is read by measuring the level of mercury on the inner column. The mercury rises and falls to indicate the temperature value. The markings on the glass thermometer can be either Fahrenheit (F) or centigrade (C). Most thermometers begin with 94°F (34°C). Each long line on the thermometer is one degree. Every other long line (or degree) is marked with a number. There are four short lines between each long line. Each short line indicates two-tenths of a degree, or 0.2.

To read the thermometer, hold it at eye level. Rotate it gently between your thumb and index finger until you can clearly see the mercury column. Find the sharp edge where the mercury ends. Take the temperature reading at the point where the mercury ends (Figure 13-4). When taking temperatures with a glass thermometer, the value is recorded as an even number.

Electronic Thermometers. Many health care agencies use electronic thermometers (Figure 13-5). These thermometers are battery-operated and stored in a

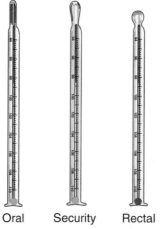

Oral   Security   Rectal

Figure 13-2 Clinical thermometers (left to right): oral, security, rectal

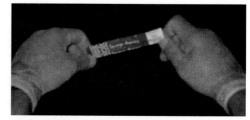

Figure 13-3 This thermometer is covered with a disposable plastic sheath.

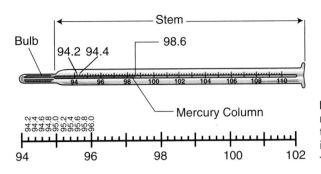

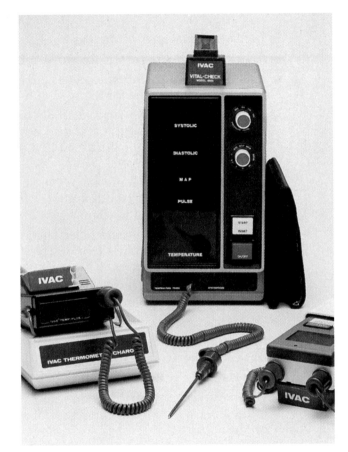

Figure 13-4 This thermometer reads 98.6°F. Most glass thermometers have an arrow to indicate 98.6°F.

Figure 13-5 Different types of electronic thermometers. The unit in the center will measure all vital signs.

■ **probe:** *the attachment on an electronic thermometer that senses temperature*
■ **probe cover:** *the plastic, disposable cover used on the thermometer probe when taking a patient's temperature*
■ **tympanic thermometer:** *instrument used to measure temperature inside the ear*

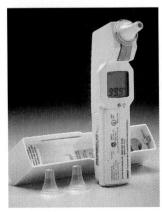

Figure 13-6 An aural (tympanic) thermometer

charger when not in use. They are quick, easy, and accurate. Electronic thermometers usually have a plastic neck strap on the end. This is worn around your neck when taking temperatures or walking in the hallway. The unit is very sensitive and can be damaged if it is dropped or bumped. Wearing it around your neck frees your hands and helps avoid accidents. The electronic thermometer displays the temperature digitally on a screen. The unit will beep or blink when the temperature reading is completed.

The electronic thermometer consists of a main thermometer unit. You will attach an oral or rectal **probe** to record the temperature. The oral probe is color-coded blue and the rectal probe is red. The probe is covered by a disposable **probe cover**, which is used for one patient and then discarded. The unit can be used by many different patients by changing the probe cover.

Tympanic Membrane Thermometers. The **tympanic thermometer** (Figure 13-6), is also a battery-operated unit. It is held in your hand and inserted into the patient's ear. The ear piece of the thermometer is also covered with a protective sheath or cover for infection control purposes. The sheath is discarded after a single use. The temperature reading is displayed digitally on the handset screen.

Tympanic thermometers can be set to provide the equivalent of either an oral or rectal reading. They can also be set for a Fahrenheit or centigrade value.

Other Types of Thermometers. Other types of thermometers are available, but they are not as widely used or as accurate as the others described here. Another type of thermometer is a paper or plastic, chemically treated, disposable unit. Dots on the thermometer are read to obtain the temperature value. This ther-

General Guidelines for Measuring Temperature

- Apply the principles of standard precautions.
- Check glass thermometers for chips and cracks.
- Make sure electronic thermometers are fully charged and you have the correct probe for the type of temperature you are taking.
- If a glass thermometer is accidentally broken, follow your facility policy for cleaning and disposing of it. Mercury is poisonous and must be discarded in a puncture-resistant container. Wear gloves.
- Use the correct thermometer for the scale (Fahrenheit or centigrade) that your facility uses. If the thermometer has both scales, be sure to read it accurately.
- When using a glass thermometer, shake the mercury down below 96°F before inserting the thermometer. Stand away from the patient or surfaces you may hit when shaking the thermometer.
- Use a probe cover or disposable sheath, depending on the type of thermometer you are using.
- Use a clean probe cover for each patient.
- Lubricate the rectal thermometer before insertion.
- Hold the oral electronic thermometer probe in place; the probe is heavy and the patient may not be able to hold it between the lips.
- When using the tympanic thermometer, make sure it is securely inside the ear canal. If it is not placed correctly, the reading will not be accurate.
- Hold the rectal thermometer in place with your gloved hand. Some agencies also require you to hold the axillary thermometer in place.
- Leave the glass thermometer in place for the length of time specified by your facility for the type of temperature you are taking.
- Follow your facility policy for cleaning, disinfecting, and storing glass thermometers.
- A glass thermometer is used for one patient only, then is disinfected. This is true even if a plastic thermometer sheath is used. Thermometers with probe covers may be used for more than one patient if the cover is changed.
- Use cold water to clean a mercury thermometer. Hot water may cause it to break.
- The containers used for clean and soiled glass thermometers must be disinfected regularly. Your facility will have policies and procedures for cleaning them.

Table 13-5 Situations in Which Oral Temperatures Are Not Taken

Patients under the age of six	Cannot keep the mouth closed around the thermometer
Mentally confused	Unable to breathe through the nose
Uncooperative	Receiving oxygen
Combative	On seizure precautions
Chilled or shivering	Has had surgery or an injury to the nose or mouth
Coughing or sneezing	Patients with a nasogastric tube
Unconscious	Some patients with dentures
Restless	
Patients who are receiving heat treatments about the neck or face	

mometer is used following the same guidelines for taking an oral temperature. A disposable sheath is not necessary, because the thermometer is discarded after use. Small, hand-held, battery-operated thermometers are also available. These are usually covered with a plastic sheath. The guidelines for taking the temperature with this thermometer are the same as those for using an electronic thermometer. Follow facility policies for disinfecting the thermometer between uses.

Oral Temperature

Oral temperature is taken by placing the thermometer in the patient's mouth. If the patient has recently had something to eat or drink, this may affect the temperature reading. Temperature is also affected by smoking. Before taking an oral temperature, always ask if the patient has had something to eat or drink, or has smoked a cigarette. If the answer is yes, instruct the patient not to have anything further, and return in 15 minutes to check the temperature.

Oral temperatures are usually taken in alert, cooperative adults and children over the age of six. (The age guideline in some facilities is eight). Table 13-5 lists situations when an oral temperature should not be taken. If you are in doubt, check with the supervisor. The oral thermometer is left in place for a minimum of three minutes.

PROCEDURE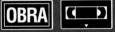

59 MEASURING AN ORAL TEMPERATURE WITH A GLASS THERMOMETER

1. Perform your beginning procedure actions.
2. Gather supplies needed: glass thermometer, disposable plastic sheath, pad and pen, disposable gloves, container for used thermometers.
3. Rinse the disinfectant off thermometer and dry.
4. Shake the thermometer down to 96°F.
5. Cover the thermometer with a plastic sheath.

continues

PROCEDURE **59** *continued*

6. Place the bulb under the patient's tongue and instruct the patient to close lips.

7. Leave the thermometer in place for three minutes, or according to facility policy.

8. Remove the thermometer.

9. Discard the sheath according to facility policy.

10. Hold the thermometer at eye level and read the mercury column (Figure 13-7). Record the reading.

11. Shake the thermometer down to 96°F.

12. Place the thermometer in the container for used thermometers or disinfect according to facility policy.

13. Perform your procedure completion actions.

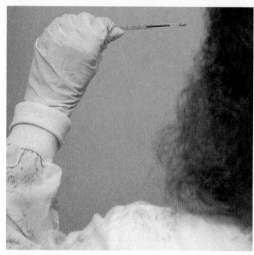

Figure 13-7 Rotate the thermometer slightly until you can see the mercury and read the thermometer at eye level.

PROCEDURE

60 MEASURING AN ORAL TEMPERATURE WITH AN ELECTRONIC THERMOMETER

1. Perform your beginning procedure actions.

2. Gather supplies needed: electronic thermometer, oral probe, plastic probe cover, pad and pen, disposable gloves.

3. Insert the probe into the probe cover.

4. Place the tip of the probe under the patient's tongue and instruct the patient to close the lips.

5. Hold the end of the probe in place.

6. When the alarm sounds, remove the probe.

7. Dispose of the probe cover according to facility policy.

8. Insert the probe into the side of the thermometer.

9. Record the reading.

10. Perform your procedure completion actions.

Rectal Temperature

Rectal temperature is commonly taken in infants, children, and adult patients when the oral method cannot be used. The rectal temperature registers one degree higher than the oral value. If the oral temperature is 98.6°F, the rectal temperature in the same patient would be 99.6°F. Table 13-6 lists times when a rectal temperature should not be taken.

Gloves are always worn when taking a rectal temperature. The thermometer is lubricated before insertion. The glass thermometer must be held in place for three full minutes, or according to facility policy.

Table 13-6 Situations in Which Rectal Temperatures Are Not Taken

Patients having diarrhea	Patients who are combative
Patients with constipation or fecal impaction	Patients with rectal bleeding, hemorrhoids, rectal surgery, and some other rectal conditions
Patients with a colostomy	Some patients with severe heart disease

PROCEDURE

61 MEASURING A RECTAL TEMPERATURE WITH A GLASS THERMOMETER

1. Perform your beginning procedure actions.
2. Gather supplies needed: glass (rectal) thermometer, disposable plastic sheath, lubricant, pad and pen, disposable gloves, container for used thermometers.
3. Rinse the disinfectant off thermometer and dry.
4. Shake the thermometer down to 96°.
5. Cover the thermometer with a plastic sheath.
6. Position the patient in Sims' position.
7. Apply gloves.
8. Place a small amount of lubricant on a tissue or paper towel. Use the tissue to lubricate the bulb of the thermometer. (Some plastic sheaths are pre-lubricated).
9. Separate the buttocks with one hand.
10. Insert the bulb into the rectum one inch.
11. Hold the thermometer in place for three minutes, or according to facility policy.
12. Remove the thermometer.
13. Discard the sheath according to facility policy.
14. Hold the thermometer at eye level and read the mercury column.
15. Place the thermometer in the container for used thermometers or disinfect according to facility policy.
16. Remove gloves and discard according to facility policy.
17. Record the temperature reading.
18. Perform your procedure completion actions.

PROCEDURE

62 MEASURING A RECTAL TEMPERATURE WITH AN ELECTRONIC THERMOMETER

1. Perform your beginning procedure actions.
2. Gather supplies needed: electronic thermometer, rectal probe, plastic probe cover, lubricant, pad and pen, disposable gloves.
3. Position the patient in Sims' position.
4. Apply gloves.
5. Insert the probe into the probe cover. Lubricate the end.
6. Separate the buttocks with one hand.
7. Insert the tip of the probe cover into the rectum one inch, or according to manufacturers' directions. (Some manufacturers recommend inserting it one-quarter to one-half inch).
8. Hold the probe in place until the alarm sounds.
9. Remove the probe.

continues

PROCEDURE **62** *continued*

10. Discard the probe cover according to facility policy.

11. Insert the probe into the side of the thermometer.

12. Wipe excess lubricant from the anal area.

13. Remove gloves and discard according to facility policy.

14. Record the reading.

15. Perform your procedure completion actions.

Axillary Temperature

Axillary temperatures are not taken as commonly as oral and rectal temperatures because they are not as accurate. They are used only when the temperature cannot be obtained by other methods. The axilla must be dry. An oral thermometer is placed in the center of the armpit and held in place for 10 full minutes. The axillary value is normally one degree less than the oral reading. If the oral temperature in a patient is 98.6°F, the axillary temperature in the same patient would be 97.6°F.

PROCEDURE

63 MEASURING AN AXILLARY TEMPERATURE WITH A GLASS THERMOMETER

1. Perform your beginning procedure actions.

2. Gather supplies needed: oral glass thermometer, disposable plastic sheath, towel, pad and pen, disposable gloves, container for used thermometers.

3. Rinse the disinfectant off thermometer and dry.

4. Shake the thermometer down to 96°.

5. Cover the thermometer with a plastic sheath.

6. Apply gloves, if this is your facility policy.

7. Dry the axilla with the towel.

8. Insert the thermometer into the center of the axilla, then lower the patient's arm and bend it across the abdomen. Hold the thermometer in place, if this is your facility policy.

9. Leave the thermometer in place for 10 full minutes.

10. Remove the thermometer.

11. Discard the sheath according to facility policy.

12. Hold the thermometer at eye level and read the mercury column.

13. Remove gloves, if worn, and discard according to facility policy.

14. Record the reading.

15. Place the thermometer in the container for used thermometers or disinfect according to facility policy.

16. Perform your procedure completion actions.

PROCEDURE

64 MEASURING AN AXILLARY TEMPERATURE WITH AN ELECTRONIC THERMOMETER

1. Perform your beginning procedure actions.

2. Gather supplies needed: electronic thermometer, oral probe, plastic probe cover, pad and pen, disposable gloves.

3. Insert the probe into the probe cover.

4. Apply gloves, if this is your facility policy.

5. Dry the axilla with the towel.

continues

PROCEDURE **64** *continued*

6. Insert the probe into the center of the axilla, then lower the patient's arm and bend it across the abdomen. Hold the probe in place, if this is your facility policy.

7. When the alarm sounds, remove the probe.

8. Dispose of the probe cover according to facility policy.

9. Insert the probe into the side of the thermometer.

10. Record the reading.

11. Perform your procedure completion actions.

Tympanic Membrane Temperature

The temperature inside the ear is the most accurate temperature in the body. This method is often preferred by health care workers because it is quick and convenient. It is particularly useful in infants, children, and restless adults. The temperature reading is taken by holding the thermometer next to the tympanic membrane, which is close to the core of the body. It takes one to three seconds to obtain a tympanic temperature. The end of the thermometer is covered with a plastic sheath or cover before it is inserted into the ear.

The tympanic, or aural, thermometer is inserted into the ear by gently lifting the top of the outer ear to straighten the ear canal. The end of the thermometer is inserted as far as it will go. For the temperature to be accurate, the detector at the end of the thermometer must be flat against the tympanic membrane. If it is tipped to the side, the reading may not be accurate. The thermometer is held in place until the display flashes, indicating that the temperature reading is complete. The thermometer is removed and the protective cover discarded.

■ PULSE

The pulse is a measurement of how fast the heart is beating. Each time the heart beats, the arteries in the body expand and contract, forcing blood through the system. The pulse is taken in locations where arteries can be easily compressed against the bones underneath. These areas are called **pulse points** (Figure 13-8). The **radial pulse** is used by most health care workers for counting the pulse. The pulse can also be heard by placing a **stethoscope** directly over the heart. This procedure is usually done by the licensed supervisor or advanced care provider.

Observations of the Pulse

Counting the pulse reveals things about the condition of the heart and circulatory system. When we take a pulse, we are doing more than counting the number of beats per minute. Other information gained from feeling the pulse is important in treating the patient's condition. Some electronic blood pressure devices count the pulse and display the rate. Feeling the pulse is still necessary, however, to make other important observations.

Pulse Rate. We count the number of beats in the pulse to determine how fast the heart is beating. The number of beats per minute is called the **pulse rate**. The normal pulse rate in an adult is between 60 and 100 beats per minute. Pulse rates outside this range may indicate a problem and should be reported to the supervisor immediately. Pulse rates lower than 60 beats per minute are called **bradycardia**. Pulse rates above 100 beats per minute are called **tachycardia**. Normal pulse rates for children are listed in Table 13-7. In infants and small children, the pulse is usually counted by listening with a stethoscope over the heart.

Pulse Rhythm and Force. The **rhythm** of the pulse is an indication of how regularly the heart is beating. The rhythm should always be regular. Pulse beats

■ ***pulse points:*** *locations on the body where the pulse can be felt*

■ ***radial pulse:*** *the pulse felt on the thumb side of the wrist*

■ ***stethoscope:*** *instrument used to listen to sounds inside the body*

■ ***pulse rate:*** *the number of pulse beats per minute*

■ ***bradycardia:*** *slow pulse rate, usually under 60 beats per minute*

■ ***tachycardia:*** *rapid pulse rate, usually over 100 beats per minute*

■ ***rhythm:*** *a recurring action or movement*

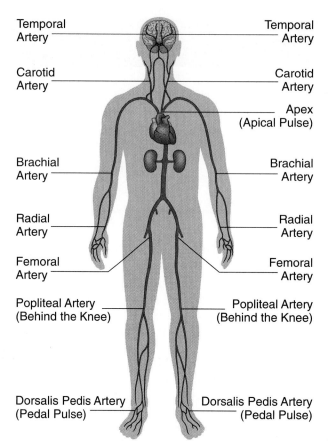

Temporal Artery

Temporal Artery

Carotid Artery

Carotid Artery

Apex (Apical Pulse)

Brachial Artery

Brachial Artery

Radial Artery

Radial Artery

Femoral Artery

Femoral Artery

Popliteal Artery (Behind the Knee)

Popliteal Artery (Behind the Knee)

Dorsalis Pedis Artery (Pedal Pulse)

Dorsalis Pedis Artery (Pedal Pulse)

Figure 13-8 Locations where the pulse can be felt

■ **force:** *energy, strength, or power*

should repeat at approximately the same time interval. There should be no missed or skipped beats, or beats that appear to come early in the cycle. If you observe that the pulse is irregular, count it for one full minute and report your findings to the supervisor immediately for assessment.

The force of the pulse is the strength of the beat. The normal pulse beat is strong and full. A pulse that is weak and hard to feel may indicate a problem. Report this information to the supervisor.

Counting the Pulse

The radial pulse is located on the thumb side of the wrist (Figure 13-9). It is easily accessible and commonly used to take vital signs. To count the radial pulse, put the first three fingers of your hand on top of the pulse. Never count the pulse beat with your thumb, which has a pulse of its own. With the second hand of your watch, count the beat for 30 seconds. If the pulse is strong and regular, you may stop after 30 seconds. Multiply the number of beats counted in 30 seconds by 2 to obtain the pulse rate for one minute. The pulse rate documented on the medical record is always recorded in number of beats per minute. If the pulse is

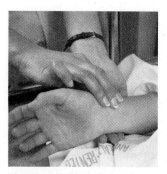

Figure 13-9 Radial pulse site

Table 13-7			
Age	**Normal Pulse Rate Per Minute**	**Age**	**Normal Pulse Rate Per Minute**
Infants	120-140	School-age children	75-100
Toddlers	90-40	Teenagers	60-90
Preschool children	80-110		

PROCEDURE

65 TAKING THE RADIAL PULSE

1. Perform your beginning procedure actions.
2. Gather needed supplies: watch with second hand, note pad, and pen.
3. Locate the radial pulse and gently place the first three fingers of your hand on it. Avoid pressing too hard.
4. Look at your watch and begin counting.

5. Count the number of pulse beats for 30 seconds.
6. Multiply the number of beats in 30 seconds by 2. Record this figure.
7. If you are taking respirations, you will leave your fingers on the pulse.
8. If you are not counting the respirations, perform your procedure completion actions.

weak, irregular, very slow, or very rapid, count the pulse for one full minute and do not multiply the number. Report the abnormality to the supervisor.

RESPIRATIONS

■ **inhalation:** breathing air into the lungs
■ **exhalation (expiration):** breathing air out of the lungs

Respiration is the act of breathing air into and out of the lungs. **Inhalation** is the act of taking air in. **Exhalation** or **expiration** is the act of breathing air out. One respiration is counted as one inhalation and one exhalation. Normal adult respirations are smooth, regular, and unlabored. The normal respiratory rate in adults is about 14 to 20 per minute. If you observe a patient with a respiratory rate under 12 or over 20, report this information to the nurse. Normal respiratory rates for children are found in Table 13-8.

Respiratory Distress

■ **dyspnea:** difficulty breathing; labored respirations
■ **Cheyne-Stokes respirations:** periods of dyspnea alternating with periods of apnea
■ **apnea:** absence of respirations

Difficulty breathing, or **dyspnea**, means labored respirations. **Cheyne-Stokes respirations** are seen in critically ill and dying patients. They are irregular and are followed by periods of apnea, or no respirations, before the patient starts breathing again. If you observe abnormal or difficult respirations, notify the supervisor immediately.

Because respiration involves bringing fresh oxygen into the body, the skin in a Caucasian patient who is breathing normally is pink. If the skin or nail beds appear cyanotic—that is, blue, gray, or dusky in appearance—this indicates a serious problem with the intake and use of oxygen. In dark-skinned patients, problems with oxygenation are noted by looking at the nail beds, lips, and mucous membranes inside the mouth. If you observe an abnormal color in any of these areas, notify the supervisor immediately.

Table 13-8

Age	Normal Respiratory Rate Per Minute	Age	Normal Respiratory Rate Per Minute
Infants	30–60	School-age children	18–30
Toddlers	24–40	Teenagers	12–16
Preschool children	22–34		

PROCEDURE

66 COUNTING RESPIRATIONS

1. Perform your beginning procedure actions.

2. Count the patient's pulse and remember the number.

3. After you have counted the patient's pulse, glance at the chest while continuing to look at your watch.

4. Count one inhalation and one exhalation as one respiration.

5. Count the number of respirations in 30 seconds and multiply this number by 2.

6. Record the patient's pulse and respirations on your note pad.

7. Perform your procedure completion actions.

Counting Respirations

Respiration is under the patient's voluntary control. The patient should not be aware that you are counting the respirations. Placing the patient's arm across the chest or abdomen when counting the pulse is helpful. After you have counted the pulse for 30 seconds, glance at the patient's chest to count respirations. Continue looking at your watch while you count. Remember, one respiration consists of one inhalation and one exhalation. If you are unable to see the patient breathing, count how many times the abdomen rises and falls when the patient breathes.

When counting respirations, you may count for 30 seconds and multiply this number by two. Like the pulse, the respiratory rate recorded on the medical record is for one full minute. If the respirations are slow, labored, irregular, or unusual, count them for one full minute and report this information.

■■■ USING A STETHOSCOPE

A *stethoscope* is a medical instrument used to listen to sounds inside the body. It intensifies sounds so they can be heard clearly. The parts of the stethoscope are shown in Figure 13-10. Many health care workers use stethoscopes on many pa-

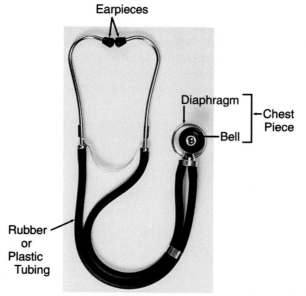

Figure 13-10 This stethoscope has a diaphragm on one side and a bell on the other.

General Guidelines for Using a Stethoscope

- Clean the ear pieces and diaphragm of the stethoscope before using it.
- Clean the stethoscope tubing if it contacts the patient or bed linen.
- Check the ear pieces of the stethoscope for wax, and remove it if present.
- Check the stethoscope tubing. Do not use if it has cracks or holes in it.
- The ear pieces of the stethoscope should face forward.
- The diaphragm of the stethoscope should not come in contact with the patient's clothing, blood pressure cuff, or other device.
- Place the diaphragm of the stethoscope flat against the patient's skin and hold it in place. If the diaphragm is at an angle, you will not be able to hear the sounds.
- Apply firm but gentle pressure when holding the diaphragm in place. If you press too hard, you may be unable to hear sound.

tients. This creates the potential for infection to be passed to both workers and patients. Before and after using the stethoscope, wipe the ear pieces and diaphragm with an alcohol sponge or other disinfectant. If the tubing of the stethoscope contacts the patient or bed linen, wipe the tubing as well.

You will use the stethoscope to take blood pressures. Your health care facility may teach you other procedures with the stethoscope, including taking an **apical pulse.** You may also use the stethoscope to listen to the apical pulse in infants and children. Taking the pulse apically in infants is easier than palpating the pulse at the wrist or other location.

■ *apical pulse: the pulse taken at the apex of the heart*

PROCEDURE

67 USING THE STETHOSCOPE

1. Perform your beginning procedure actions.
2. Gather needed equipment: stethoscope, alcohol sponges, note pad and pen, watch with second hand.
3. Wipe the ear pieces and diaphragm of the stethoscope with the alcohol sponge.
4. If the diaphragm is cold to touch, rub it against your clothing to warm it.
5. Feel the pulse you will be listening to with your fingers.
6. Place the ear pieces of the stethoscope in your ears.
7. Place the diaphragm of the stethoscope over the pulse.
8. Listen to the sound and count, if necessary.
9. Remove the stethoscope from your ears and record your findings.
10. Wipe the ear pieces and diaphragm of the stethoscope with the alcohol sponge.
11. Perform your procedure completion actions.

BLOOD PRESSURE

■ *systolic blood pressure:* the first sound heard when taking the blood pressure; taken during the contraction phase of the heartbeat

■ *diastolic blood pressure:* the last sound heard when taking the blood pressure; taken during the relaxation phase of the heartbeat

■ *hypertension:* high blood pressure, usually 140/90 or above

■ *hypotension:* low blood pressure, usually 100/60 or below

■ *sphygmomanometer:* instrument used to measure blood pressure

■ *aneroid gauge:* a gauge that operates with a spring-loaded dial

Blood pressure is a measurement of how the heart is working. It measures the force of the blood on the inside of the arteries. The systolic blood pressure is a sound you hear during the working phase of the heart cycle. The systolic sound is the first sound heard when the heart contracts and forces blood through the body. The diastolic blood pressure is the sound you hear when the heart is resting. This sound is heard when the heart relaxes and refills with blood. Blood pressure is often called the fourth vital sign. If the supervisor instructs you to obtain the vital signs, you will take the patient's TPR and blood pressure. Sometimes the doctor will order two blood pressure readings, one taken when the patient is sitting and one when standing. Most of the time, the patient should be seated and relaxed when the blood pressure is taken.

In adults, the normal blood pressure range is between 100/60 and 140/90. Blood pressure values outside of this range must be reported to the supervisor. Hypertension is the medical term for high blood pressure, or values over 140/90. Hypotension is the medical term for low blood pressure, or values below 100/60.

Measuring Blood Pressure

Blood pressure is recorded with an instrument called a sphygmomanometer. Several different types of sphygmomanometers are used in health care facilities (Figure 13-11). The technique for measuring blood pressure is the same for most units. Many blood pressure units use an aneroid gauge, a dial marked with numbers to display the reading. The mercury blood pressure cuff also has numbers marked on it. With this unit, the blood pressure is measured by reading the level of a column of mercury. When a mercury unit is used, it must be placed on a flat surface and must be read at eye level for readings to be accurate. Some health care facilities use electronic units.

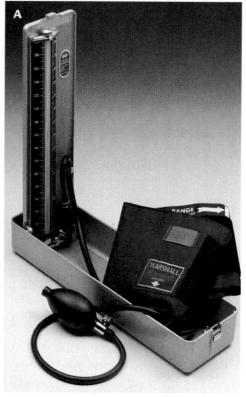
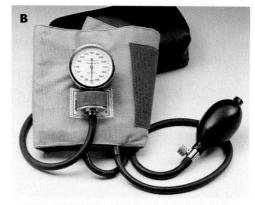
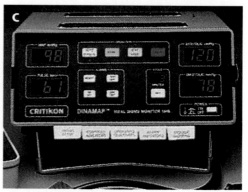

Figure 13-11 Three types of sphygmomanometers: A. mercury gravity sphygmomanometer; B. dial (aneroid) sphygmomanometer; C. electronic sphygmomanometer

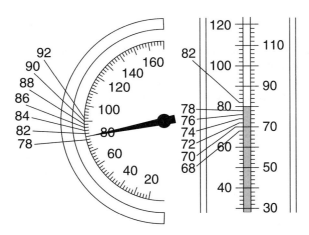

Figure 13-12 Read the blood pressure at the closest line. The blood pressure on both of these gauges is 80.

■ *brachial artery:* the artery in the antecubital space, in front of the elbow
■ *popliteal artery:* the artery behind the knee in which the pulse can be felt

The fabric blood pressure cuff is wrapped around the patient's upper arm about one inch above the brachial artery. An alternate method is to wrap a large-size cuff around the patient's thigh. This is used only for patients whose arms cannot be used for blood pressure, such as those with severe burns. After the cuff is wrapped around the arm, a stethoscope is placed over the brachial artery (popliteal artery in the thigh) to obtain the reading.

Reading the Blood Pressure Gauge. The gauge on the sphygmomanometer is marked with a series of lines. A number is marked on the gauge in increments of 10 or 20, depending on the unit you are using. If the gauge is marked in increments of 20, a long line appears in the center of each 20 units. The long line represents a value of 10. Each short line on the gauge represents a value of 2. Figure 13-12 demonstrates how to read the gauge in both aneroid and mercury blood pressure units. The number on the gauge is 80 for both units. If the dial or mercury was one small line above 80, the reading would be 82. If the dial or mercury was one small line below 80, the value would be 78. Blood pressure is always recorded in even numbers.

When measuring blood pressure, you will use your vision and hearing. Inflate the cuff and then release it slowly, so the gauge falls in increments of 2mm Hg. Place the stethoscope over the brachial artery and listen for a sound while simultaneously looking at the gauge. The first sound you hear is the systolic value. The last sound you hear is the diastolic value. The difference between the two numbers is called the pulse pressure. In healthy adults, the difference is about 40mm Hg. The normal range is between 30 and 50mm Hg. For example, if the systolic pressure is 120 and the diastolic pressure is 80, 120 minus 80 equals 40. The pulse pressure in this case is 40.

■ *pulse pressure:* the difference between the systolic and diastolic blood pressure

Accuracy of Blood Pressure. The physician uses the blood pressure value to measure the patient's progress and determine treatment. Thus, it is important that blood pressure values be accurate. Blood pressure should not be measured in an arm with an IV, on the side of the body from which a breast has been removed, or has a shunt in a dialysis patient. Some facilities require you to take the blood pressure in the left arm, which is closest to the heart. If a patient has a paralyzed or edematous arm, take the blood pressure on the opposite side.

Ask the patient not to talk when taking the blood pressure. Talking makes it difficult for you to hear and may change the reading. The temperature in the room should be comfortable. Changes in temperature may affect the reading.

■ *shunt:* a passage between two blood vessels, commonly under the forearm skin in patients who are receiving hemodialysis
■ *dialysis:* a process of removing waste products from the blood in patients with kidney disease

The technique you use for measuring the blood pressure affects the accuracy of the reading. The cuff must fit the patient correctly. Although there is a standard size adult cuff, some patients require an extra large cuff. Very small patients require a pediatric cuff. A cuff that is too large or small will give an incorrect reading. To check the size of the cuff, compare the length of the rubber bladder (Figure 13-13), inside with the patient's arm circumference. The bladder should be at least 80% of the circumference of the arm. If it is larger or smaller, obtain a different size cuff.

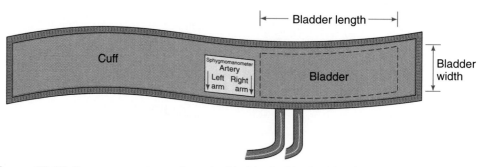

Figure 13-13 For an accurate reading, the bladder inside the blood pressure cuff should be 80% the circumference of the patient's arm. The arrows on the cuff should be placed over the brachial artery.

The cuff must be wrapped snugly around the patient's arm. If it is too loose or tight, the reading will be affected. Many cuffs have arrows marked on the fabric near the tubing (Figure 13-13). The arrows and markings show you where to place the cuff in relation to the brachial artery. When reading the value on the blood pressure gauge, be sure the gauge is flat and not tipped. Always read the gauge at eye level.

■ *antecubital space: the space in front of the elbow*

Documenting Blood Pressure. Blood pressure is recorded in millimeters of mercury. The abbreviation for this is mm Hg. Blood pressure is recorded in fraction

---

PROCEDURE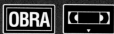

68   MEASURING THE BLOOD PRESSURE

1. Perform your beginning procedure actions.
2. Gather supplies needed: sphygmomanometer, stethoscope, alcohol sponges, note pad, pen.
3. Wipe the ear pieces and diaphragm of the stethoscope with the alcohol sponge.
4. Locate the brachial artery on the thumb side of the inner upper arm.
5. Wrap the cuff around the arm, centering the bladder over the brachial artery. The cuff should be one inch above the artery in the antecubital space.
6. Locate the radial pulse on the thumb side of the wrist. Keep your fingers on it.
7. Close the screw on the handset of the cuff and inflate the bladder (using the bulb) until you can no longer feel the radial pulse. Mentally add 30 to this number.
8. Open the screw and deflate the cuff.
9. Wait 30 seconds.
10. Place the stethoscope in your ears. Place the diaphragm of the stethoscope over the brachial artery.
11. Close the screw and inflate the cuff to 30 points higher than where the radial pulse was last palpated.
12. Slowly release the screw so the pressure in the cuff falls at 2mm Hg increments.
13. Listen for a sound. When you hear it, note the closest number on the gauge. This is the systolic pressure.
14. Continue to listen until the sound stops. Note the closest number on the gauge. This is the diastolic pressure. Continue to listen for 10 to 20mm Hg below this sound.
15. Open the screw completely and rapidly deflate the cuff.
16. Remove the stethoscope from your ears.
17. Remove the cuff from the patient's arm.
18. Record your findings.
19. If you are unsure of the blood pressure and must recheck it, wait one to two minutes before reinflating the cuff.
20. Wipe the ear pieces and diaphragm of the stethoscope with the alcohol sponge.
21. Perform your procedure completion actions.

General Guidelines for Taking Blood Pressure

- Blood pressure cuff:
  - Be sure the cuff is the correct size to fit the patient.
  - Check the screw valve release to be sure it closes and opens easily.
  - Close the valve and pump the cuff. Make sure the gauge rises.
  - Place the center of the bladder in the cuff over the brachial artery, or use the arrows on the cuff to guide you in placement.
- Aneroid sphygmomanometer
  - Check the placement of the needle on the gauge. It should be exactly at zero. The needle is very delicate and will change position if the gauge is bumped or dropped.
  - Place the manometer flat against the cuff where you can see it.
- Mercury sphygmomanometer
  - Check to be sure you can see the mercury in the glass tube.
  - Make sure the glass tube is clear, not cloudy.
  - Check the mercury level. It should be at zero.
  - Place the unit on a flat surface where you can read it at eye level.
  - When you inflate the cuff, the mercury should rise readily. If it responds slowly, there may be a problem with the unit that will result in an inaccurate reading.
- Patient
  - Have the patient sit and relax.
  - Remove clothing or pull up the sleeve of the clothing. Do not roll up the sleeve and constrict the arm. This will alter the reading. The cuff must be wrapped around the bare arm.
  - Ask the patient not to talk while you are taking the blood pressure.
  - Notify the supervisor if the patient is in pain or was uncomfortable when the reading was taken. Pain, anxiety, and discomfort will affect the accuracy of the reading.
  - Ask the patient to turn the radio or television off to avoid distracting sounds
  - Flex the patient's arm slightly and support it at the level of the heart while you are taking the blood pressure. If the arm is not supported, or is above or below heart level, this will affect the accuracy of the reading.
- Environment
  - The temperature should be comfortable.
  - Environmental noise should be eliminated whenever possible.

form. Because the systolic sound is the first sound you hear, it is the first number recorded. The diastolic reading is the second number recorded. An example of how to record the blood pressure is 120/80. 120 is the systolic value, 80 is the diastolic value. Facilities use different forms for recording blood pressure values.

Facility policies vary in the order in which to record vital signs. For example, some facilities require you to record the blood pressure first. In these facilities, the vital signs would be recorded in this order:

- blood pressure
- temperature
- pulse
- respirations

In this example, a sample reading would be recorded as 120/80-98.6°F(O)-88-16. Other facilities require health care workers to record the blood pressure last. Know and follow your facility policy.

■■■ MEASURING AND RECORDING HEIGHT AND WEIGHT

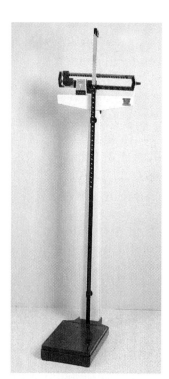

Figure 13-14 The standing balance scale is used for weighing ambulatory patients.

Measuring the patient's height and weight is often the responsibility of the patient care technician. Many members of the interdisciplinary team need the height and weight to perform their assessments and plan care. The dietitian uses the information to plan the diet. The physician uses the information to calculate doses of medications. Most health care facilities get the height and weight upon admission, then periodically thereafter. This gives the team members baseline information to compare with. Patients who have heart and kidney disease are usually weighed frequently to monitor for rapid weight gain, which may indicate a fluid balance problem.

Methods of Weighing Patients

Many different scales are used by health care facilities. Some are mechanical balance scales. Others are electronically operated. Most of the balance scales must be leveled or balanced before they are used. This assures an accurate reading. Check your facility policy and learn how to balance the type of scale you are using.

The Standing Balance Scale. The standing balance scale (Figure 13-14) is commonly used in offices and clinics. Patients must be able to stand and balance unassisted to use this scale. Shoes are usually removed and the patient stands on a paper towel.

To weigh a patient on the balance scale, you must understand how to calculate the weight by adding the readings on the two bars. The lower bar is marked with lines every 50 pounds. The upper bar has single-pound readings. Even numbers are marked on the bar every two pounds. Each long line indicates an odd-numbered pound. Each short line on the upper bar is one quarter of a pound. You will adjust the weights on each balance bar until the rod hangs free on the end. Add the number of pounds on each bar to obtain the total weight.

Chair Scales. The chair scale is manufactured with a chair permanently attached to it. The patient is transferred to the chair to be weighed. Some chair scales use a balancing mechanism similar to the standing balance scale. Others read the weight electronically and print a digital readout on a screen.

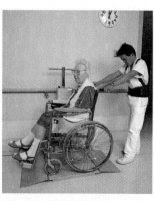

Figure 13-15 Subtract the weight of the empty wheelchair from the total weight.

Wheelchair Scales. The wheelchair scale (Figure 13-15) requires a three-step procedure to obtain an accurate weight. First, the wheelchair is weighed empty. The weight of the chair is recorded. The patient is transferred to the chair and weighed. The weight is recorded. The empty weight of the chair is subtracted from the total weight. This figure gives you the patient's weight. Most wheelchair scales are balance scales. Some facilities have removable ramps that are placed over the standing balance scale so it can be used for wheelchairs. Some wheelchair scales are electronically operated.

Bed Scales. There are several types of bed scales. The electronic bed scale has a sling attached. The patient is placed in the sling, which is then suspended from the bed. To obtain an accurate weight, both the patient and the sling must be lifted completely off the surface of the bed. After the patient is removed from the bed, the scale electronically records the weight.

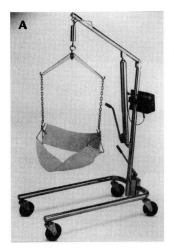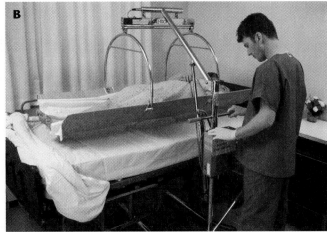

Figure 13-16 The mechanical lift with a scale attachment is used for weighing bedfast patients.

Another type of bed scale is attached to a mechanical lifting device (Figure 13-16A). The patient is transferred to the mechanical lift using the guidelines in Procedure 25. To obtain the weight, the lift is elevated until the patient is above the surface of the bed. This type of scale usually has a dial, balance mechanism, or electronic gauge to record the weight. A similar electronic bed scale (Figure 13-16B) is used for patients who must remain supine.

Methods of Measuring Height

Knowing the patient's height is important to determine if the patient is within the ideal weight range. The height is usually taken on admission. It is not checked again because it does not change. You must learn several methods of measuring the patient's height. Height may be measured in either centimeters or inches, depending on your facility policy.

Standing Height. The standing balance scale has a height bar that can be used for patients who can stand. Height is usually measured when weight is taken. An adjustable height bar is lifted up from the scale and the height is measured.

Measuring Height in Non-Ambulatory Patients. There are several methods of measuring a patient who cannot stand. The simplest is to use a tape measure while the patient is lying supine in bed. Straighten the patient's back, arms, and legs so she is lying as straight as possible. Make a small mark on the sheet with your pen at the top of the patient's head. Make another mark at the level of the patient's heels. Measuring the distance between the two marks with the tape measure will give you the height.

General Guidelines for Weight and Height Measurements

- Weigh patients at the same time of day.
- Use the same scale each time.
- Balance the scale before weighing the patient.
- Have the patient wear similar clothing each time he is weighed.
- Have the patient empty the bladder before being weighed.
- If you are taking a standing weight and height on a balance scale, have the patient remove his shoes and stand on a paper towel.

69 MEASURING WEIGHT AND HEIGHT

1. Perform your beginning procedure actions.
2. Gather supplies needed: scale, paper towels, note pad and pen.
3. Standing scale:
   a. Balance the scale.
   b. Place a paper towel on the scale platform.
   c. Assist the patient to remove shoes and stand on the platform.
   d. Adjust the weights on the scale until the bar hangs freely on the end.
   e. Add the weight on the two bars to determine the weight. Write this down on your note pad or remember it.
   f. Assist the patient to turn around, facing away from the scale.
   g. Raise the height bar until it is level with the top of the patient's head.
   h. Record the height measurement in the center of the height bar (Figure 13-17).
   i. Assist the patient to step down from the scale and to put on shoes.
   j. Remove and discard the paper towel according to facility policy.

4. Chair scale:
   a. Balance the scale.
   b. Assist the patient to transfer from the wheelchair to the chair scale.
   c. Place the feet on the footrest of the chair.
   d. Move the weights until the balance bar hangs freely, or read the electronic display screen. Remember this number or write it down on your note pad.
   e. Transfer the patient back to the wheelchair.

5. Wheelchair scale:
   a. Balance the scale.
   b. Obtain a wheelchair. Take it to the scale and weigh it. Write down the weight.
   c. Take the wheelchair to the patient's room and assist the patient to transfer to the wheelchair.
   d. Take the patient to the scale. Roll the wheelchair up the ramp and lock the brakes.
   e. Adjust the weights until the balance bar hangs freely on the end. Write down this number.
   f. Unlock the brakes and slowly guide the wheelchair down the ramp.
   g. Return to the patient's room and assist the patient to transfer out of the wheelchair.
   h. Subtract the weight of the empty wheelchair from the total weight of the patient and chair and record this number.

6. Bed scale (follow the guidelines in Procedure 25 for assisting the patient into the lift seat or sling):
   a. Balance the scale. The scale should be balanced with the canvas seat, chains, or straps attached.
   b. Remove the sling from the scale and position the patient on the sling.
   c. Connect the straps and elevate the lift above the level of the bed. Lift the patient so the patient's body and the sling hang freely over the bed.
   d. Adjust the weights until the balance bar hangs freely on the end, or read the electronic display screen. Remember this number.
   e. Lower the patient back into the bed and remove the sling.

7. Perform your procedure completion actions.

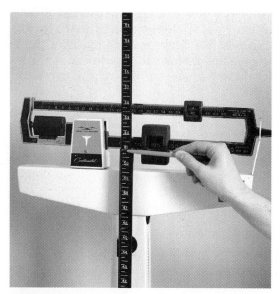

Figure 13-17 Read the height at the movable part of the ruler.

KEY POINTS IN CHAPTER	*Vital signs tell you how well the body's vital organs are working.*

Vital signs tell you how well the body's vital organs are working.

Body temperature can be measured orally, rectally, axillarily, or aurally.

The site used most often for taking the pulse is the radial artery.

Because respirations are under voluntary control, the patient should not know when you are counting them.

The systolic blood pressure is the first sound heard when the heart is contracting.

The diastolic blood pressure is the last sound heard when the heart is resting.

Abnormal vital signs must be reported to the supervisor immediately.

Accuracy is very important when taking and recording vital signs.

The PCT is responsible for obtaining and accurately recording the patient's height and weight.

REVIEW QUIZ

Multiple Choice Questions

1. The supervisor assigns you to take vital signs on Mr. Vasquez. You know this means you will take the:
   a. TPR.
   b. B/P.
   c. TPR and B/P.
   d. B/P and mm Hg.

2. The aural temperature is taken:
   a. in the ear.
   b. rectally.
   c. under the arm.
   d. in the mouth.

3. The normal rectal temperature is:
   a. 97.6°F.
   b. 98.6°F.
   c. 99.6°F.
   d. 100.6°F.

4. The normal oral temperature is:
   a. 97.6°F.
   b. 98.6°F.
   c. 99.6°F.
   d. 100.6°F.

5. The normal axillary temperature is:
   a. 97.6°F.
   b. 98.6°F.
   c. 99.6°F.
   d. 100.6°F.

6. You are assigned to take Mr. Washington's rectal temperature with a glass thermometer. After lubricating the thermometer, you will insert it into the anus:
   a. one-quarter inch.
   b. one-hale inch.
   c. three-quarters inch.
   d. 1 inch.

7. The oral thermometer is marked with a:
   a. blue dot.
   b. red dot.
   c. green dot.
   d. pink dot.

8. The rectal thermometer is marked with a:
   a. blue dot.
   b. red dot.
   c. green dot.
   d. pink dot.

9. When taking an axillary temperature, you should use a:
   a. green probe.
   b. red probe.
   c. rectal thermometer.
   d. oral thermometer.

10. Before taking a temperature with a glass thermometer, shake the thermometer down to:
    a. 96°F.
    b. 97°F.
    c. 98°F.
    d. 99°F.

11. The most commonly used site for taking the pulse in adults is the:
    a. temporal artery.
    b. apex of the heart.
    c. brachial artery.
    d. radial artery.

12. When palpating the pulse, always use your:
    a. thumb.
    b. stethoscope.
    c. first three fingers.
    d. third and fourth fingers.

13. Which of the following pulse rates should you report to the nurse?
    a. 60
    b. 72
    c. 96
    d. 112

14. A pulse rate that is abnormally slow is called:
    a. tachycardia.
    b. hypotension.
    c. bradycardia.
    d. pulse pressure.

15. The normal respiratory rate in adults is:
    a. 14 to 20.
    b. 16 to 24.
    c. 10 to 20.
    d. 20 to 30.

16. You are assigned to take vital signs on Unit A. Which of the following would you report to the nurse?
    a. 98.4°F(O)-80-18
    b. 97.6°F(Ax.)-64-16
    c. 100.2°F(R)-110-24
    d. 99.2°F(O)-96-20

17. Which artery is used for taking blood pressure?
    a. carotid
    b. brachial
    c. radial
    d. femoral

18. Hypertension is blood pressure:
    a. under 140/90.
    b. over 140/90.
    c. under 90/60.
    d. over 90/60.

19. Hypotension is blood pressure:
    a. under 140/90.
    b. over 140/90.
    c. under 100/60.
    d. over 90/60.

20. The instrument used to take a blood pressure is the:
    a. sphygmomanometer.   c. aneroid.
    b. thermometer.   d. mercury probe.

21. When weighing a patient on the balance scale, you know that each marking on the large bar represents:
    a. 1 pound.   c. 25 pounds.
    b. 5 pounds.   d. 50 pounds.

22. Oral temperatures should not be taken on:
    a. patients over the age of 50.
    b. patients with colostomies.
    c. infants and small children.
    d. teenagers.

23. Rectal temperatures should not be taken on:
    a. children under the age of 6.
    b. patients with fecal impaction.
    c. patients using oxygen.
    d. all of the above.

24. The normal pulse rate in preschool children is:
    a. 120–140.   c. 80–110.
    b. 90–140.   d. 60–90.

25. Which of the following is the *least accurate* method of taking the temperature?
    a. Rectal   c. Oral
    b. Aural   d. Axillary

14 Admission, Transfer, and Discharge

OBJECTIVES:

After reading this chapter, you will be able to:

Spell and define key terms.

Explain why first impressions are important and describe how they set the tone for the patient's hospital stay.

Describe the PCT's responsibilities in the admission, transfer, and discharge process.

Demonstrate admitting, transferring, and discharging a patient.

■ **admission:** *procedure for checking a patient into the health care agency and getting him or her settled*
■ **discharge:** *procedure for helping a patient to leave the health care agency*

■ **IV standard:** *a metal pole used to hang an IV bag, bottle, or pump above the infusion site*

ADMITTING, TRANSFERRING, AND DISCHARGING A PATIENT

One responsibility of the patient care technician is to assist patients with admission, transfer, and discharge in the health care facility. You are expected to gather information, meet the patient's basic needs, and make the process as smooth and comfortable as possible. Your pleasant, courteous manner will set the tone for the admission process. During transfer, calm and understanding will ease any fears the patient may have. Upon discharge, the professionalism you have shown throughout the patient's stay will be remembered and appreciated.

Admission

The patient care technician is frequently the person who admits patients to the health care facility. This may be a difficult, frightening time for the patient. A common expression says that "first impressions are usually lasting ones." The patient's perception of what is happening may be affected by illness, pain, and fear. Making a good first impression on the patient and family members is important. A negative first impression of the health care provider affects the patient's impression of all health care providers and even the health care facility. Think about this; remember the patient's fears during the admission process and do your best to provide a positive, professional impression (Figure 14-1).

Each health care facility has policies and procedures for patient admissions. Usually you will be aware of the admission in advance, and can prepare the room by opening the bed (Figure 14-2) and checking to see if the call signal works properly. If the patient will require special equipment, such as an IV standard (Figure 14-3), the equipment should be taken to the room prior to admission. When you meet the patient, introduce yourself by name and title. Ask the patient what he prefers to be called. Avoid addressing adults by their first names without their permission. Your responsibility is to make the patient feel secure and welcome.

Assist the patient to undress and get into bed, if necessary. You will begin gathering information that will be used by members of the interdisciplinary team. You may be responsible for gathering information for the admission checklist (Figure 14-4), checking and listing the patient's belongings, and obtaining vital signs, height, and weight.

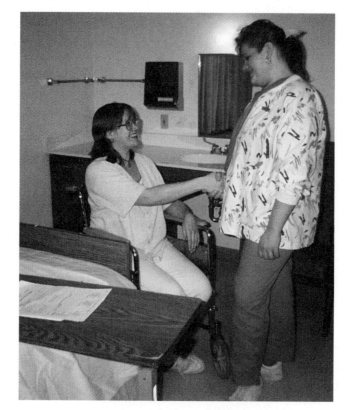

Figure 14-1 First impressions are important.

■ **assess:** *gather information and facts to identify the patient's problems and needs*
■ **nursing process:** *the four-step process of assessment, planning, implementation, and evaluation of the patient and care provided to meet the patient's needs*
■ **planning:** *deciding what to do with information gathered in an assessment*
■ **implementation:** *the process of carrying out a plan*
■ **evaluation:** *the determination of how the patient's plan of care is working*

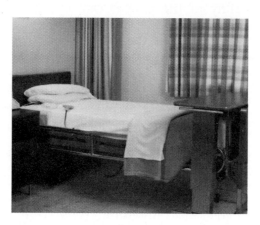

Figure 14-2 Open the bed and prepare the unit before the patient arrives.

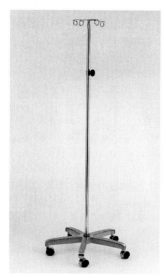

Figure 14-3 An IV standard is used for intravenous feeding solutions, tube feedings, and some irrigations. (Courtesy Medline Industries, Mundelein, IL)

Provide information about the health care facility to the patient and visitors. Before you leave the room, provide fresh drinking water, if allowed, and make sure the patient knows how to use the call signal, telephone, television, and electric bed controls. Label disposable equipment, such as the water pitcher, drinking glass, bedpan, urinal, emesis basin, and other personal care items, with the patient's name according to facility policy. Ask the patient if he needs anything else, and do what he asks, if possible.

After you have completed your part of the admission, the supervisor will **assess** the patient. Assessment is the first step of the **nursing process**. **Planning** is the next step. Assessment and planning involve gathering information to determine the patient's problems and needs, then planning care to meet them. The supervisor will begin to develop the care plan based on his assessment and the information you provide. **Implementation** is the next step. The interdisciplinary team will implement the care plan. **Evaluation** is the final step of the nursing process. The patient's response to the care plan is evaluated and the plan is revised continuously throughout the patient's stay to ensure that her needs are met.

PATIENT PREFERS TO BE ADDRESSED AS:

_____

FROM: ☐ E.R.   ☐ E.C.F.   ☐ HOME   ☐ M.D.'S OFFICE

COMMUNICATES IN ENGLISH: ☐ WELL   ☐ MINIMAL

☐ INTERPRETER (NAME PERSON)   ☐ NONE

_____

MODE OF TRANSPORTATION:

☐ AMBULATORY   ☐ OTHER   **SMOKER:** ☐ Y ☐ N

☐ WHEELCHAIR   _____

☐ STRETCHER   _____

☐ NOT AT ALL   ☐ OTHER LANGUAGE (SPECIFY) _____

HOME TELEPHONE NO. (   ) _____

WORK TELEPHONE NO. (   ) _____

ORIENTATION TO ENVIRONMENT:

☐ ARMBAND CHECKED   ☐ CALL LIGHT

☐ BED CONTROL   ☐ PHONE

☐ TV CONTROL   ☐ SIDE RAIL POLICY

☐ BATH ROOM   ☐ VISITATION POLICY

☐ PERSONAL PROPERTY POLICY ☐ SMOKING POLICY

PERSONAL BELONGINGS: (CHECK AND DESCRIBE)

☐ CLOTHING _____

☐ JEWELRY _____

☐ MONEY _____

☐ WALKER _____

☐ WHEELCHAIR _____

☐ CANE _____

☐ OTHER _____

DENTURES: **CONTACT LENSES:**

☐ UPPER   ☐ PARTIAL ☐ HARD   ☐ LT   ☐ RT

☐ LOWER   ☐ NONE   ☐ SOFT

GLASSES: ☐ Y ☐ N   **HEARING AID:** ☐ Y ☐ N

PROSTHESIS: ☐ Y ☐ N

(DESCRIBE) _____

DISPOSITION OF VALUABLES:

☐ PATIENT

☐ HOME   GIVEN TO: _____

                    RELATIONSHIP: _____

☐ PLACED

  IN SAFE _____

              (CLAIM NO.)

IN CASE OF EMERGENCY NOTIFY:

NAME: _____

RELATIONSHIP: _____

HOME TELEPHONE NO. (   ) _____

WORK TELEPHONE NO. (   ) _____

VITAL SIGNS

TEMP: _____ ☐ ORAL   ☐ RECTAL   ☐ AXILLARY

PULSE: _____ ☐ RADIAL   ☐ APICAL   RESPIRATORY

                              RATE _____

         ☐ RT

B/P: _____ ☐ LT ☐ STANDING ☐ SITTING   ☐ LYING

HEIGHT: _____ WEIGHT: _____ ☐ BEDSIDE

                                 ☐ STANDING

ALLERGIES:

MEDICATIONS: ☐ NONE KNOWN   FOOD: ☐ NONE KNOWN

☐ PENICILLIN ☐ TAPE   (SHELLFISH, EGGS, MILK, ETC.)

☐ SULFA   ☐ OTHER (LIST)   _____

☐ IODINE   _____ _____

☐ ASPIRIN   _____ _____

☐ MORPHINE _____ _____

☐ DEMEROL   _____ _____

(PRESCRIPTIVE & NON PRESCRIPTIVE)
MEDICATIONS: _____   **DOSE/FREQUENCY**   (DATE/TIME) **LAST DOSE**   **DISPOSITION OF MEDICATIONS:**

1. _____ _____ _____   ☐ NONE BROUGHT TO HOSPITAL

2. _____ _____ _____   ☐ SENT HOME _____

3. _____ _____ _____   WITH _____

4. _____ _____ _____   ☐ TO PHARMACY: (LIST)

5. _____ _____ _____   _____

6. _____ _____ _____   _____

ADMITTING DIAGNOSIS: _____

NURSE'S SIGNATURE: _____ RN/LVN   DATE _____ TIME _____

CHARTER SUBURBAN HOSPITAL
16453 SOUTH COLORADO AVENUE
PARAMOUNT, CALIFORNIA 90723
NURSING ADMISSION ASSESSMENT PAGE 1 of 6

Figure 14-4 The nurse may ask you to gather information for the initial patient assessment.

PROCEDURE

70 ADMITTING THE PATIENT

1. Perform your beginning procedure actions.

2. Gather supplies needed: admission checklist, pen and paper, urine specimen cup, transport bag, lab requisition, disposable gloves, hospital gown, clothing inventory list, scale, tape measure for height, sphygmomanometer, stethoscope, thermometer, standard agency admission kit (Figure 14-5), if used.

3. Open the bed by fanfolding the covers to the foot of the bed.

4. Lay the hospital gown at the foot of the bed.

5. Remove contents of the admission kit and put them away.

6. Bring permanent equipment to the room, if needed for patient care.

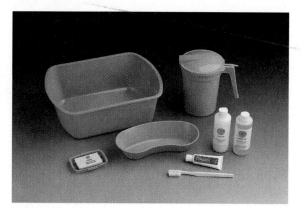

Figure 14-5 The standard admission kit. (Courtesy of Medline Industries, Mundelein, IL)

7. Upon patient arrival, introduce yourself by name and title.

8. Introduce the patient to roommates.

9. Provide privacy and inform family members where they can wait.

10. Assist the patient to undress, and put on own pajamas or gown, if necessary.

11. Obtain the patient's height and weight, following the guidelines in Procedure 69.

12. Ask the patient to provide a urine specimen, if required. Apply the principles of standard precautions. Follow the guidelines in Procedure 52.

13. Assist the patient to put personal articles and toilet items away, if necessary.

14. Transfer the patient into bed.

15. Obtain the vital signs. Follow the guidelines in Procedures 60 through 68.

16. Complete the information on the admission checklist.

17. Familiarize the patient with his surroundings. Show the patient how to use the call signal and explain the intercom system. Explain the use of the telephone, bed controls, and any other equipment in the room.

18. Provide water, if the patient is not NPO.

19. Make the patient comfortable.

20. Perform your procedure completion actions.

Transfer

There are two types of health care facility transfers. The patient care technician usually assists with both types. Performing this procedure correctly will ease the patient's fears about going to a new, unfamiliar unit or location. You are responsible for moving the patient and her belongings, making the patient comfortable in the new unit, and introducing her to the staff who will be caring for her.

After the initial admission to the health care facility, the patient's needs may change, requiring a transfer to another unit within the facility. For example, the patient is admitted to a medical unit for diagnostic tests. The tests reveal that surgery is necessary. The patient is transferred to the surgical unit for care and follow-up.

Patients with chronic diseases may require a transfer to another health care facility when their condition has stabilized. For example, a patient who has suffered a stroke is admitted to the acute care hospital. After the medical symptoms of the stroke have stabilized, the patient is transferred to a subacute care unit,

PROCEDURE

71 TRANSFERRING THE PATIENT

1. Perform your beginning procedure actions.

2. Gather supplies needed: wheelchair or stretcher, cart for patient's belongings, chart, and other medical supplies as instructed by nurse.

3. Gather the patient's belongings and other items to be transferred and place them on the cart.

4. Assist the patient to transfer to the wheelchair or stretcher for transportation to the new unit. Reassure the patient that family and visitors will be given information about the new location.

5. Transport the patient and belongings to the new unit.

6. Assist the patient to transfer to bed in the new room.

7. Introduce the patient to the roommate and nursing staff.

8. Put away the patient's belongings, if this is your facility policy.

9. Make the patient comfortable.

10. Before leaving the unit, make sure that the call signal is within reach and that the patient knows how to use it.

11. Return to your unit.

12. Inform the supervisor that the transfer has been completed, the patient's reaction, and any observations.

13. Strip the patient's unit and remove any permanent equipment from the room, according to facility policy. Notify the **environmental services department** that the unit is ready to be cleaned.

14. Perform your procedure completion actions.

■ *environmental services department:* the housekeeping department; the department responsible for cleanliness and sanitation in most health care agencies; in some facilities, this department also includes maintenance

■ *discharge planner:* a social worker who is responsible for helping the patient make the transition between the health care facility and the community

rehabilitation center, or skilled nursing facility to complete the recovery. In this case the patient is discharged from one facility and admitted to another facility. This process is also called a *transfer,* although you will be performing the procedure in the same manner as a discharge.

Discharge

Discharge planning begins at the time of admission. Many members of the interdisciplinary team are involved with this process. Most health care facilities have full-time **discharge planners,** many of whom are social workers. They are responsible for making arrangements with other community agencies, assisting with social and financial concerns, and providing continuity of care between the health care agency and the community. Discharge planners fill an important role throughout the patient's stay and during the discharge process.

When a patient is ready to leave the health care facility, you will perform the discharge procedure. This involves assisting the patient to gather his belongings and escorting him to a waiting car or ambulance outside the facility. The supervisor is responsible for patient teaching and providing discharge instructions before the patient leaves. You may be asked to assist with this process during routine care to ensure that the patient understands the instructions. For example, a patient who has a paralyzed arm needs to learn how to perform basic activities of daily living using the non-paralyzed arm. You will assist the patient to perform these procedures when you are assisting with bathing and other personal care. A correctly performed discharge will increase the patient's confidence to manage and adjust in his new location.

The physician must write an order for discharge. If the patient advises you that she is leaving without a physician order, report this information to the supervisor immediately. In some health care agencies, the patient must make arrangements with the business office before leaving. Know and follow your facility policy.

PROCEDURE

72 DISCHARGING THE PATIENT

1. Perform your beginning procedure actions.

2. Gather supplies needed: wheelchair, cart for patient's belongings, discharge slip (if used by your agency), instructions and supplies provided by the supervisor.

3. Collect and pack the patient's belongings.

4. Assist the patient to dress, if necessary.

5. Complete and have the patient sign the clothing inventory, if used.

6. Assist the patient to transfer to the wheelchair.

7. Check with the supervisor to see if prescriptions, medications, or other supplies will be given to the patient before she leaves the unit.

8. Transport the patient to the business office, if required, or to the door of the facility. Help the patient into the car.

9. Say goodbye to the patient.

10. Return to your unit.

11. Inform the supervisor that the transfer has been completed, the patient's reaction, and any observations.

12. Strip the patient's unit and remove any permanent equipment from the room, according to facility policy. Notify the environmental services department that the unit is ready to be cleaned.

13. Perform your procedure completion actions.

KEY POINTS IN CHAPTER

- *The first impression that the patient has of the health care agency and its workers is a lasting one.*

- *The patient's perception of the admission process may be clouded by pain, illness, and fear.*

- *The PCT is responsible for admitting the patient, gathering information, and making the patient comfortable.*

- *The nursing process involves assessment, planning, implementation, and evaluation. The PCT makes valuable contributions to the nursing process.*

- *The PCT is responsible for transferring the patient to a new unit within the health care facility and ensuring the patient's comfort before leaving the unit.*

- *A physician's order is required for discharge from the health care facility.*

- *The PCT is responsible for gathering the patient's belongings and safely escorting the patient from the facility.*

REVIEW QUIZ

Multiple Choice Questions

1. Which of the following is true?
   a. Sick patients do not care about first impressions.
   b. First impressions are important for family members only.
   c. First impressions are often lasting ones.
   d. Illness does not affect the patient's fear of admission.

2. An IV standard is the:
   a. pump used to administer an intravenous feeding.
   b. metal pole that supports the IV pump, bottle, or bag.
   c. standard of care for administering IVs.
   d. bag that contains the intravenous fluid.

3. The admission process includes the following assessment information:
   a. vital signs.
   b. height.
   c. weight.
   d. all of the above.

4. After you have admitted a patient, what should you do before leaving the room?
   a. Show the patient how to use the call signal.
   b. Call the supervisor and inform her that the admission is complete.
   c. Always provide fresh water.
   d. All of the above.

5. Which step of the nursing process involves gathering information?
   a. Planning
   b. Implementation
   c. Assessment
   d. Evaluation

6. Which step of the nursing process involves providing care to meet the patient's needs?
   a. Planning
   b. Implementation
   c. Assessment
   d. Evaluation

7. Which step of the nursing process involves analyzing information and developing a care plan?
   a. Planning
   b. Implementation
   c. Assessment
   d. Evaluation

8. Which step of the nursing process involves determining whether the care plan is working?
   a. Planning
   b. Implementation
   c. Assessment
   d. Evaluation

9. Discharge planning begins:
   a. at admission.
   b. at discharge.
   c. several days before discharge.
   d. none of the above.

10. When discharging the patient, the patient care technician is responsible for:
    a. taking vital signs, height, and weight.
    b. safely escorting the patient from the health care agency.
    c. giving the patient instructions on medications to use at home.
    d. all of the above.

CHAPTER

15

Restorative Care

OBJECTIVES:

After reading this chapter, you will be able to:

Spell and define key terms.

Describe restorative care and the restorative environment.

Explain why promoting independence is important in restorative care.

List and describe common restorative programs.

List three types of range-of-motion exercises and describe how each is different.

Describe how a bowel and bladder management program is established and list the PCT's responsibilities for the program.

Describe the PCT's role in using restorative equipment.

▬▬ INTRODUCTION TO RESTORATION

Restorative care is given to assist the patient to attain and maintain the highest level of function possible in the patient's individual situation. A **restorative environment** allows the patient to function as independently as possible. Being **dependent** on others has a negative effect on self-esteem. You learned in Chapter 5 that persons with disabilities do not want to be treated different from anyone else. Most can do the same things you do, but they may do those things differently, because their bodies work differently. Being **independent** is important for most people. This is especially true with personal care. Imagine how frustrated you would feel if someone had to bathe you and feed you. Your self-esteem might suffer. Feeling helpless causes feelings of hopelessness.

The Restorative Team

Many departments assist in providing restorative care to patients. All members of the interdisciplinary team provide restorative care. The therapy departments usually take the lead role in patient restoration. Rehabilitation is designed by a therapist to help patients regain lost skills or teach new skills. Therapists teach patients, families, and staff members techniques for reinforcing and maintaining what the patient has learned. When you follow the restorative program established by the therapist to complement the rehabilitation program, it reinforces what the therapists are teaching and the patient masters the skill more quickly. This process is called **restoration**. Some agencies use the terms *rehabilitation* and *restoration* interchangeably, but rehabilitation really refers to a higher level of care provided by licensed therapy personnel. Restoration is delivered by both unlicensed and licensed caregivers in many departments. A licensed nurse may also develop restorative programs. The interdisciplinary approach provides **continuity of care**, because all staff members are working on the same goals 24 hours a day to benefit the patient.

Complications of Bed Rest

Years ago, putting sick patients to bed for long periods was common. After childbirth, women were often kept on **bed rest** for at least seven days. We now know

■ **restorative environment:** *an environment that has been modified so the patient can function as independently as possible*
■ **dependent:** *unable to care for oneself*
■ **independent:** *self-reliant, able to care for self*

■ **restoration:** *basic nursing care measures designed to maintain or improve a patient's function and assist the patient to return to self-care*
■ **continuity of care:** *all staff working on the same goals and providing the same approaches to the patient 24 hours a day*
■ **bed rest:** *a medically prescribed treatment in which the patient cannot get out of bed*

Table 15-1 Effects of Immobility by Body System

System	Complication
Respiratory	Patient has more difficulty expanding the lungs. Fluid and secretions collect in the lungs, increasing the risk of pneumonia and other lung infections.
Circulatory	Blood clots caused by pooling of blood and pressure on the legs. Edema may be caused by lack of movement. Heart must work harder to pump blood through the body.
Integumentary (Skin)	Pressure sores may develop in a short time due to lack of oxygen to the tissues.
Muscular	Weakness and atrophy from lack of use. Contractures (deformities) develop because of patient's position. Contractures may be painful and are difficult or impossible to reverse.
Skeletal	Calcium drains from bones when patient is inactive. This may contribute to fractures, non-healing, osteoporosis, and other complications.
Genitourinary	The extra calcium in the system from bones promotes the development of kidney stones. Retention of urine is common and is often caused by the patient's position in bed. Overflow of a full bladder leads to incontinence.
Gastrointestinal	Indigestion and heartburn may result if patient is not positioned properly for meals. Loss of appetite may occur from lack of activity, illness, and boredom. Constipation and fecal impaction result from immobility.
Nervous	Weakness and limited mobility. Insomnia may result from sleeping too much during the day, then being unable to sleep at night.
Mental	Irritability, boredom, lethargy, and depression result from patient's frustration and feelings of helplessness.

that early activity is best for the patient. Rest is essential to the treatment of many illnesses. Nevertheless, the physician and other members of the interdisciplinary team will assess the patient and determine how much activity the patient can tolerate. This assessment forms the basis for the restorative program. Like the nursing process, the patient's response to the program is continuously evaluated, and the program modified to meet the patient's individual needs. Keep in mind that bed rest, inactivity, and immobility affect every system in the body (see Table 15-1).

■ **inactivity:** *being still, quiet, sedentary, or immobile*
■ **immobility:** *being motionless, the inability to move*

▆▆▆ PROMOTING INDEPENDENCE

Promoting independence is part of restorative care. Independence is relative to the patient. No one is 100% independent. We all depend on others for some things. Independence for the patient, then, means being as self-sufficient as possible. Preventing total dependence on others is important both physically and psychologically. It is better for the patient to complete part of a task than it is to complete the entire task yourself. Allowing the patient to do what she is able makes the patient feel useful and worthwhile. It may take longer for the patient to complete a task than it takes you. However, maintaining the patient's ability to perform the skill and the effect of personal independence on the patient's self-esteem is worth the investment of your time.

Some patients have medical problems that cause physical dependence. For example, a patient who suffered a neck injury in an accident may be paralyzed from the neck down. This patient is physically dependent. However, if the patient is allowed to set the care routine, and tell you what she wants, she is psychologically independent. Psychological independence is also very important.

Principles of Restoration

The principles of restoration and rehabilitation are the same, and apply to all patients:

■ *Begin treatment early.* If restorative care is started early in the patient's disease, the outcome of the process will be better.

■ *Activity strengthens and inactivity weakens.* The goal should be to keep the patient as active as possible, considering the medical condition. The patient should do an activity whenever possible. For example, passive range-of-motion exercises given by the care provider will prevent deformity and complications. However, active range-of-motion exercises done by the patient will also strengthen muscle.

■ *Prevent further disability.* Follow the care plan to prevent injury and deformity. Practice safety.

■ *Stress what the patient can do. Minimize what the patient cannot do.* Emphasizing what the patient is still able to do is better than saying, "You cannot feed yourself."

■ *Treat the whole person.* Restorative care works on the principle that patients are complex individuals with many strengths and needs. You cannot isolate the medical problem from the rest of the person. Consider all of the patient's strengths and needs when delivering restorative care. Use and build on the patient's strengths to overcome the needs. The program must be individualized for the patient. The care plan will guide you in approaches to use. If you discover something that works for the patient, share this information with your supervisor.

Providing Restorative Care. When providing restorative care, always follow the care plan. The amount and type of activity allowed are ordered by the physician. The care is supervised by the licensed nurse. The care plan will guide you in the type of restorative care to deliver.

Providing restorative care takes a great deal of patience. We did not learn to care for ourselves overnight. Think about how long it takes a small child to learn to take a bath and get dressed. When adults lose the ability for self-care, it takes time to restore. The process can be frustrating for both the patient and the care provider. Being patient, positive, and supportive is the best approach.

Monitoring the Patient's Response to Restorative Care. It is important to observe how the restorative program affects the patient. This is particularly true in the early stages of illness. The patient may become easily frustrated. Allow the patient to struggle, but intervene before she reaches the point of frustration. Encourage the patient and remind her that learning takes time. Practice empathy. Tell the patient you understand how frustrated she feels. Be aware of the patient's fears. Sometimes fear of falling or spilling prevent the patient from participating in the restorative program.

Early in the restorative program, the patient may also have a physical response. Bed rest, even for a short period, can have a negative effect on the body. Any movement or exertion may cause a change in the patient's physical condition. Monitor for signs of fatigue. Be alert for changes and report them to the supervisor. A good practice is to take the patient's pulse before you begin restorative care. Then perform the activity. Monitor the pulse every five minutes during the activity. Normally, the pulse will increase. If the rate is more than 100, or if the patient shows signs of other problems, such as pain, shortness of breath, nausea, or perspiration, stop the activity and notify the supervisor. After you complete the activity, check the pulse again. It should return to within 10 beats of the resting pulse rate within 5 minutes.

Maintaining a Restorative Attitude. Your attitude affects the patient. You must believe that restorative care works and that it is good for the patient. Do not judge the value of restorative care by tomorrow's outcome—you will see little to no change in only one day. Restorative care should be viewed as a positive process that is best for the patient over the long term. Be patient, sincere, tactful, sensitive, and empathetic. Explain the importance of the program to the patient and provide encouragement. Good communication is part of restorative care.

■■■■ APPLYING THE PRINCIPLES OF RESTORATIVE CARE TO ACTIVITIES OF DAILY LIVING

Most of the restorative care you provide will be done when you assist patients with activities of daily living. Observe the patient carefully. Learn which activity of daily living the patient is most interested in accomplishing. Share this information with the supervisor. The information you contribute to the interdisciplinary team based on your observations of the patient is very important.

Role of the PCT in Assisting with Restorative Programs

The care plan will guide you in implementing restorative programs. Each program is designed specifically by the therapist or licensed nurse to meet the patient's individual needs. You must develop a sensitivity to the patient's abilities. Provide what the patient needs, but do not do more than necessary. Be available to assist, but do not help until you are certain the patient cannot accomplish the task. This may be difficult, but the only way the patient will relearn the skill is by doing it.

■ **task analysis:** *analyzing the steps of a procedure and determining which steps the patient can complete independently*

Bathing and Personal Hygiene Programs. Patients with many different illnesses lose the ability to bathe themselves and perform routine hygienic measures. This is very difficult and frustrating for the patient. The occupational therapist often develops restorative programs to assist in this area. The care plan will provide directions for each program. The therapist does a task analysis (see sample in Table 15-2) of the steps in each procedure. For example, part of the task analysis for brushing one's teeth involves turning on the faucet, wetting the toothbrush, removing the lid from the toothpaste, and squeezing the toothpaste onto the brush. If the patient cannot do any of these steps, she will be unable to brush her teeth. The therapist will assess the patient to determine which steps the patient can do, then instruct you to work on the next step. After the patient accomplishes this step, the therapist will instruct you to add another step until the entire task is accomplished.

Common hygiene and grooming ADL programs include bathing and dressing, applying makeup, styling hair, and shaving. You will assist the patient to perform small parts of a skill, then build on his accomplishments. For example, a patient may be unable to wash his face. You will assist him to wash one cheek. When he accomplishes this, assist him to wash the other cheek. Build on this ability until he is able to wash his entire face. All ADL skills start with small tasks. Like building blocks, each new step is built on mastery of the previous step. It may take a long time to accomplish the entire task.

Feeding Programs. Eating is a social activity. Patients who eat alone may not eat as well as those who eat with others. Being spoon-fed also takes some of the pleasure out of eating. A patient may be able to eat finger foods, but need to be spoon-fed the remainder of the meal. Restorative feeding programs frequently involve teaching the patient to use adaptive feeding equipment. The goal of restorative feeding is to assist the patient to be as independent as possible with meals. Your responsibility is to set up the tray by uncovering containers, opening milk cartons, buttering bread, cutting meat, or seasoning foods. Do only what the patient needs. If the patient is able to do some of these things for her-

Table 15-2 Toothbrushing Task Analysis

Key:
+   = Patient can complete task
0   = Patient cannot complete task
N/A = Not applicable

Date	Key	Initial	Step
			1. Identifies equipment for toothbrushing.
			2. Gathers equipment.
			3. Removes cap from toothpaste.
			4. Turns on cold water.
			5. Wets toothbrush.
			6. Squeezes tube slowly and applies toothpaste to toothbrush.
			7. Places cap on toothpaste.
			8. Fills a cup with water for rinsing mouth.
			9. Turns off water.
			10. Grasps toothbrush handle.
			11. Turns bristles upward and brushes chewing surface of upper teeth.
			12. Brushes upper teeth beginning at one side, moving across front teeth, and ending on opposite side.
			13. Turns toothbrush and brushes inside of upper teeth.
			14. Brushes lower teeth beginning at one side, moving across front teeth, and ending on opposite side.
			15. Turns toothbrush and brushes inside of lower teeth.
			16. Brushes tongue.
			17. Turns bristles upward and gently brushes roof of mouth.
			18. Takes a sip of water from the cup.
			19. Rinses mouth.
			20. Spits water from mouth.
			21. Turns on cold water.
			22. Rinses toothbrush.
			23. Turns water off.
			24. Dries face with towel.
			25. Returns toothbrushing supplies to storage area.

General Guidelines for Restorative Care

- Practice good body mechanics for yourself and the patient.
- Provide restorative care at the usual time of day for the activity.
- Remember that all ADLs have many steps. If the patient cannot complete one step, he will not be able to do the activity.
- Do not rush the patient.
- Give verbal **cues**, if necessary. Make your directions as clear and simple as possible. If the patient does not understand, demonstrate.
- Practice safety, and teach the patient safety measures.
- Allow the patient to do as much self-care as possible. Show the patient that you are confident in her ability.
- Use **adaptive devices** (Figures 15-1A and 15-1B) if necessary.
- Apply **orthotic** and **prosthetic** devices as ordered by the therapist and described on the care plan.

cues: *brief verbal hints to tell the patient what you want him or her to do*

adaptive devices: *pieces of equipment used to help a patient perform a task independently*

orthotic or orthosis: *a device that restores or improves function and prevents deformity*

prosthetic: *a device that takes the place of a body part*

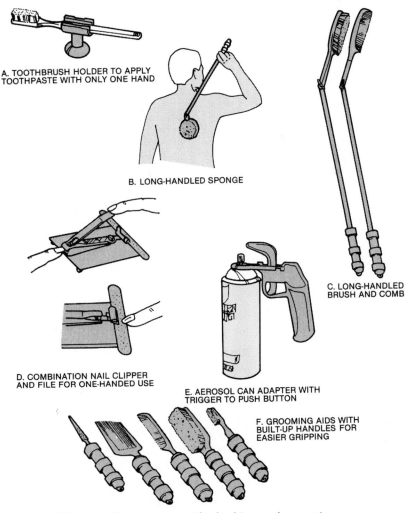

A. TOOTHBRUSH HOLDER TO APPLY TOOTHPASTE WITH ONLY ONE HAND

B. LONG-HANDLED SPONGE

C. LONG-HANDLED BRUSH AND COMB

D. COMBINATION NAIL CLIPPER AND FILE FOR ONE-HANDED USE

E. AEROSOL CAN ADAPTER WITH TRIGGER TO PUSH BUTTON

F. GROOMING AIDS WITH BUILT-UP HANDLES FOR EASIER GRIPPING

Figure 15-1A Adaptive equipment for bathing and grooming

continues

General Guidelines for Restorative Care, *continued*

■ Modify the environment to promote independence, if necessary.

■ If the patient cannot complete an ADL, praise her accomplishment and complete the task for her.

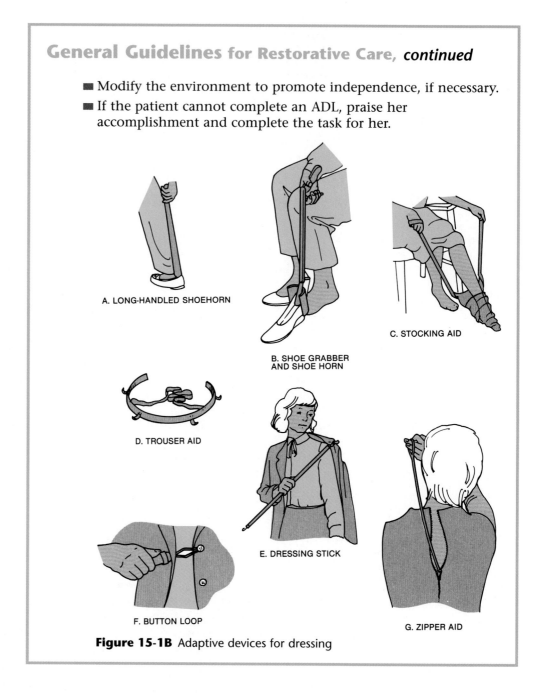

A. LONG-HANDLED SHOEHORN

B. SHOE GRABBER AND SHOE HORN

C. STOCKING AID

D. TROUSER AID

E. DRESSING STICK

F. BUTTON LOOP

G. ZIPPER AID

Figure 15-1B Adaptive devices for dressing

self, allow her to do so. You will also help the patient use adaptive dishes, cutlery, and cups.

■ **mobility:** *the ability to move about*

Restorative Mobility Programs. Mobility means the ability to move about. Walking is the most common means of mobility. However, patients may be mobile enough to move about in bed, or in a wheelchair or other device. Restorative mobility programs are prescribed for many patients. You may be asked to assist patients to move themselves in bed by using the side rails or other equipment. Teaching a patient to use a wheelchair is also a mobility program. Patients in wheelchairs may be taught to lean over, shift their weight, or do push-ups in the chair to relieve pressure and prevent skin breakdown.

Restorative Ambulation Programs. These programs are designed for patients who have completed an intensive therapy rehabilitation program. Restorative ambulation further strengthens the patient and ensures that he will maintain the ability to ambulate. In most cases, you will support the patient by using a gait belt. You may also assist with the use of a cane, crutches, or walker.

▰▰▰ RANGE OF MOTION

■ *range of motion:*
normal joint movements

Maintaining a patient's range of motion is a very important part of restorative care. *Range of motion* is the normal movement of the joints, and is affected by age, body size, genetics, and the presence or absence of disease. We use the range of motion many times each day during our normal activities of daily living and at work.

Reasons for Range-of-Motion Exercises

■ *atrophy: weakness and muscle wasting from lack of use*
■ *contractures: permanent shortening and deformity of muscles from lack of use*
■ *deformity: disfigurement of the body*

People who are ill or have been confined to bed do not move as actively, so the joints are not exercised normally. Weakness occurs quickly. Weakness and muscle wasting from lack of use are called atrophy. Over time, the muscles become rigid and the joints do not move as freely as they once did. Contractures (Figure 15-2) and deformities develop. These are serious and painful complications of inactivity. Joint movement may become painful because the muscles shorten from lack of use. When the joint is moved, the muscle is stretched, and this is uncomfortable or painful. Doing range-of-motion exercises also stimulates circulation and improves the patient's sense of well-being. Patients' joints must be moved regularly to prevent complications. If patients cannot move independently, the patient care technician is often responsible for exercising the joints several times each day.

If you are assigned to assist patients with range-of-motion exercises, take this responsibility very seriously. Sometimes the physical or occupational therapist will prescribe a special routine. The care plan will describe your responsibilities. All patients, including those with no potential for rehabilitation, should be exercised regularly to prevent deformities. Like pressure sores, contractures and deformities are much easier to prevent than to reverse. Sometimes contractures become permanent and cannot be reversed. Your facility will have a policy for how often to perform range-of-motion exercises on patients. Most facilities exercise patients twice a day. Each joint is taken through its normal range of motion three to five times.

Precautions and Special Situations

■ *osteoporosis: a decrease in bone mass that leads to fractures with minimal trauma*

Patients with certain conditions require special care and handling. Avoid exercising extremities with fractures or dislocations. Patients with osteoporosis or bone cancer have bones that break very easily. Check with the supervisor before proceeding. If the patient has a wound or open area on the joint you are exercising, check with the supervisor to see if exercise will be harmful to the healing tissue. If a patient is combative or resists exercise, try to explain why it is important and coax her into participating. However, do not force the patient. Notify the supervisor if the patient continues to refuse.

■ *active range of motion: moving all joints through their normal movements independently*

Active Range of Motion. Active range-of-motion exercises are done by the patient each day during movement and ADLs. Some patients cannot move all of their joints independently. However, they may be able to use a strong extremity to exercise a weaker extremity. For example, a patient who has had a stroke has a strong right arm and a weak left arm. This patient can be taught to move the

Figure 15-2 This patient's hand is severely contracted.

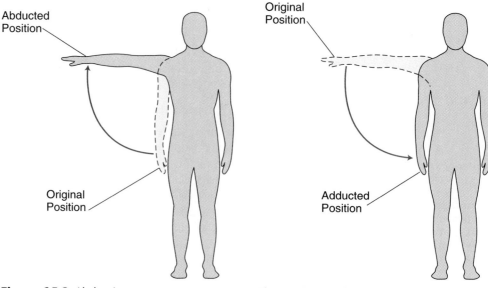

Figure 15-3 Abduction   **Figure 15-4** Adduction

weak left arm with the stronger right arm. Active range of motion maintains movement, prevents deformity, and strengthens muscles.

Active Assistive Range of Motion. Active assistive range-of-motion exercises are either started or completed by the patient. The care provider assists with the exercise. Sometimes a piece of equipment, such as a pulley, is used to exercise the joint.

Passive Range of Motion. Passive range-of-motion exercises are performed by the care provider. The joint is taken through the normal range of movement. Passive range-of-motion exercises maintain movement and prevent deformities, but do not strengthen the muscles.

Range-of-Motion Terminology. Range of motion involves taking the joint through its normal movements. Some important terms are used to describe common joint movements. Abduction (Figure 15-3) is moving an extremity away from the body. Adduction (Figure 15-4) is moving an extremity toward the body. Flexion (Figure 15-5) is bending a joint. Extension (Figure 15-6) is straightening a joint. Supination is moving a joint so it faces upward. Pronation is moving a joint to face downward. Rotation (Figure 15-7) means moving a joint in, out, and around. Inversion is turning a joint inward. Eversion is turning a joint outward.

■ *active assistive range of motion:* exercises that are started or completed by the patient with some assistance from the care provider

■ *passive range of motion:* joint exercises performed on the patient by the care provider

■ *abduction:* moving an extremity away from the body

■ *adduction:* moving an extremity toward the body

■ *extension:* straightening a joint

■ *supination:* moving a joint to face upward

■ *pronation:* moving a joint to face downward

■ *rotation:* moving a joint in, out, and around

■ *inversion:* turning a joint inward

■ *eversion:* turning a joint outward

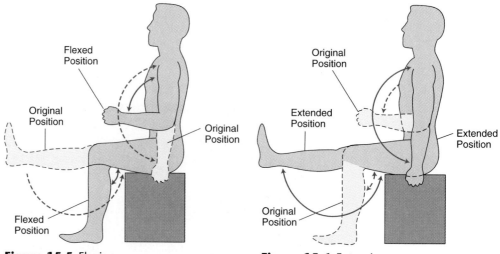

Figure 15-5 Flexion   **Figure 15-6** Extension

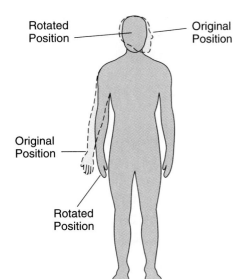

Rotated Position — Original Position

Original Position — Rotated Position

Figure 15-7 Rotation

General Guidelines for Assisting Patients with Range-of-Motion Exercises

- Check the care plan for limitations and guidelines for each patient.
- In some facilities, the neck is not exercised without a physician's order. Follow your facility policy.
- Perform each joint motion five times, or according to facility policy.
- Make sure you have enough space for full movement of the extremities.
- Use good body mechanics and position the patient on the back, in good body alignment, before beginning.
- Expose only the part of the body you are exercising.
- Work systematically from the top of the body to the bottom.
- Never push the patient past the point of joint resistance. Move each joint as far as it will comfortably go.
- Stop the exercise and report to the supervisor if the patient complains of pain. Watch the patient's face for an indication of pain or discomfort.
- Support each joint while you exercise it by placing one hand above and one hand below the joint.
- Move each joint slowly and consistently. Stop briefly at the end of each motion before repeating it.
- Be alert for any changes in the patient's condition during the activity. If you feel that the activity is harming the patient, stop the exercise and notify the supervisor. Changes that indicate a potential problem are pain, shortness of breath, sweating, and change in color.
- Help the patient relax during exercise.
- Use the time spent during range-of-motion exercises as quality time to communicate with the patient.

PROCEDURE

73 PASSIVE RANGE-OF-MOTION EXERCISES

1. Position the patient in good alignment in the supine position.

2. Exercise each extremity as indicated on the care plan, supporting the extremity above and below the joint.

Head and neck (if this is your facility policy or if you have a physician's order)

3. Tip the head forward, bringing the chin to the chest.

4. Tip the head backward, with the chin up.

5. Move the head from side to side.

6. Move the head back and forth in a circular motion.

Shoulders, arms, and elbows

7. Raise the arm over the head, then return the arm to the side.

8. Move the arm from side to side (Figure 15-8), as far away from the body as possible, then return to the side.

9. Move the arm across the chest until the fingers touch the opposite shoulder. Return the arm to the side.

10. With the arm straight out at the side, bend at the elbow and rotate the shoulder (Figure 15-9). Return the arm to the side.

11. Bend at the elbow and bring the hand to the chin or shoulder. Return the arm to the side.

Wrists, fingers, and forearms

12. Support the elbow.

13. Grasp the hand as in a handshake. Turn the palm up, then down.

14. Bend the hand backward at the wrist, then return to the neutral position (Figure 15-10).

15. Bend the hand forward at the wrist, then return to the neutral position.

16. Move the hand from side to side, first toward the thumb, then outward.

17. Move the hand in a circle.

18. Clench the fingers and thumb as if making a fist.

19. Extend the fingers and thumb (Figure 15-11).

20. Move fingers and thumb together and then apart.

21. Flex and extend joints in the thumb and fingers.

22. Move each finger and thumb in a circular motion.

Legs, hips, and knees

23. Keeping the knee straight, raise the leg up and down.

24. Bend and straighten the knee (Figure 15-12).

25. With the leg resting on the bed, roll it inward and outward.

26. Stretch the leg out from the body. Return the leg to touch the other leg.

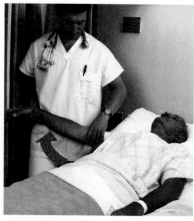

Figure 15-8 The arm is abducted to exercise the shoulder.

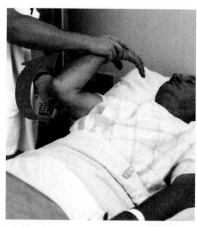

Figure 15-9 Flexion of the elbow

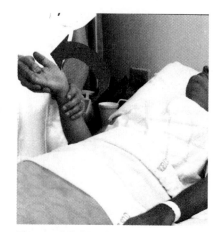

Figure 15-10 The wrist is extended.

continues

PROCEDURE **73** *continued*

Ankles, feet, and toes

27. With the leg straight on the bed, push foot and toes toward the knee, then back down (Figure 15-13).

28. Push the foot and toes out straight, pointing toward the foot of the bed.

29. With the leg straight, turn the foot and ankle from side to side.

30. Bend the toes downward and upward.

31. Spread each toe apart, then back together again.

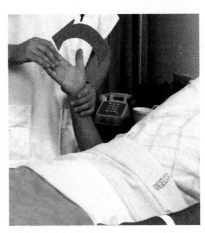

Figure 15-11 Extension of the fingers

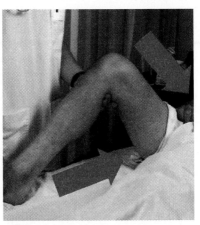

Figure 15-12 Flexion of the knee

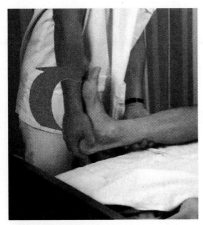

Figure 15-13 The foot and toes are moved toward the head.

■ BOWEL AND BLADDER MANAGEMENT

The OBRA legislation for long-term care facilities specifically addresses the prevention of declines. Acute illness and deterioration in mental status may cause a loss of bowel or bladder control. Incontinence is a decline, not a normal consequence of aging. Incontinence should be prevented and treated aggressively. Managing incontinence is difficult and unpleasant for the care provider, and affects the patient's self-esteem. Incontinence also greatly increases the risk of skin breakdown. Apply the principles of standard precautions when assisting patients with incontinence and bowel and bladder management programs.

Incontinence Management Programs

■ *incontinence management program: a routine in which the patient is taken to the toilet at regular intervals*

Incontinence management programs are not active restorative programs. Rather, they are designed for patients who are mentally confused and unable to communicate the need to use the toilet. However, if the patient is placed on the toilet, she will use it correctly. The toileting schedule in a typical management program is every two hours. The care provider will take the patient to the bathroom according to the schedule. This prevents incontinence most of the time. A trial of incontinence management should be used on all mentally confused patients who are physically able to use a toilet or commode. Although the patient is not actually "trained" to use the toilet, a successful incontinence management program benefits the patient and health care facility staff in many ways.

Bowel and Bladder Retraining Programs

Bowel and bladder retraining programs are individually designed for patients who have become incontinent due to acute illness, trauma, infection, medications, and other factors. Patients do not have to be mentally alert to participate but they need some ability to follow directions and cooperate with the program.

For the best results, bowel and bladder programs should be developed as early in the illness as possible. Members of the interdisciplinary team assess the patient's physical condition, mental status, and ability to participate in the program. An environmental assessment is also completed to determine access and distance to the toilet, whether the patient can get out of the bed or chair independently, and so forth. The patient care technician contributes important information to this assessment. After all data are collected, an individual program is developed to meet the patient's specific needs.

Part of the bowel and bladder assessment involves identifying factors that contribute to or cause incontinence. After these factors are identified, the nurse manager will develop a plan to eliminate them. The nurse manager will take a history of the patient's previous bowel and bladder habits. A detailed analysis of the patient's incontinent episodes over a period of 3 to 14 days is completed. The patient care technician is usually responsible for checking the patient hourly and recording information about incontinence or patient requests to use the toilet (Figure 15-14). Accurate completion of this analysis is very important, because the patient's individual toileting schedule will be developed based largely on this information. You are more aware of the patient's habits and patterns than many other care providers, so notify the nurse manager if you believe the patient shows a pattern of urge incontinence, stress incontinence, or overflow incontinence.

Following the initial assessment period, the nurse analyzes all the information collected and develops a plan for the patient. The plan is based on the patient's previous routines and habits and information about times when the patient was incontinent during the assessment. The nurse writes a specific schedule with times to toilet the patient. There may or not be a pattern to this schedule; it is based on the patient's individual needs. Some people can wait for eight hours before urinating. Others urinate every hour or two. The patient's medical condition, specific habits, and needs are considered when the schedule is written. Some environmental modification may be necessary.

The schedule is implemented and reassessed by the nurse every few days. During this time, you will continue to record each time the patient eliminates. The nurse reviews the information and readjusts the schedule as necessary until success is obtained. Treat the patient with dignity at all times. Flexibility in your schedule, consistency, and punctuality in being available at the scheduled toileting times will help guarantee success. In addition, believe that the program will succeed and maintain your motivation to help the patient.

Scheduled Toileting. **Scheduled toileting** is used for patients who require physical assistance to get to the bathroom. You will be assigned to assist the patient to the bathroom according to a fixed schedule, usually every two to four hours.

Prompted Voiding. Some patients know that the bladder is full, but do not communicate the need to use the toilet. The nurse may instruct you to use **prompted voiding** for these patients. In a prompted voiding program, you will check the patient frequently to determine if he is wet or dry. Each time you are in the room, you will ask the patient if he needs to use the toilet. Assist the patient to the bathroom, or use the commode, bedpan, or urinal. Praise the patient for remaining dry and for trying to use the toilet. Inform the patient when you will return to take him to the bathroom again.

Habit Training. **Habit training** is done for patients who are mentally confused and urinate at fairly predictable times. The patient is taken to the toilet at those times. Praise the patient for being dry and for using the toilet.

Special Situations. Some patients are placed on bladder retraining programs because they have an indwelling catheter. Facilities manage these programs differently. Some facilities completely remove the catheter and begin the retraining assessment. Other facilities clamp and unclamp the catheter at intervals so the patient gets used to the sensation of urine in the bladder. You may be asked to clamp and unclamp the catheter during the retraining process. This does not in-

■ *scheduled toileting:* a bladder management program used for patients who cannot use the bathroom without physical help; the patient is taken to the bathroom on a fixed schedule developed by the nurse
■ *prompted voiding:* a bladder management program used for patients who know that the bladder is full, but do not communicate the need to use the toilet
■ *habit training:* a type of bladder management program used for mentally confused patients who urinate at the same time every day

ASSESSMENT FOR BOWEL & BLADDER TRAINING

PATIENT: _Frank Martin_   ROOM NO: _629C_

	DAY 1	DAY 2	DAY 3	DAY 4	DAY 5	DAY 6	DAY 7
DATE	10/2/XX	10/3/XX	10/4/XX	10/5/XX	10/6/XX	10/7/XX	10/8/XX
7 AM	D	IU	IU	D			
8 AM	IU	D	D	D			
9 AM	D	IU	D	IU			
10 AM	D	D	D	D			
11 AM	D	D	IU	IU			
12 AM	IU	D	D	D			
1 PM	IU	IU	IU	IU			
2 PM	D	D	D	D			
3 PM	D	D	D	D			
4 PM	IBM	D	D	IU			
5 PM	IU	IBM	D	IBM			
6 PM	D	IU	IU	D			
7 PM	D	D	D	IU			
8 PM	IU	IU	IU	D			
9 PM	D	D	D	D			
10 PM	D	D	D	IU			
11 PM	D	IU	IU	D			
12 AM	D	D	D	D			
1 AM	IU	D	D	D			
2 AM	D	IU	IU	IU			
3 AM	IU	D	D	IU			
4 AM	D	D	D	D			
5 AM	D	D	IU	D			
6 AM	IU	IU	D	D			
CODE:	D = DRY IBM = INCONTINENT BM IU = INCONTINENT URINE		TBM = TOILET BM TU = TOILET URINE				

Figure 15-14 The patient is checked hourly. At the end of the assessment period, the nurse develops an individual toileting schedule based on this information.

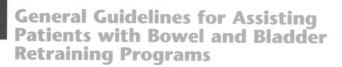

General Guidelines for Assisting Patients with Bowel and Bladder Retraining Programs

- Follow the care plan exactly.
- Answer the call signal promptly.
- Do not rush the patient when toileting.
- Provide privacy by closing the door and privacy curtain. Close the bathroom door even if you must remain in the bathroom with the patient for safety.
- Avoid scolding the patient for accidents. Tell the patient that she can try again next time. Praise the patient for using the toilet and for staying dry.
- If the patient cannot physically use the toilet, assist with the bedpan, urinal, or commode.
- Keep the path to the bathroom well lit and free from obstacles.
- If used, keep the wheelchair, walker, or cane close to the bed.
- Keep the patient's skin clean and dry.

volve opening the closed system. While the catheter is clamped, urine remains in the bladder. Report patient complaints of pain or discomfort to the nurse. Be punctual in the scheduled times to unclamp the catheter to prevent the bladder from overfilling.

■ **Kegel exercises:** *exercises used to make the muscles around the bladder stronger*

Kegel Exercises. Some patients must do exercises, **Kegel exercises**, to make the bladder muscles stronger. Nurses with special training work with these patients initially. Later in the program, you may be instructed to assist and remind the patient to perform these exercises.

Intake and Output. You may also be asked to record the patient's intake and output during the retraining period. The overall fluid intake for the patient may be increased during retraining. In some facilities, fluids are limited during the evening and night hours. The retraining program may take several months. You must be patient, supportive, and encouraging of the patient's success.

■■■■ RESTORATIVE EQUIPMENT

Special restorative equipment is used for many patients to prevent contractures and deformities, which can develop very quickly as a result of immobility. Follow the care plan and use common sense in using restorative equipment. The patient care technician is usually responsible for placing and applying the equipment. Some items, such as splints, are worn according to a schedule. Other equipment, such as handrolls, are used at all times. If the equipment is fastened to the patient's body, you are responsible for keeping the skin clean and dry under the device. Usually, the equipment is removed to perform range-of-motion exercises, then replaced. Follow the care plan and your facility policy.

Handrolls

■ **handrolls:** *props that are placed in the hands to prevent contractures*

Handrolls prevent the fingers from contracting into a tight fist. Although some devices can be fashioned from common items in the health care facility, using commercially manufactured handrolls is best. Years ago, we used rolled washcloths for handrolls. We now know that the softness and texture of a rolled

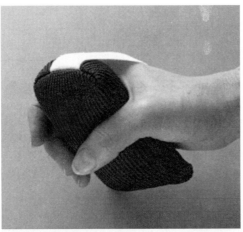

Figure 15-15A The soft handroll attaches to the hand with a Velcro® strap. (Courtesy of Skil-Care Corp.)

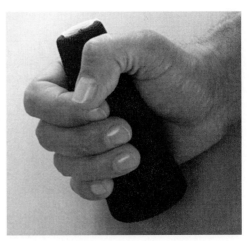

Figure 15-15B The cone hand grip. (Courtesy of Skil-Care Corp.)

washcloth promotes squeezing and actually worsens contractures! Handrolls should be used in all dependent patients. Soft handrolls (Figure 15-15A) are the most comfortable and commonly used. Most commercial varieties have a Velcro® strip attached that is fastened around the hand. Semi-rigid, cone-shaped handrolls (Figure 15-15B) are also available. These are used in patients who may have early contractures and those whose fingers are rigid. The cones are fastened to the hand with the large end by the little finger.

Splints

■ *splints:* devices used to maintain position of an extremity or joint.

Splints (Figure 15-16) are rigid devices used on the hands, arms, legs, and feet. They are used to maintain good alignment, prevent and reverse early contractures, and maintain the extremity in a fixed position. Sometimes splints are used to maintain good alignment of a fracture until the area is casted or an operation is performed. The physical or occupational therapist usually fabricates or orders splints for a specific medical purpose. The care plan will describe the reason for the splint and provide instructions for applying and removing the splint. Splints used to support broken bones are usually not removed by the patient care technician. Splints used to prevent or reverse contractures are usually worn according to a schedule. For example, the splint may be worn during the day and removed at night. Keeping the extremity under the splint clean and dry is very important. The splint must be removed at least once each 24 hours for bathing. Check the area under the splint for signs of redness, irritation, and breakdown. Report your observations to the supervisor.

Footboards

Footboards are used to prevent *foot drop*, a severe contracture that is difficult to reverse. It occurs quickly in patients who are confined to bed. The toes of a pa-

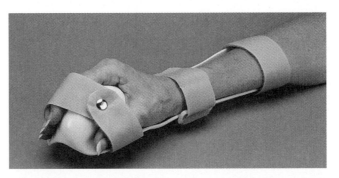

Figure 15-16 The hand splint keeps the hand in a position of function to prevent contractures.

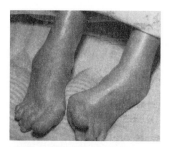

Figure 15-17 This patient has severe foot drop.

tient with foot drop (Figure 15-17) point downward, similar to the position of a woman's foot in high heels. The muscles in the foot become stiff and rigid and the patient is unable to pull the ball of the foot and toes toward the shin. This will prevent the patient from standing normally on the foot with the heel flat on the floor.

Footboards are positioned at the end of the mattress. The heels hang over the end of the mattress so there is no pressure on them. The ball and sole of the foot are positioned flat against the footboard to prevent the toes from pointing downward. Other commercial devices that fasten to the foot may be used as a substitute for a footboard. Preventing contractures of the feet is a very important responsibility.

Other Positioning Devices

Sometimes it is hard to differentiate positioning devices from restraint alternatives. Many devices are used for both purposes. Restraints are commonly used because the patient has a particular positioning problem. When trying to decide how to meet the patient's positioning needs, consider the restraint alternatives mentioned in Chapter 12. These devices can be used for support and to keep patients positioned comfortably in good body alignment.

KEY POINTS IN CHAPTER

- *Restorative care is given to assist patients to attain and maintain their highest level of function.*
- *Promoting independence is part of restorative care.*
- *Restorative care is most effective if it is started early in the patient's illness.*
- *Activity strengthens patients and inactivity weakens them.*
- *When providing restorative care, stress what the patient can do. The PCT should look at the entire person and not just the illness.*
- *Many restorative programs involve assisting patients to relearn ADL skills.*
- *Range of motion is normal movement of joints. If a patient's joints do not move through the normal range of motion each day, contractures and deformities may develop.*
- *Bowel and bladder retraining programs are individualized to the patient's needs based on an assessment.*
- *The PCT is responsible for applying, removing, and assisting patients with many types of restorative equipment.*

REVIEW QUIZ

Multiple Choice Questions

1. Being dependent on others may cause feelings of:
   a. helplessness.
   b. hopelessness.
   c. decreased self-esteem.
   d. all of the above.

2. Restorative care is:
   a. highly skilled.
   b. designed to maintain and improve patients.
   c. always given by licensed personnel.
   d. all of the above.

3. Continuity of care involves:
   a. being assigned to different patients each day.
   b. providing total care to all patients.
   c. all caregivers using the same approaches with the patient.
   d. all of the above.

4. Which of the following is true?
   a. Bed rest, immobility, and inactivity affect every system of the body.
   b. All sick patients should remain on bed rest.
   c. The cardiopulmonary system is not affected by bed rest.
   d. All of the above.

5. You are assigned to care for an alert patient who is paralyzed and cannot perform self-care. You should:
   a. perform total care as quietly as possible.
   b. allow the patient to determine the care routine.
   c. provide the care you think is best.
   d. all of the above.

6. Principles of restoration include:
   a. beginning treatment early.
   b. knowing that activity strengthens and inactivity weakens.
   c. stressing what the patient can do.
   d. all of the above.

7. You are assisting a patient with a restorative ADL program. The patient is struggling to squeeze the water out of a washcloth. You should:
   a. allow the patient to struggle for a few seconds.
   b. intervene immediately.
   c. complete the procedure for the patient.
   d. get the supervisor immediately.

8. The therapist who develops bathing, hygiene, and grooming programs is the:
   a. physical therapist.
   b. occupational therapist.
   c. speech therapist.
   d. respiratory therapist.

9. Weakness and muscle wasting caused by immobility are called:
   a. range of motion.
   b. edema.
   c. atrophy.
   d. adduction.

10. Contractures are:
    a. extensions of the joints.
    b. pressure sores.
    c. blood clots.
    d. painful deformities.

11. You are assigned to do passive range-of-motion exercises on Mr. King. He had knee surgery yesterday and his left knee is bandaged. You should:
    a. consult the supervisor before performing range of motion on the left knee.
    b. not do the range-of-motion exercises because of the surgery.
    c. exercise all of Mr. King's joints.
    d. perform only flexion and extension exercises on the left knee.

12. When performing range-of-motion exercises, you should:
    a. stretch all joints as far as you can.
    b. move each joint as far as it will comfortably go.
    c. ask the patient to tolerate discomfort.
    d. none of the above.

13. An incontinence management program:
    a. is an individual bladder retraining program.
    b. is an assessment of the patient's ability to void.
    c. involves toileting patients on a fixed schedule.
    d. all of the above.

14. You will assist with the assessment for a bowel and bladder retraining program by:
    a. taking the patient to the bathroom every two hours.
    b. writing down the times the patient is incontinent.
    c. administering suppositories and enemas daily.
    d. all of the above.

15. Handrolls are used to:
    a. prevent contractures of the hands.
    b. promote squeezing.
    c. increase strength.
    d. all of the above.

Death and Dying

After reading this chapter, you will be able to:

Spell and define key terms.

Examine your personal feelings about death, dying, and terminal illness.

List the five steps in the grieving process and describe what happens in each.

List 14 signs and symptoms of impending death.

Describe the care of a dying patient.

Demonstrate the postmortem care procedure.

Explain why standard precautions are used when providing postmortem care.

INTRODUCTION

Health care professionals deal with life-and-death situations daily. Caring for patients who are dying, and caring for the body after death, will probably be part of your responsibility. Death is expected in some patients. Other patients die suddenly, without warning. The patient care technician plays an important role in the care of the dying patient. Although you can do nothing to prolong the patient's life, you can do a great deal to make the patient's remaining time as comfortable as possible.

All staff members must be aware of what the patient has been told about her or his condition. In some situations patients are not told of their impending death. This is a medical decision made by the physician. If this is the case, you must respect the decision and abide by it, whether you agree or not. In other cases patients are told of their impending death and may wish to discuss it. Your listening and communication skills are especially important when caring for the dying patient.

Resuscitation Orders

■ **do-not-resuscitate (DNR) order:** *a physician order indicating that no CPR or life-sustaining measures will be performed*

Resuscitation is performed on all patients unless the physician has written a **do-not-resuscitate (DNR) order**. Patients with DNR orders are usually terminally ill and have signed an advance directive indicating that they do not want life-sustaining procedures performed in the event of death. In the absence of a DNR order, cardiopulmonary resuscitation (CPR) is performed if a patient shows signs of clinical death. In many facilities, the patient care technician is trained to perform CPR and may initiate and assist with this procedure.

■ **code blue:** *an emergency designation to alert staff and summon help when a cardiac arrest occurs*
■ **cardiac arrest:** *a condition that occurs when the heartbeat and respirations cease*

Each health care agency has an emergency code designated for resuscitation. Many agencies use the term **code blue** to signify a **cardiac arrest**. Announcing a resuscitation event (or code blue) on the public address system will alert the emergency response team to respond to the unit. CPR and other aggressive measures will be performed to save the patient's life.

EXAMINING YOUR FEELINGS ABOUT DEATH AND DYING

As a whole, society in the United States avoids meaningful discussions about death and dying. As a result, we may be very uncomfortable speaking about this subject.

■ terminal illness: an illness for which there is no cure

Some people avoid making wills because it reminds them of their own mortality. For some, discussing death and dying is painful because it reminds them of personal experiences with friends and loved ones. The AIDS epidemic of the 1980s and 1990s has evoked strong feelings about death and dying. Most AIDS victims were young, in the prime of their lives. The scientific community is beginning to view AIDS in a new light, as a chronic, manageable disease. However, many people are fearful of the disease and continue to consider it a **terminal illness**. A terminal illness is a condition from which the patient is not expected to recover. Young people tend to see themselves as invincible, and receiving a terminal diagnosis is traumatic and painful. A nurse who died of AIDS summed up her feelings about the disease and about dying. She explained that before she developed AIDS, she felt it was a disease for "them." After she became ill, it was difficult for her to accept care given to her by other nurses. As a nurse, she felt she should be giving care, not receiving it. It was embarrassing to lose control of her body functions. She said that the disease caused her to realize that "them is us." There is a great deal of wisdom and insight in this statement. The "them is us" philosophy can be applied to many different diseases in addition to AIDS.

Factors That Influence Your Feelings About Death and Dying

As a care provider, you will care for both young and old patients who are dying. It is never your responsibility to inform them that they are dying. However, once the information has been delivered, you must be prepared to assist the dying patient meet physical, emotional, psychological, social, and spiritual needs. In some cases, you will also be a source of strength and support for the family.

You may feel that death in infants, children, and young adults is unfair. Health care workers often have different views of death and dying in the elderly, who have lived long lives. Your body begins to age as soon as you are born. Death is a natural extension of life. Your feelings and beliefs about death and dying will affect the care you give. To care for dying patients effectively, you must examine and understand your own feelings about death. Sometimes we feel that we have failed in our job if the patient dies. As long as you have done all you can for the dying patient, you have succeeded in your responsibilities. Learn to take comfort in that.

Your age, culture, experiences, religion, values, and personal losses all influence your feelings about death and dying. Sometimes your attitude about death changes because of your personal experiences. As we age, we also may view death differently. Many elderly patients see death as a relief from pain and suffering. Some people fear death. It is a journey into the unknown. They are afraid that it will be lonely and painful. Studies of people who have had near death experiences have shown that death is not unpleasant or frightening. Patients may also worry about dying alone. Many people worry about unfinished personal business, and what will happen to cherished family members and pets after their death.

■ hospice: an organization that cares for dying patients

Hospice. There is no cure for some diseases. Sometimes trauma and injuries to the body are severe and the patient cannot recover. Some patients do not respond to traditional medical treatment. Some patients die soon after receiving a terminal diagnosis. Others live for extended periods of time. We cannot predict when death will occur.

A **hospice** is an agency that cares for patients who are dying. Hospice workers are members of an interdisciplinary team who work to meet the patient's and family's physical, emotional, psychological, social, and spiritual needs. Hospice care is delivered in many different settings. Sometimes care is given in a hospital or nursing home. Many patients use hospice services in their own home. Hospice care is not designed to be aggressive or to prolong life. It is designed to make the patient and family as comfortable as possible as death approaches. The quality of care given is as good as the care given to all other patients. Family members may participate in patient care if they wish. Hospice care is designed to ensure that the patient dies in comfort, with dignity and respect.

■ coping mechanisms: responses to stress and loss that people use to protect feelings of self-esteem

Coping Mechanisms. **Coping mechanisms** are responses to stress and losses that people use to protect feelings of self-esteem. An understanding of some common coping mechanisms will help you understand patient and family reactions to dealing with terminal illness. Coping mechanisms develop throughout a person's life. Success or failure in developing coping skills depends on how well the developmental tasks of earlier life were mastered. When a person's ability to cope is inadequate, the following reactions may be seen:

- Chronic complaining
- Anger
- Irritability
- Crying and tearfulness
- Agitation
- Restlessness
- Fatigue or insomnia
- Muscle tension and headaches
- Depression
- Withdrawal
- Weight loss or gain
- Sleep disturbances

Patients may criticize and blame you for things that are not your fault. Do not take their comments personally. These patients usually need additional emotional support. Your understanding of basic human needs, normal developmental tasks, and coping mechanisms will help you provide quality care. The following are other ways you can provide this support:

- Offer choices over routines and as much control as possible.
- Realize that angry outbursts may be the result of feelings of hopelessness, loss, and unmet needs.
- Direct the patient's emotional energy in positive ways.
- Avoid responding to the patient in a negative manner.
- Report any change in the patient's behavior to the supervisor.

THE GRIEVING PROCESS

■ *grieving process: five steps that people go through when they anticipate or suffer a loss*

When we anticipate or experience a loss, we go through a series of emotional changes and behaviors called the **grieving process**. This process was first described by Dr. Elisabeth Kübler-Ross. Loss of someone or something you love is very difficult. The patient, family, friends, and care providers each go through the grieving process, which involves five steps. The grieving process varies with each of us, so not all persons experience each step. The steps are not always obvious to others. Sometimes we recognize the steps in other people, but fail to recognize them in ourselves. Some people move from one stage to another and back again. It may take a long time to complete all the steps in the grieving process. The patient may die before going through the entire process. Throughout the grieving process, the care provider must offer honesty, reassurance, understanding, caring, and empathy. Helping a patient die in comfort and dignity is very important. Table 16-1 gives examples of typical patient reactions and appropriate PCT responses in each stage of the grieving process.

Denial

■ *denial: the first stage in the grieving process, in which the patient denies the terminal diagnosis*

The first stage in the grieving process is **denial**. This occurs when a person first learns of a terminal diagnosis. The patient may feel that the diagnosis is incorrect. He may exhibit false hope, tell untrue stories, and spend a tremendous amount of effort to keep denial alive. He may refuse to participate in his care and may not follow the directions of the physician and other staff. The patient and family need strong emotional support during this process in order to move through this stage. Allow them to express their feelings, but do not provide false hope. Conversations should be reality-based. Spend time with the patient to show him he will not be left alone. Later in the denial stage, the patient may isolate himself from others.

	Table 16-1	
Stages of Grief	**Response of the PCT**	
Denial	Reflect patient's statements, but try not to confirm or deny the fact that the patient is dying. *Example: "The lab tests can't be right—I don't have cancer."* *"It must have been difficult for you to learn the results of your tests."*	
Anger	Understand the source of the patient's anger. Provide understanding and support. Listen. Try to meet reasonable needs and demands quickly. *Example: "This food is terrible—not fit to eat."* *"Let me see if I can find something that would appeal to you more."*	
Bargaining	If it is possible to meet the patient's requests, do so. Listen attentively. *Example: "If only God will spare me this, I'll go to church every week."* *"Would you like a visit from your clergy person?"*	
Depression	Avoid cliches that dismiss the patient's depression ("It could be worse—you could be in more pain"). Be caring and supportive. Let the patient know that it is okay to be depressed. *Example: "There just isn't any sense in going on."* *"I understand you are feeling very depressed."*	
Acceptance	Do not assume that, because the patient has accepted death, she or he is unafraid, or that she or he does not need emotional support. Listen attentively and be supportive and caring. *Example: "I feel so alone."* *"I am here with you. Would you like to talk?"*	

Anger

■ **anger:** *the second step in the grieving process, in which the patient is angry because of a terminal diagnosis*

The second stage of the grieving process is **anger**. The patient feels angry with himself, family and staff, the doctor, and God. He may use abusive language and refuse care and nutrition. Recognize that the patient is not angry with you personally. Practice empathy and let him know you understand how he feels.

Bargaining

■ **bargaining:** *the third stage in the grieving process, in which the patient attempts to buy more time*

The third stage of the grieving process is **bargaining**. The patient hopes he can live to see a certain event, such as a graduation or birth of a grandchild. Sometimes he bargains with God and makes promises, such as attending church every Sunday in return for more time. Bargaining is an attempt to postpone the inevitable. This stage is usually short. Realize that the patient still needs time to accept the impending death. Spend as much time as you can with the patient to show that you sincerely care.

Depression

■ **depression:** *the fourth stage in the grieving process, in which the patient is trying to deal with the loss of everything he or she has*
■ **apathy:** *indifference; lack of feeling or emotion*

Depression is the fourth stage in the grieving process. The patient is dealing with the loss of everything that he has. His physical ability may decline. He is losing his home, possessions, loved ones, hopes, and dreams. He may also be feeling regrets for things he has said or done throughout his life. The patient may experience **apathy**, decreased ability to concentrate, insomnia, fatigue, constant crying, poor appetite, and lack of interest in people and the environment. In this stage, the patient is beginning to separate himself from life. Do not attempt to humor or cheer him. Allow him to express his feelings and be available to sit quietly and offer support.

Acceptance

The final stage in the grieving process is **acceptance**. The patient may feel empty and peaceful. This stage usually brings less emotional pain and discomfort, and the patient calmly waits for the end. The patient may not want to be alone during this stage. If he does not object, allow others with whom he is comfortable to assist with care. Allow the patient to express his needs in his own time and way. Communication may be limited in this stage.

■ SIGNS OF APPROACHING DEATH

Signs of death may appear slowly or rapidly. Always report changes in the patient's condition to the supervisor. Some patients are alert until the moment of death. Others have a period of unconsciousness first. After the patient dies, a physician will examine the patient and pronounce death. In some states, registered nurses may pronounce death. This is never the responsibility of the patient care technician. The supervisor or physician are also responsible for notifying the family after death has been established.

Signs of approaching death are:

■ Level of responsiveness decreases.

■ Movement, muscle tone, and sensation decrease until they are eventually lost.

■ The lower jaw relaxes and the mouth falls open.

General Guidelines in Caring for the Dying Patient

■ Practice empathy for the patient, friends, and family

■ Check the care plan for special patient care instructions.

■ Consider and respect the religious beliefs of the patient and family even if they are different from your own.

■ Learn the patient's cultural and religious practices regarding death.

■ Keep the patient clean and comfortable.

■ Keep the lips and mouth moist and give frequent oral care.

■ Turn the patient every two hours, or more often. Position with props and pillows for comfort.

■ Keep the skin clean. Apply lotion as needed.

■ Change the linen immediately if it is wet or soiled. Provide blankets for warmth.

■ Provide perineal care after each episode of incontinence.

■ The room should be well lighted and as comfortable and pleasant as possible.

■ Allow privacy if the family is present, but check on the patient frequently.

■ Touch and continue to talk to the patent as you normally would.

■ Avoid saying things that you do not want the patient to hear. Explain all procedures before doing them. The patient may appear unconscious, but may still be able to hear.

■ Support family members. Allow them to be involved in care, if appropriate.

■ Make the family as comfortable as possible by providing coffee, pillows, blankets, or other needed items.

- The skin appears pale and is moist and cool to touch.
- The lips, fingernails, and mucous membranes take on a dusky, gray, or blue color.
- The pulse becomes rapid, weak, or thready.
- Respirations become slow, labored, irregular, or noisy. Cheyne-Stokes respirations may be present. Mucus collects in the throat.
- Blood pressure decreases. Sometimes blood pressure can no longer be heard at the brachial artery, even though the patient remains alive.
- The patient may become incontinent of urine and feces.
- Eyes stare and pupils do not respond to light.
- The skin takes on a blue or dusky appearance, beginning in the lower extremities and moving upward. The skin feels cool or cold to touch.

Care of the Dying Patient

Care of the dying patient is a continuation of care that shows support, dignity, and respect. The Dying Person's Bill of Rights (Figure 16-1) provides guidelines and should be used as a basis for care.

The Dying Person's Bill of Rights

I have the right to be treated as a living human being until I die.

I have the right to maintain a sense of hopefulness, however changing its focus may be.

I have the right to be cared for by those who can maintain a sense of hopefulness, however changing this may be.

I have the right to express my feelings and emotions about my approaching death, in my own way.

I have the right to participate in decisions concerning my care.

I have the right to expect continuing medical and nursing attention even though "cure" goals must be changed to "comfort" goals.

I have the right not to die alone.

I have the right to be free from pain.

I have the right to have my questions answered honestly.

I have the right not to be deceived.

I have the right to have help from and for my family accepting my death.

I have the right to die in peace and dignity.

I have the right to retain my individuality and not be judged for my decisions, which may be contrary to the beliefs of others.

I have the right to discuss and enlarge my religious and/or spiritual experiences, regardless of what they may mean to others.

I have the right to expect that the sanctity of the human body will be respected after death.

I have the right to be cared for by caring, sensitive, knowledgeable people who will attempt to understand my needs and will be able to gain some satisfaction in helping me face my death.

Figure 16-1 The Dying Person's Bill of Rights (Barbus, A.J.: *American Journal of Nursing* 75 (1):99 (1975). Used with permission of Lippincott-Raven Publishers)

POSTMORTEM CARE

■ **postmortem care:** *physical care of the body after death*

■ **rigor mortis:** *a condition that occurs two to four hours after death in which the muscles and limbs become stiff*

■ **shroud:** *a cloth, paper, or plastic covering used to wrap the body after death*

Your facility will have a policy and procedure for postmortem care, which is care given after death. In most cases, the patient care technician delivers this care. Some facilities have a morgue to which the body is taken. In some facilities the body is left in the room until it can be transferred to a mortuary. Within two to four hours after death, a condition called rigor mortis develops. In this condition, the body becomes rigid and stiff. Position the body in good alignment before this condition occurs.

Always use standard precautions when providing postmortem care. The body can be infectious after death. Handle the body very gently. Show the same respect that you would if the patient were alive. Respect the religious beliefs of the deceased. Spiritual beliefs vary and people of some faiths and cultures have special religious requirements for preparation of the body (Table 16-2).

Table 16-2 Cultural/Religious Beliefs Affecting Care at the Time of Death

Culture/Religion	Religious Belief
Adventist (Seventh Day, Church of God)	Some believe in divine healing, anointing with oil, and prayer.
American Indian	There are many different tribes, and beliefs vary with each. Some believe an owl is an omen of death. Some tribes have family members prepare the body for burial. Some tribes will not touch the dead person's belongings after death. Some tribes believe the dead are happy in the spirit world. Others believe the body is an empty shell. Some have extensive preparation of the body and visitation of the deceased. If a member of some tribes dies at home, the house is abandoned forever, or may be burned.
Armenian Church	Holy Communion may be given as a form of last rites; laying on of hands is practiced.
Baptist	Pastor, patient, and family counsel and pray. Some practice healing and laying on of hands.
Black/African American	The deceased is highly respected. Health care providers usually prepare the body. Cremation and organ donation are usually avoided.
Black Muslim	Practices for washing the body, applying the shroud, and funeral rites are carefully prescribed.
Brethren	Anointing with oil is done for physical healing and spiritual guidance.
Buddhist Churches of America	The priest is contacted. Chanting may be done at the bedside after death.
Cambodian (Khmer)	Monks recite prayers. Family wants to be present at time of death and may want to care for the patient. Incense may be burned. Death is accepted in a quiet, passive manner. Family and monks may wish to prepare the body. A white cloth is used as a shroud and mourners wear white.
Central American	Catholics may want a priest to administer Sacrament of the Sick. Candles may be used if oxygen is not in use in the room. Family members may wish to prepare the body. *continues*

Table 16-2, *continued*

Culture/Religion	Religious Belief
Chinese American	Family may prefer that patient not be told of impending death, or may prefer to inform the patient themselves. Some may not want to talk about the terminal illness with anyone. Some believe that dying at home is bad luck. Others believe that the spirit gets lost if the patient dies in the hospital. Family members may place special cloths and amulets on the body. Some prefer to bathe their own family members after death.
Christian Scientist	A Christian Science Practitioner may be called for spiritual support.
Church of God	Believes in divine healing through prayer. Speaking in tongues may be used.
Colombian	Catholic prayer and Anointing of the Sick common. Family may practice Catholic prayer at bedside. Family members may cry loudly or become hysterical. All family members may want to see the body before it is taken to the morgue. In Colombia, the deceased are usually buried within 24 to 36 hours. The supervisor may need to inform them that in the U.S. the body may not be buried this quickly.
Cuban	Family may not want patient told of impending death (varies according to Cuban culture). Family members may stay with patient 24 hours a day during terminal phase of illness.
Eastern Orthodox	Last rites are given. Anointing of the sick is performed as a form of healing with prayer.
Episcopal	Last rites are available, but not mandatory.
Ethiopian	Friends are told of death before family so they can be present when family is informed. Female family members are never told first. Great displays of feelings are encouraged at death. They may cry loudly and hysterically. Women may tear their clothing and beat their chests. Men may cry out loud. Some families may want to say goodbye to the deceased before the body is removed from the room.
Filipino	Head of family is informed away from patient's room. Catholic priest is called to deliver Sacrament of the Sick. Do-not-resuscitate decisions may be made by the entire family. Religious objects may be placed around the patient. Family may pray at the bedside when patient is dying. After death, may cry loudly and hysterically. Family may wish to wash the body. Death is considered a very spiritual event. All family members may say goodbye before body is removed from the room.
Friends (Quaker)	Do not believe in afterlife.
Greek Orthodox	The priest should be called while the patient is still conscious. Practices last rites and administration of Holy Communion.
Gypsy	In general, discussion of death is avoided. Eldest in authority is informed of death first. A priest may be present for body purification. Family may want the window open at the time of death and afterward so the spirit can leave the room. May ask for special personal items in room at the time of death. An older female relative may remain at the window to keep spirits out of room. The

continues

Table 16-2, *continued*

Culture/Religion	Religious Belief
Gypsy, *continued*	moment of death and the patient's last words are very significant. The body after death may represent a source of spiritual danger to the family. Family may want body embalmed immediately after death to remove blood. They may sit with the body around the clock after death, and will eat and drink at this location.
Haitian	Elaborate rituals after death. When death is imminent, family will cry hysterically and uncontrollably. Family members may bring religious symbols and medallions. They have a deep respect for the dead. Family members may wish to wash the body and participate in postmortem care.
Hindu	Specially prescribed rites. The family washes and dresses the body and only certain persons may touch the dead.
Hmong	Important to wear fine traditional Hmong clothing at the time of death. Family may put amulets on body, which should not be removed. The family usually prepares the body at the funeral home. The body cannot be buried with hard objects, buttons, or zippers against the body.
Iranian	Death is seen as the beginning of a spiritual relationship with God, not end of life. Family may wish to be present at all times when patient is dying, and may cry and pray at bedside. Families may wish to wash the body.
Islam (Muslim)	Begging forgiveness and confession of sins must be done in presence of family members before death. There are five steps to prepare the body for burial. The first step involves washing of the body by a Muslim of the same gender. May offer special prayers at bedside to ease pain and suffering. Some have spiritual leader give patient holy water to drink prior to death to purify body. After death, arms and legs are straightened and the toes tied together with a bandage.
Japanese	Patient and family may be aware of impending death, but will not speak about it. Family may wish to remain at bedside during terminal stage of illness. Cleanliness and dignity of the body are very important.
Judaism (Orthodox and Conservative)	Church members wash and prepare the body.
Korean	Chanting, incense, and praying may be used. Family crying and mourning may be extreme. Family may want to spend time alone with patient after death. Some may wish to wash the body.
Lutheran	Last rites optional; the patient may request anointing of the sick.
Mexican American	Entire family may be obligated to visit the sick and dying. Pregnant women may be prohibited from visiting. Spiritual items may be important. May want to die at home because of the fear that the spirit will get lost in the hospital. Crying loudly and wailing are culturally accepted and a sign of respect. A Catholic priest is called for the Sacrament of the Sick. A family member may wish to assist with postmortem care. Family will want time alone with the body before it is removed from the room.
Orthodox Presbyterian	Scripture reading and prayer.

continues

Table 16-2, *continued*

Culture/Religion	Religious Belief
Puerto Rican	If death is imminent, family may stay around the clock. Some believe that all immediate family members must be present at time of death. Believe that the body must be treated with great respect.
Roman Catholic	The Rite for Anointing of the Sick is desired. Patient or family may request anointing if prognosis is poor.
Russian	Family may not want patient to know of terminal diagnosis. Depending on religion, family may wish to wash the body and dress it in special clothes.
Russian Orthodox	Many wear a cross necklace, which should not be removed, if at all possible. After death, the arms are crossed and fingers set in the form of a cross. Clothing must be of a natural fiber so the body changes to ashes sooner.
Samoan	Patient and family prefer to be told of terminal diagnosis as early as possible. Family would prefer to care for patient at home, if possible. Family members usually prefer to prepare the body.
Sikh	Believe that the soul remains alive after death. Family washes the body and dresses it in new clothing.
Vietnamese	DNR decisions are made by entire family. For Catholic families, religious items are kept close to patient. For Buddhist families, incense is burned. Families prefer time alone with the deceased before body is moved. The body is highly respected, and the family may prefer to wash it. Some may prefer the body left as it is.
West Indian	When death is near, close family and friends wish to remain at the bedside to pray. Family members may wish to view the body exactly as the patient was at the time of death. Most wish to be alone with the deceased.

PROCEDURE

74 POSTMORTEM CARE

1. Perform your beginning procedure actions.
2. Gather supplies needed: shroud kit or morgue pack with gown and identification tags, a basin of warm water, soap, washcloth, towels, swabs for oral care, linen, and gloves.
3. Apply gloves.
4. Position the patient on the back with a pillow below the head and shoulders.
5. Close the eyes by gently pulling eyelids down.

6. Provide mouth care using moistened oral care swabs or sponges.
7. Place cleaned dentures in the mouth, or follow your facility policy. If the dentures are not replaced, they should be sent to the funeral home with the body.
8. Close the mouth. A rolled-up washcloth may be placed under the chin to keep the jaw closed.

continues

PROCEDURE 74 *continued*

9. Remove all tubing from the body as instructed by the nurse.

10. Bathe the body, straighten the arms and legs, and comb the hair.

11. Apply clean dressings to wounds, if necessary.

12. Place a bed protector or underpad under the buttocks. Urine and stool may continue to seep out after death.

13. Put a gown on the body.

14. Attach identification tags to the body according to facility policy.

15. Replace soiled linen and cover the body to the shoulders with a sheet.

16. Remove gloves and discard according to facility policy.

17. Wash your hands.

18. Straighten the room and remove unnecessary equipment.

19. Wash your hands.

20. Provide privacy and allow family members to be alone with the body.

21. Collect the patient's personal belongings, place them in a bag and label them correctly. Usually these are given to the family. If no family members are present, follow facility policy. Complete and sign the inventory sheet according to your facility policy.

22. After the family leaves, wash your hands and put the shroud on the body. Wear gloves if contact with blood or body fluid is likely.

23. Remove gloves and discard according to facility policy.

24. Follow facility policy to take the body to the morgue or close the door until the funeral home arrives.

25. Notify the supervisor when the funeral home arrives.

26. Assist the funeral home to move the body if necessary.

27. Strip and clean the unit according to your facility policy after the body has been removed.

28. Perform your procedure completion actions.

KEY POINTS IN CHAPTER

- *The patient care technician is expected to provide care to patients who are dying and to care for the body after death.*

- *When caring for patients who are dying, the PCT will assist patients and families to meet physical, emotional, psychological, social, and spiritual needs.*

- *Patients with terminal illness are not expected to recover, but the exact time of death cannot be predicted.*

- *The care provider's personal beliefs about death and dying will affect the care given to the patient.*

- *A hospice is an agency that cares for dying patients. Hospice care focuses on keeping patients comfortable and allowing them to die with dignity and respect.*

- *Coping mechanisms are responses to stress and loss that are used to protect self-esteem.*

- *The five steps in the grieving process are denial, anger, bargaining, depression, and acceptance.*

- *The patient and family's cultural and religious beliefs about death and dying must be respected.*

- *Standard precautions are used when caring for the deceased, because the body can be infectious after death.*

REVIEW QUIZ

Multiple Choice Questions

1. Our feelings about death and dying are influenced by:
   a. age.
   b. culture.
   c. experiences.
   d. all of the above.

2. Hospice care is designed to:
   a. treat the patient aggressively.
   b. keep the patient comfortable.
   c. prolong life.
   d. all of the above.

3. Coping mechanisms are:
   a. responses to stress.
   b. used to protect self-esteem.
   c. learned throughout life.
   d. all of the above.

4. In the first stage of the grieving process, the patient shows signs of:
   a. denial.
   b. bargaining.
   c. depression.
   d. all of the above.

5. The patient is beginning to separate himself from life during the:
   a. denial stage.
   b. anger stage.
   c. depression stage.
   d. bargaining stage.

6. Signs of approaching death include:
   a. cooling of the skin, beginning with the lower extremities.
   b. constricted pupils.
   c. steady, slow pulse.
   d. all of the above.

7. When caring for the dying patient:
   a. be as quiet as possible and do not speak when providing care.
   b. always explain procedures before doing them.
   c. do not move the patient in bed, as this is painful and disturbing.
   d. all of the above.

8. Which of the following is true about providing postmortem care?
   a. There is no need to provide privacy.
   b. The dentures are always removed from the mouth and given to the family to take home.
   c. Standard precautions are used because the body can be infectious.
   d. All of the above.

9. The condition in which the muscles become stiff and rigid is:
   a. algor mortis.
   b. liver mortis.
   c. muscle mortis.
   d. rigor mortis.

10. When a patient is dying, the room should be:
    a. dark and cold.
    b. well lighted and ventilated.
    c. dark and hot.
    d. well lighted and cold.

MENTAL HEALTH AND SOCIAL SERVICE NEEDS

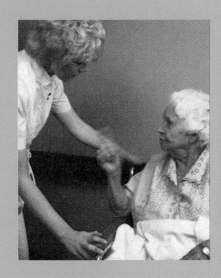
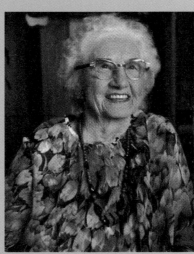
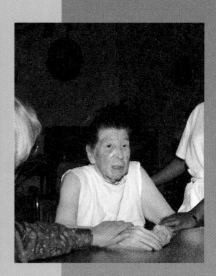

Special Behavioral Problems

After reading this chapter, you will be able to:

Spell and define key terms.

Identify common causes of behavior problems in alert and confused patients.

Explain why physical and chemical restraints are not desirable in the management of behavior problems.

Describe the effect of losses and unmet needs on patients' behavior.

List the three steps in the ABC method of behavior management, and explain how this method is used to eliminate undesirable behavior.

Describe how to assist patients with specific behavior problems.

Differentiate cognitive impairment from dementia and delirium.

Describe methods of caring for and communicating with patients with cognitive impairment and dementia.

List the three stages of Alzheimer's disease and describe signs and symptoms of each stage.

BEHAVIOR PROBLEMS

■ **cognitive impairment:**
a decline in intellectual functioning

Behavior problems frequently have medical, social, or emotional causes that create great stress. Typical behavior problems include physical or verbal aggression (Figure 17-1), wandering, yelling or calling out, and other socially inappropriate behaviors. Some behavior problems are related to cognitive impairment. Problem behaviors may present a danger to the patient, staff, and other patients on the unit. Other behaviors, though harmless, may be annoying or distressing to the staff. Care providers often have difficulty caring for patients with behavior problems. Sometimes this results in overuse of physical restraints or sedation with chemical restraints. Both interventions may have serious consequences and do not always solve the underlying problem. They often worsen physical dependence and may increase confusion. Although both forms of treatment are useful sometimes, other methods of dealing with the behavior should be tried first. If they are ineffective, physical and chemical restraints are the last resort. *Behavior management* is a technique commonly used to modify patient behavior. Dealing with patients with behavior problems requires patience, common sense, good communication skills, and a great deal of empathy. The trend in health care is moving away from using physical and chemical restraints, and toward employing other methods to manage behavior.

The Effect of Losses on Behavior

When people are sick or injured, they suffer losses. The most obvious is loss of health, which causes loss of independence. Loss of health and independence cause inability to work. The inability to work causes loss of income and security. The loss of health, independence, income, and security may affect the patient's relationships with others. Family and friends may be lost. The patient may feel

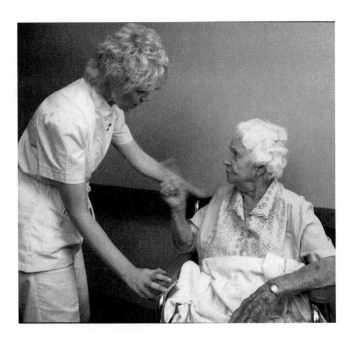

Figure 17-1 Aggressive behavior often indicates an unmet need.

like a bother, unloved, or both; she often feels that she has lost control. Changes in relationships and losses often affect the patient's self-esteem. A job often gives people a sense of identity. People are proud to say they are bankers, mechanics, actors, or care providers. When the patient is unable to work, this identity is lost. Although the loss may be only temporary, the patient may fear that the loss will be permanent.

The patient may have to relocate to a hospital, subacute unit, or nursing facility. The loss of home and the comfort of belongings, even if temporary, is a difficult adjustment. When this is combined with other losses, the patient may feel overwhelmed. Many people go through the grieving process (see Chapter 16) when they suffer the types of losses described here. Sadness and grief are normal when people suffer a loss. You will be caring for patients in various stages of the grieving process.

The patient may also be fearful and anxious. This is caused in part by fear of the unknown. The patient does not know what the outcome of the illness will be. She may fear a negative outcome. She may also be afraid of treatments and procedures used to manage the illness. The patient may begin to feel helpless and hopeless. She may also become frustrated and angry. The anger may be internal, that is, directed toward herself. It is difficult to maintain your self-esteem when you are angry with yourself. The anger may also be external, directed toward family, friends, and caregivers.

Unmet Needs

Many people develop behavior problems in response to unmet needs. Think about the needs in Maslow's hierarchy. Patients with behavior problems who are mentally alert are often expressing or responding to an unmet psychosocial need. They also may be responding to a feeling of lack of control over their body, their situation, or the environment. Get to know the patient and respect his uniqueness as a person. Promote and reward independence, decision making, and assertive behavior. If you are able to identify the patient's need, share this information with the supervisor and other members of the interdisciplinary team.

Behavior problems in patients who are mentally confused are a response to fear, loneliness, boredom, or an unmet physical need. The behavior may be the only way the patient has to express herself. For example, a mentally confused patient screams frequently throughout the day. The patient is alone in bed in her room. This patient presents a particular challenge because there are so many potential reasons for the screaming. She may be hungry or thirsty, in pain, scared, lonely, or bored. She may need to use the bathroom, but be unable to tell you. There may be too much noise or stimulation in the environment, causing her to be agitated. The only way to find out why the patient is screaming is by using common sense and experimenting with different approaches. Offer her a drink or something to eat. Take her to the bathroom. Sit quietly with her and hold her hand. If you find an approach that calms her, share this information with other members of the interdisciplinary team.

The Meaning of Behavior Problems. All behavior has a meaning, though the meaning may not be evident to you. The patient may not even realize that she is demonstrating a behavior that you consider abnormal. This is particularly true if the patient is from a different culture. Behavior that is acceptable in one culture may be considered abnormal by persons from other cultures. Behavior patterns develop throughout a person's lifetime and are affected by heredity, culture, environment, and lifetime experiences. Behavior problems usually develop in response to stress, loss, or unmet needs that exceed the patient's ability to cope.

Normal Coping and Defense Mechanisms. Patients compensate for losses using methods they have learned over their lifetime. Several common defense mechanisms are:

■ Denial—refusing to admit there is a problem

■ Rationalization—providing an acceptable but untrue reason for the illness or behavior

■ Compensation—using strength and overachieving in one area to overcome a weakness in another area of life

■ Projection—placing the blame for the illness or situation on someone or something else

The patient care technician must use good communication and listening skills when dealing with patients who have suffered losses. Understand that when patients use coping mechanisms, they are responding to stress. Do not take angry outbursts or other behavior personally. Although the patient may say she is angry with you, this is not always the case. She is usually angry because of the situation she is in. You may need to modify your behavior. Monitor how the patient responds to you, then adjust your approach to achieve better results. Practice empathy. Put yourself in the patient's shoes and try to understand what is happening.

■ THE ABCS OF BEHAVIOR MANAGEMENT

An effective technique of behavior management is the ABC plan (Table 17-1). This plan is useful with many patients, both alert and mentally confused. The theory behind this program is that if the antecedent or consequences of the behavior are eliminated or modified, the behavior will change or cease.

Glossary (left margin):

■ **rationalization:** *providing an acceptable but untrue reason for the illness or behavior*

■ **compensation:** *using strength and overachieving in one area to overcome a weakness in another area of life*

■ **projection:** *placing the blame for an illness or situation on someone or something else*

■ **antecedent:** *an event that causes or triggers a behavior*

■ **consequences:** *the outcome of a behavior*

Table 17-1	
Identify the ABCs	**Definition**
A = Antecedent	The cause or trigger of the behavior
B = Behavior	The behavior itself
C = Consequences	The consequences, effect, or results of the behavior

The Three Steps of Behavior Management

There are three steps in the ABC method of behavior management.

1. Attempt to determine the cause of or trigger for the behavior. Does the behavior occur in specific environmental conditions, at a certain time of day, or during a certain activity? Does the presence or absence of other persons trigger the behavior?

2. Eliminate the cause of the behavior. If the cause can be identified and eliminated, the behavior will cease or change.

3. Examine the consequences of the behavior. They may also have to be eliminated or changed in order to change the behavior. Modifying the consequences of behavior requires practice. For example, a mentally confused patient yells and cries. You discover that if you sit and hold the patient's hand, the behavior stops. Sitting and holding the hand serves as a reward for the behavior. To modify the consequences, sit and hold the patient's hand *before* the yelling and crying start. Pay attention to the patient on a regular basis. In this case, modifying the consequences changes the behavior. If the patient's behavior has been rewarded for a long period of time, do not expect to see immediate results. All team members will have to practice the new approach consistently before results become evident.

Using the ABC Method. A common problem occurs in mentally alert patients who use the call signal frequently. When you answer the signal, the requests seem unimportant. The patient may ask you to turn on the light or position the window blinds. Within minutes after you leave the room, the patient signals again. Patients who display this type of behavior are often lonely and scared. They may be using the call signal to get attention. An effective approach is to tell the patient what time you will return when you leave the room. Be sure to return at that time. Keeping your word shows the patient you can be trusted. Stop by the room and check on the patient as often as you can. When the patient knows she can depend on you to check on her regularly, unnecessary use of the call signal will gradually decrease.

This simple example shows how the ABCs of behavior management are used effectively. In this case:

A, or antecedent, is the patient's loneliness and fear.

B, or behavior, is using the call signal frequently for requests that seem unimportant to you.

C, or consequence, is attention and companionship when you are in the room.

By checking on the patient frequently and keeping your promise to return, you have changed the consequences. You are already providing companionship and attention regularly. This eases the patient's loneliness and fear, so there is no reason for her to continue the problem behavior.

In the preceding examples, the consequences were modified to change the behavior. Sometimes the antecedent must be changed. For example, a mentally confused patient is quiet all day, but begins to scream every night at bedtime after you have done H.S. care. You discover that she stops screaming when you enter the room and turn on the light. When it is dark, the patient is frightened. Leaving a light on in the room or bathroom will cause the patient to stop screaming.

Role of the PCT in Assisting with Behavior Management Programs. If a patient demonstrates a behavior problem, members of the interdisciplinary team will develop a care plan for all team members to use. If you have identified a possible cause for the problem behavior, or know of an effective approach, inform the supervisor. It is very important to include this information in the care plan, which is based on the patient's individual strengths and needs. Behavior management is a form of restorative care, so the principles of restoration are followed. The plan may have to be modified several times, depending on the patient's response. For

> ## General Guidelines for Assisting Patients with Behavior Problems
>
> - Follow the approaches listed on the care plan.
> - Maintain control of your own responses and reactions.
> - Remove the irritant or cause of the behavior, if possible.
> - Protect the safety of the patient and others in the environment.
> - If the care plan calls for you to respond when a patient demonstrates a specific behavior, implement the approaches at the first sign of distress. Do not wait for the patient to lose control.
> - Use good communication and listening skills.
> - Practice empathy.
> - Attempt to learn the cause of the behavior and communicate this information to other team members.
> - Communicate effective approaches to other team members.
> - Monitor the patient's response to your approaches. Adjust your approach if necessary.
> - Discuss family, friends, or other pleasant information with patients. This can provide a source of strength and support.
> - Make sure that the patient's physical needs are met.
> - For alert patients, give as much control as possible. Offer choices in care and routines.

■ **consistent:** *same; approaches to care that are the same with all care providers*

the plan to be effective, all team members must be **consistent** in their approaches to the patient.

Implementing the Behavior Management Plan. After the care plan has been developed, become familiar with it and implement the approaches listed. Your objective observations of the patient's response to the plan are important and should be reported to the supervisor. The plan may call for you to modify your own behavior in response to the patient's behavior. Appropriate patient behavior is usually reinforced or rewarded. If the behavior is rewarded, the patient tends to repeat it. Verbal praise, positive feedback, and other signs of approval are rewards. Nonverbal reinforcement, such as a hug, smile, or pat on the back, may also be used. Sometimes snacks and privileges are used as rewards.

The care plan will describe how to reduce the patient's inappropriate behavior. Sometimes this is done by ignoring the behavior, if it is safe to do so. Other non-punitive responses may also be used as specified in the care plan. The goal is not to punish the patient, but to show her a more positive way of directing her energy.

Assisting Patients with Specific Behavior Problems

It is hard to make generalizations about behavior management, because each person is a unique individual. However, certain conditions are often seen in patients in health care facilities. The general care you provide to patients with these conditions is similar. Always follow the care plan for specific patient information, goals, and approaches.

Depression. Depression may occur because of stress and loss, but sometimes it occurs for unknown reasons. The signs and symptoms of depression vary widely. Decreased concentration, memory loss, fatigue, insomnia, sadness, crying, loss of appetite, overeating, apathy, and loss of self-esteem are all symptoms of depression.

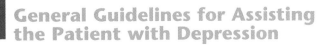

General Guidelines for Assisting the Patient with Depression

- Be honest, supportive, and caring with the patient.
- Be a good listener (Figure 17-2). Encourage the patient to express feelings. Do not pass judgment or criticize. Avoid interrupting or changing the subject.
- Give positive feedback on the patient's strengths and successes.
- Do not make comments like, "Cheer up. Things could be worse."
- Encourage physical activity as stated on the plan of care.
- Monitor the patient's appetite and report over- or undereating to the supervisor.
- Report changes in behavior or talk of suicide to the supervisor immediately.

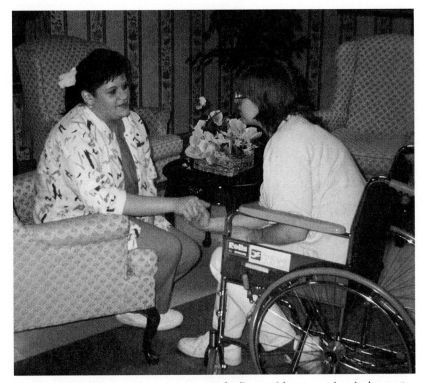

Figure 17-2 Allow patients to express feelings without passing judgment.

Sleep Disturbances. Sleep problems may be related to physical, emotional, or environmental causes. Some patients complain of being unable to sleep. Others appear to sleep all the time. Look for causes of the sleep disturbance, such as excessive caffeine intake, pain, fear, anxiety, room temperature, or noise.

Complaining, Demanding Behavior. Listening to patient complaints requires a great deal of tact. Sometimes patient complaints are justified, but at times they are not. Listen objectively to what the patient says. Report the information to the supervisor objectively. If the complaint is about something simple that you can correct, do so immediately.

Yelling and Screaming. Yelling and screaming may be the only way the patient can communicate or express displeasure. Most screaming behavior is seen in confused patients, but occasionally alert patients also yell and scream. Dealing with this type of behavior is done by trial and error.

General Guidelines for Assisting the Patient with Sleep Problems

- Offer H.S. care by making the patient comfortable, giving a back rub, controlling room temperature, adjusting the lights, and eliminating noise in the environment.
- If the patient wakes up frightened during the night, provide support and reassurance. Make her comfortable.
- If the patient wakes up confused, provide orientation to person, place, and time.
- If the patient wants to stay awake during the night, provide diversional activities and comfort measures that will not disturb others.

General Guidelines for Assisting the Patient with Complaining/Demanding Behavior

- Reassure the patient that you understand the complaint or problem and will report it to the appropriate person.
- Use good listening skills and support the patient.
- If the complaints are about care, remain neutral and do not criticize other workers. If the complaints are about your care, listen but do not argue or become defensive.
- Attempt to determine the cause of unjustified complaints and correct it, if possible.
- Give the patient as much control as possible. For example, ask the patient what time he would like to have his bath or other care.
- Offer the patient choices when possible. Offering choices gives the patient control and shows that you respect him as a person and value his opinion.

General Guidelines for Assisting the Patient Who Is Yelling/Calling Out

- Look for the cause of the behavior. If you can identify it, correct it.
- If the patient is alert, ask what the problem is. Use your listening skills and provide comfort.
- Realize that screaming with pain and grief is socially acceptable in the some patients' cultures.
- Offer the patient something to eat or drink.
- Monitor body language to see if the patient grimaces or shows other signs of pain.
- Try to distract the patient.
- Provide physical comfort measures, such as turning, positioning, or a back rub.

General Guidelines for Assisting the Aggressive Patient

- Attempt to identify the cause of the behavior and eliminate it, if possible.
- Respect the patient's need for personal space.
- Take physical threats seriously and keep your distance.
- Remain calm.
- Do not make the patient feel trapped or cornered.
- Do not turn your back on the patient.
- Avoid touching the patient, as this may cause further agitation.
- Reassure the patient. Do not argue or try to reason with the patient.
- Monitor your body language to be sure it is not threatening.
- If aggressive behavior occurs in a public area, move the patient if it is safe to do so. If not, move others out of the way.
- Call for assistance from others, if necessary.

■ *combative behavior:*
physically aggressive behavior such as hitting, kicking, scratching, or biting

Physical or Verbal Aggression. *Physical aggression* is hitting, scratching, kicking, biting, or fighting. This is often called **combative behavior**. *Verbal aggression* is arguing, accusing, threatening, or swearing. The patient usually does this loudly, using an angry tone of voice.

Sexual Behavior. All human beings need sexuality. Sexuality does not diminish with age (Figure 17-3). Sexual expression may be physical or psychological. Sexuality is a basic human need, according to Maslow. Always knock before entering a patient's room and wait for a response before entering.

Many health care workers feel that masturbation is inappropriate behavior. Masturbation is not harmful and is satisfying to the patient. It is an acceptable behavior as long as it is done in a private area. If you enter a patient's room and find the patient masturbating, provide privacy and leave the room.

If you enter a room and find two consenting adults engaged in a sexual act, provide privacy and leave. Adults have a legal right to do whatever is pleasing to them, as long as it is not medically contraindicated and both partners are mentally capable of consent. Do not pass judgment on the patient's choice of partner or methods of sexual expression.

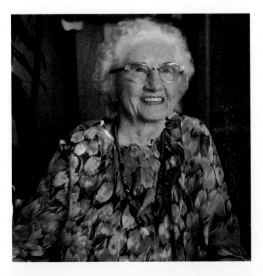

Figure 17-3 An attractive appearance is a way of maintaining sexuality.

■ *sexual abuse:* *forcing a patient to perform a sexual act*

Health care facility staff is responsible for protecting patients who are physically or mentally vulnerable to unwanted sexual contact. Sexual contact with unwilling, alert patients who are physically unable to defend themselves, or with confused patients who cannot give full informed consent, is sexual abuse. Sexual abuse is a violation of patient rights and is illegal. No health care worker, visitor, or other patient can sexually abuse others. Anyone who sexually harasses or abuses a patient or care provider should be reported to the supervisor or other appropriate person, according to your facility policy. If sexual abuse occurs, the police are notified.

Sometimes patients may make unwanted sexual advances toward care providers. Humans have a normal need to express sexuality. Realize that although the desire for sexuality is normal, the choice of person is not appropriate. Be certain your actions or words do not suggest or encourage this type of behavior. However, if a patient does make sexual advances, do not ridicule or belittle the patient. Be patient and understanding, but let the patient know tactfully that the behavior is not acceptable. Follow your facility policy for reporting sexual advances.

COGNITIVE IMPAIRMENT

Cognitive impairment means damaged or impaired thinking. It can have many causes, including disease, trauma, alcohol, street drugs, prescription medications, and anesthesia. It is not a normal part of aging. Functional changes in self-care ability are often the first sign of cognitive impairment. Patients gradually become unable to recognize familiar faces, objects, or surroundings. They lose the ability to learn new information. Decision-making ability is also affected. The most common symptoms are memory loss, mental confusion, and poor judgment (Figure 17-4). In early stages of cognitive loss, the patient often realizes that there is a problem. She may spend a tremendous amount of energy trying to hide the memory loss. If she cannot remember something, she makes up a story. Treatment is supportive. Safety is always a primary concern. Care is designed to maintain the patient's abilities—but avoid placing too many demands on the patient, which cause stress. Appropriate care of patients with cognitive impairment centers on maintaining their quality of life, functional abilities, and dignity.

Dementia

■ *dementia:* *a set of symptoms affecting the patient's thinking, judgment, memory, and ability to reason*

Dementia is a mental disorder that causes cognitive impairment. It can be acute or chronic. Dementia is not a disease. It occurs as the result of some diseases and medical conditions. It is a set of symptoms affecting the patient's thinking, judgment, memory, and ability to reason. Patients with dementia have a progressive decline in mental function. The rights of patients with dementia are the same as those of alert patients, but the care provider may need to assist the patient to exercise these rights.

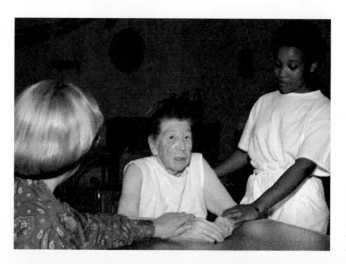

Figure 17-4 The cognitively impaired patient may not be aware of person, place, or time.

Delirium

 delirium: *an acute confusional state indicative of a treatable illness*

Delirium is an acute confusional state that is an indication of a treatable illness. There are many causes, including medications and drugs, fever, isolation, depression, use of restraints, recent relocation, and dehydration. The most

---

General Guidelines for Caring for Patients with Dementia

- Be calm, gentle, and flexible in your approach to the patient.
- Approach the patient by being matter-of-fact and non-demanding.
- Speak in a "here and now" time frame.
- If the patient is not agitated, use touch to show you care.
- Speak slowly and clearly, using short, simple sentences and words.
- Offer simple choices, but do not overwhelm the patient with options. Best results are obtained if you ask the patient to select one of two choices.
- Break each large task down into a series of smaller tasks.
- Give the patient familiar, orienting cues for performing ADLs.
- Follow the same routine each day.
- If the patient does not understand your instructions, demonstrate what you are trying to say. For example, put the brush in the patient's hand. Simulate brushing your hair and tell the patient to imitate you.
- Use good eye contact.
- Make sure your body language matches your words.
- Use one-step commands. If the patient does not respond, count to five before repeating. After the patient completes one step, move to the next.
- Allow adequate time for the patient to complete a task. Avoid rushing the patient.
- Avoid words such as "don't," or "no," whenever possible. Instead use words like "do," or "let's."
- Alternate periods of activity with rest periods.
- Monitor for signs of increasing frustration or anxiety.
- Accept communication that does not make sense. Do not argue with the patient. For example, the patient tells you that her mother ate lunch with her. A good response is, "Are you thinking about your mother?"
- Concentrate on what the patient is telling you, even if it does not seem sensible. Respond positively to what you think the patient is saying.
- Do not argue with the patient about fixed, false beliefs.
- Avoid situations that you know are upsetting to the patient.
- Keep the environment simple.
- Maintain a safe environment. Do not make changes in the environment unnecessarily.
- Provide activities at the time of day the activity would normally be done.
- Reduce excessive noise and stimulation in the environment.

common causes are infection and circulatory, respiratory, and metabolic disorders. Often two or three different causes contribute to the delirium. If one cause is eliminated, the delirium will remain until all contributing factors have been discovered and eliminated. Delirium is characterized by changing states of consciousness, disorganization, mental disorientation, behavioral changes, and lack of awareness of the environment. It usually develops quickly, over several hours or several days. Rapid development of symptoms is a key indicator that there is an underlying medical problem, compared with dementia, which develops gradually over a much longer period of time. When the treatable medical condition is managed properly, the patient's mental status clears. This may occur quickly or take several weeks.

■ *disorientation: lack of awareness of person, place, or time*

Sensory Losses

Sensory losses often produce signs of cognitive impairment. The problem is worsened if the patient has an existing dementia. If the patient cannot see, hear, feel, or otherwise communicate with others and the environment, he may appear cognitively impaired. Besides the inability to communicate with others, the patient may misinterpret noises, people, or other images. This may cause him to have behavior problems. Sometimes simple measures, such as putting the patient's glasses on or using the hearing aid, are enough to improve the condition.

■ *sensory losses: difficulty seeing, hearing, smelling, or touching*

Observing the Patient

Careful assessment and observation of the patient by the interdisciplinary team is necessary to differentiate these conditions. Sometimes delirium, medical problems, or sensory losses worsen existing dementia. Because the patient care technician spends more time with the patient than other team members, your observational skills are very important in patients with mental confusion. Small, seemingly minor changes may be important. Sometimes we think that certain behaviors are "normal for the patient." For example, each night when you give a patient H.S. care, the patient hits and fights. You accept this as normal for that patient, complete your care, and continue your assignment. Because you are the only person in the room with the patient, others may not know of this behavior. The behavior is not normal and may be important. Report your observations of the patient's physical and mental status to the supervisor and be alert for changes. Some health care facilities keep a log of behaviors so they can study the time of day, type of behavior, and triggering events. This helps to determine if there is a pattern to the behavior.

■■■ ALZHEIMER'S DISEASE

Alzheimer's disease is the most common form of dementia. The cause of it is unknown, but it is believed that heredity plays a significant role in its development. Most cases of Alzheimer's disease occur in patients over the age of 65, but it can occur in middle-aged individuals. Alzheimer's disease causes physical and chemical changes in the brain. The brain atrophies. In muscles, atrophy is preventable, but this is not true of the brain. The disease causes progressive deterioration and is eventually fatal, though some individuals may live up to 20 years with the disease. Their physical health may be excellent in the early stages, but declines as the disease progresses. Some medications will improve the symptoms, but there is no cure.

■ *Alzheimer's disease: an incurable disease that causes loss of mental abilities and judgment*

Three Stages of Alzheimer's Disease

Persons with Alzheimer's disease go through three stages. Each stage brings progressively worse physical and mental problems. Eventually, all cognitive ability is lost. Initially, the patient can perform normal activities of daily living with verbal cues and reminders, but over time the patient becomes totally dependent on others.

Stage I: Mild Dementia. Patients in the first stage of Alzheimer's appear normal and can function with minimum assistance and supervision. The changes in this stage are in memory and personality, and include:

- Short-term memory loss
- Long-term memory retention
- Personality changes
- Indifference and apathy
- Not being outgoing and/or being generally uninterested in life
- Decreased attention span
- Decreased concentration
- Poor judgment; making bad decisions
- Lack of awareness of time
- Forgetting to eat and drink
- Moodiness
- Blaming others for mistakes and problems
- Disorientation as to location; inability to remember how to get home
- **Delusions of persecution**
- Carelessness
- Unkempt appearance
- Anxiety, agitation, and depression

Stage II: Moderate Dementia. In the second stage of illness, short-term memory continues to decline. Long-term memory loss becomes apparent. All the symptoms from the first stage continue. The person initially continues to be in good physical health. Other symptoms are:

- Loss of control over impulses and behavior
- Complete disorientation
- Inability to recognize danger
- Restlessness
- Wandering and pacing
- **Sundowning**
- Sensory and perceptual changes that cause the person to be unable to differentiate hot and cold, left and right, up or down. The ability to recognize common items such as silverware or grooming items is lost.
- Loss of ability to perform learned motor skills, such as eating, dressing, and toileting
- Gradual loss of ability to follow directions
- **Perseveration**
- Difficulty speaking, reading, and writing
- Gradual loss of ability to understand others
- Walking and motor problems; gradually develops a shuffling gait
- Incontinence of bowel and bladder
- **Hallucinating** and having **delusions**
- **Catastrophic reactions**

Stage III: Severe Dementia. The patient in stage III of Alzheimer's disease is totally dependent on others for care and develops severe physical problems. The ability to swallow is progressively lost, and the patient is at high risk for choking and aspiration. The patient becomes bedfast and unable to sit in a chair or walk. Seizures may be present. The patient progresses to coma

- **delusions of persecution:** *thinking that others are trying to cause personal harm*

- **sundowning:** *increased restlessness and confusion in the late afternoon, evening, and night*

- **perseveration:** *repetitious behavior, speech, movements, or actions*

- **hallucinating:** *seeing, hearing, or feeling something that is not real*
- **delusions:** *false beliefs*
- **catastrophic reactions:** *uncontrolled emotional outbursts in response to feeling completely overwhelmed or fearful; may include crying, sudden mood changes, anger, and combative behavior*

and death. Other signs and symptoms of the third stage of Alzheimer's disease are:

- Complete mental disorientation as to time, place, and person
- Complete loss of ability to communicate
- Inability to recognize family, friends, and care providers
- Total dependence on others for care
- Resistance to care
- Refusal to eat
- Sleep disturbances

COMMUNICATION

Good communication skills are necessary when caring for patients with Alzheimer's disease and other dementias. Try to talk to the patient in an area that is free from distractions. These patients have lost the ability to screen out distractions and noises from television, radio, or other conversations. Begin your conversation socially to win the patient's trust. One way of doing this is to sit and talk before beginning patient care. Begin your conversation with orienting information. Call the patient by name and tell her who you are. After the patient is relaxed, explain what you are going to do. Make eye contact with the patient and be sure you have her attention before beginning to speak. If the patient ignores you, wait a minute and try again. Gently touch the patient's arm to get her attention. However, avoid startling the patient, as this can cause a catastrophic reaction. Try to sit at the patient's eye level when you speak. Speak slowly and clearly, using short, simple sentences. Ask questions that require only a yes-or-no answer. Use concrete terms and familiar words. Keep your tone of voice low, and speak in a calm, warm, pleasant manner.

When performing ADL care, try to focus on familiar skills and tasks. Although the patient probably cannot learn new information, he may be able to do familiar tasks. Give the patient control by offering one of two choices. Allow enough time for the patient to process the information. If your instructions are not understood, repeat them in exactly the same way. If the instructions are still not understood, try demonstrating what you want the patient to do. Break the task down into small, simple steps. Telling the patient to "take a bath" may be overwhelming. Start by telling the patient to wash his face. After he has completed this task, instruct him in the next step. Sincerely compliment the patient for success.

Sometimes you may have difficulty understanding what the patient is telling you. Listen actively and carefully. If you do not understand, apologize and ask the patient to repeat. If you do understand, repeat what the patient says or use paraphrasing. Try to focus on a word or phrase that you understand. Repeat what you do understand and help the patient clarify it. Respond to the emotional tone of the statement. For example, say, "You sound very angry." Try to stay calm and patient. If the patient repeats certain words, ask family members if they know the meaning. Sometimes people with Alzheimer's talk by using "code" words that close friends and family understand.

Avoid arguing with the patient. Arguing always makes the situation worse. Such patients have lost the ability to reason. Do not tell the patient what she can and cannot do. Instead, use distraction. The patient may say "I'm going home to cook dinner for my children." You know that her children are grown and do not live at home. Instead of arguing with the patient, ask what she likes to cook. Then distract her by asking her to sit with you and look at a magazine. Avoid asking the patient many questions that require a good memory. People with dementia recognize that they have memory loss and feel humiliated and frustrated when they cannot remember. Do not talk about patients with dementia in front of them. We do not know what they understand, and their understanding changes from one moment to the next.

Special Problems

Alzheimer's disease is frustrating for the patient, family, and care provider. Remember, the patient is not responsible for the symptoms of the disease. Some patients say unkind things, hit, or act aggressively. The disease has triggered the problem. Because the disease also causes poor impulse control, the patient is powerless to do anything to correct the behavior. Caring for patients with Alzheimer's disease requires patience and understanding.

Catastrophic reactions occur as a result of being startled or in response to overwhelming stimulation. Anger and rage are often signs that the patient is feeling loss of control. The patient cannot control the reaction. Catastrophic reactions are marked by increased agitation and physical activity. The patient may talk, yell, or mumble. Sometimes the behavior is explosive and violent. The best way to deal with catastrophic reactions is to anticipate and prevent them. Monitor the patient's behavior closely and watch for signs of increasing restlessness or agitation. Minimize noise and confusion in the environment. Make sure the patient's physical needs are met. If a catastrophic reaction occurs, do not attempt to reason with the patient. Avoid restraints and use of physical force. Approach the patient using a soft, calm, but firm voice. Touching the patient may worsen the reaction. Remove the patient from the stressful situation, if possible. Distraction may be effective. In a calm voice, instruct the patient to calm down. Avoid responding with anger and hostility. Make every effort to calm the patient down by speaking calmly and listening to what the patient says.

If you feel that your physical safety is threatened during a catastrophic reaction, stand out of the patient's reach. Call for help. Avoid having many care providers approach the patient at one time, as this can make the patient feel trapped or cornered. Watch the patient's eyes. The patient will usually stare at the person or body part that will be attacked. Protect yourself according to your facility policy.

Problems with Bathing. Many patients with Alzheimer's disease are resistive to bathing. This may be because the patient has forgotten the purpose of bathing. Because perception to hot and cold is lost, bathing may be uncomfortable. The patient may fear the water, be fearful of washing, or find the mechanics of taking a bath too overwhelming. The patient may also be sensitive with an unfamiliar care provider, or may be modest and uncomfortable undressing in front of you.

Try making the bath schedule flexible to accommodate the patient's mood. Avoid forcing the patient. Leave and try again later if the patient refuses. Make sure the room is warm and private. Let the patient feel the water before you begin the bath. Saying something like "This feels good" may be helpful. Explain what you are going to do and what you want the patient to do, one step at a time. If you will be giving the patient a complete bath, giving the patient a washcloth or other object to manipulate may be helpful. Noise from an institutional whirlpool bath may frighten the patient. Washing the hair in the shower may also frighten the patient. Guide your actions and care according to the patient's responses.

Dressing Problems. Some patients are resistive to dressing. Others remove their clothing after they are dressed. Keep the morning routine consistent and familiar. Avoid delays or interruptions because the patient may forget the activity. Make sure the room is warm and private. Lay out clothing in the order in which it will be put on. Give the patient simple instructions and assist her to dress if needed. Make sure you do only one step at a time. Praise the patient and compliment her appearance.

If the patient removes clothing, understand that she is not doing this deliberately. Evaluate the situation and correct problems through trial and error. Is the patient dressed too warmly? Does she need to use the bathroom? Is she tired and ready for bed? Is she bored? Modifying these factors may solve the problem.

Problems with Wandering. Wandering is a very serious concern for health care providers. Patients who wander within the health care facility may become lost or injured. Patients who wander outside the facility are in danger of being hit by a car, overexposure to heat and cold, and other harmful or dangerous situations. Allowing the patient to wander in a safe area is the best approach to take. Consider physical causes for the wandering, such as pain, thirst, hunger, or looking for the bathroom. Decrease noise levels in the environment. Approach the patient from the front, then walk with the patient by falling in step at her side. If the patient leaves the unit or goes outside, walk with her and circle back in. Use distraction with food, drink, or activity. Monitor the patient for signs of fatigue and encourage her to get adequate rest. Many techniques are used to keep wanderers safe. Most important, wanderers require supervision and understanding. Restraints should be used only as a last resort.

KEY POINTS IN CHAPTER

- *All behavior has a meaning, even if the meaning is not evident to you.*
- *Losses and unmet needs affect patients' behavior.*
- *Physical and chemical restraints are treatments of last resort in the management of behavior problems.*
- *When using the ABC method of behavior management, modifying the antecedent or consequences will change the behavior.*
- *Consistency is important to the success of a behavior management program.*
- *Cognitive impairment has many causes and is not a normal part of aging.*
- *Safety is a primary concern when caring for patients with cognitive impairment and dementia.*
- *Delirium is a reversible condition with medical causes.*
- *Sensory losses may mimic cognitive impairment or worsen existing dementia.*
- *Alzheimer's disease causes atrophy of the brain and progressive mental deterioration.*

REVIEW QUIZ

Multiple Choice Questions

1. Causes of behavior problems may be:
   a. physical.
   b. mental.
   c. social.
   d. all of the above.

2. A cognitively impaired patient yells and screams loudly when she is in bed. A good first step in managing this behavior is:
   a. applying a restraint.
   b. asking the supervisor to give the patient a tranquilizer.
   c. attempting to learn the cause of the behavior.
   d. isolating the patient.

3. When an alert patient displays a behavior problem, it may be in response to:
   a. unmet psychosocial needs.
   b. cognitive impairment.
   c. dementia.
   d. delirium.

4. Defense mechanisms are:
   a. means of defending yourself against physical assault.
   b. a response to stress, loss, or unmet needs.
   c. medical problems.
   d. all of the above.

5. Projection is:
   a. refusing to admit there is a problem.
   b. placing the blame for a problem on someone else.
   c. overachieving in one area to overcome a weakness.
   d. making excuses for a problem.

6. According to the ABC method of behavior management:
   a. "A" is an abbreviation for anger.
   b. "A" is an abbreviation for anxiety.
   c. "B" is an abbreviation for behavior.
   d. "C" is an abbreviation for control.

7. When caring for patients with behavior problems:
   a. adjust your approach to the patient according to the patient's response.
   b. make sure the patient's physical needs are met.
   c. implement the behavior care plan at the first sign of distress.
   d. all of the above.

8. Masturbation is:
   a. acceptable if done in private.
   b. always inappropriate.
   c. harmful to the patient.
   d. an indication that the patient is homosexual.

9. Sexual abuse is:
   a. acceptable if done by the patient's spouse.
   b. acceptable if a confused patient consents.
   c. unwanted sexual contact.
   d. all of the above.

10. Causes of stress and agitation in cognitively impaired patients include:
    a. noise and confusion in the environment.
    b. placing too many demands on the patient.
    c. sensory losses.
    d. all of the above.

11. Dementia:
    a. is a psychiatric disorder.
    b. has social causes.
    c. is the result of mental illness.
    d. none of the above.

12. Delirium:
    a. is a mental illness.
    b. is caused by reversible medical problems.
    c. is a sign of cognitive impairment.
    d. none of the above.

13. Sundowning is:
    a. increased agitation when the patient is put to bed.
    b. restlessness early in the morning.
    c. increased restlessness in the late afternoon and evening.
    d. a form of combative behavior.

14. Perceptual changes caused by Alzheimer's disease include:
    a. inability to differentiate left from right.
    b. loss of sense of smell.
    c. deterioration in vision.
    d. all of the above.

True/False Questions

15. ___ A person's job provides a sense of identity.

16. ___ Patients who are cognitively impaired may display abnormal behavior in response to too much stimulation in the environment.

17. ___ Modifying the behavior changes the antecedent.

18. ___ When managing behavior problems, all care providers should use different approaches with the patient.

19. ___ Cognitive impairment is a normal part of aging.

20. ___ Safety is a primary concern when managing behavior problems and caring for patients with cognitive impairment and dementia.

21. ___ When caring for patients with dementia, assume that they can do nothing for themselves and provide total care.

22. ___ Patients with Alzheimer's disease may be afraid of being bathed.

23. ___ Patients in the late stage of Alzheimer's disease may lose the ability to swallow.

24. ___ Wanderers should always be restrained for their own safety.

25. ___ Patients with Alzheimer's disease can easily remember something you told them an hour ago.

SURVEY READINESS AND EMPLOYMENT INFORMATION

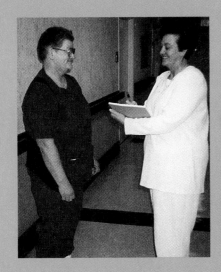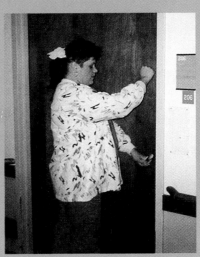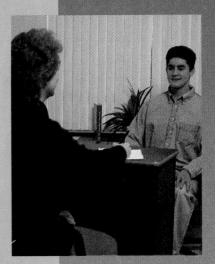

Surviving a Survey

THE SURVEY PROCESS

license: a state permit allowing the health care facility to operate

certification: an inspection process for facilities that accept state or federal funds as payment for health care

survey: a review and evaluation of a health care facility to ensure that the agency is maintaining acceptable standards

surveyor: a representative of a private or governmental agency who reviews health care facility policies, procedures, and practices

Health Care Financing Administration (HCFA): a governmental agency that sets policy and administers payment of Medicare and Medicaid money to health care facilities

accreditation: a process that health care facilities participate in voluntarily to ensure that high standards of care are maintained.

Health care facilities must meet certain quality standards to operate. Many different private and public agencies establish quality standards for health care facilities. Different types of facilities meet different levels of quality inspection standards. The health care facility holds a state license permitting it to conduct business. Some facilities also possess the certification necessary to collect Medicare and Medicaid money.

Licensure and certification surveys are done by the state health department or human service agency. A survey is a review and evaluation to ensure that facilities are maintaining acceptable standards of practice. Sometimes surveyors from the Health Care Financing Administration (HCFA) conduct the survey. This agency is a division of the federal government with regulatory authority over health care facilities that receive federal money.

Many facilities are also accredited. Accreditation is a voluntary process that health care facilities undergo to ensure they are meeting high quality standards. Gaining accreditation is difficult. There is a high degree of prestige in becoming accredited because facilities must meet such high standards. Some insurance companies will not pay medical bills from unaccredited health care facilities.

Many different governmental and private agencies survey health care facilities. Surveyors review every area of the health care facility. They observe patient care, staff preparation and training, recordkeeping, infection control, food preparation, and facility cleanliness. They also review facility policies and procedures. The purpose of a survey is to review the quality of care. In long-term care facilities, quality of life and resident rights are also reviewed. Surveys identify specific areas in which care is deficient. Surveyors are instructed not to be consultants to the facility. They are responsible for identifying deficient practices. The facility is responsible for finding ways to correct the problems noted.

In addition to licensure, certification, and accreditation visits, the Occupational Safety and Health Administration (OSHA) also surveys health care facilities. OSHA's mission is to protect the health and safety of employees. OSHA inspectors review infection control, isolation practices, employee tuberculin testing, material safety data sheets, and other policies and facility practices designed to protect the employee. The OSHA survey process involves interviews with employees, during which the inspector will ask questions about facility health and safety practices. OSHA inspectors will make recommendations for correcting unsafe conditions. If the inspector notes dangerous or unsafe conditions during the survey, the agency may receive a **citation** or fine. The employer must post the written report of each citation at or near the place the violation occurred for three days, or until the unsafe condition is corrected.

So many agencies survey health care facilities that it is impossible to prepare for a survey. Most surveyors arrive at the health care facility unannounced. Laws provide severe penalties or jail terms for individuals who alert the facility to an impending licensure, certification, or OSHA survey. Surveyors want to see patient care and facility routines on a normal day. Some accrediting bodies notify the health care facility of the survey dates several weeks in advance. However, many other surveys are completely unannounced. Knowing this, we must be survey-ready every day. This means that care is delivered in the manner in which you were taught and good infection control techniques are practiced routinely. Infection control problems are a major cause of **deficiencies** in health care facility surveys. Surveyors receive a great deal of training in infection control so they can easily identify deficiencies in this area. The reason so much emphasis is placed on infection prevention practices is because the spread of infection to patients, visitors, and workers has serious consequences.

Upon completion of a survey, surveyors conduct an **exit conference**. The health care facility is given the survey agency's findings. A formal written report is mailed to the facility after the survey. This report lists the deficiencies the facility receives. Most states require facilities to post this report in a prominent location. Facilities have a specified amount of time to correct deficiencies. They must submit a written **plan of correction** to the survey agency. The plan must state what will be done to correct the deficiencies, who will make the correction, who will monitor the deficient area, and how similar deficiencies will be prevented in the future. If deficiencies are severe, actual harm has occurred to a patient, or the potential for serious harm to patients exists, measures are taken against the facility license, certification, or accreditation. Some agencies fine the facility heavily if care is not up to the standards, or if dangers to patients or employees exist. Survey agencies can also issue a probationary license or even revoke facility approval. The fines can be as high as $10,000 per day in long-term care facilities. Facility payment for Medicare and Medicaid recipients may be withheld. Long-term care facilities can lose their approval to conduct nursing assistant training because of a negative survey. Unfavorable surveys have caused some long-term care facilities to close. JCAHO-approved facilities can lose their accreditation. Because accreditation is so closely related to the reimbursement process, insurers will not pay the facility for its services. Some agencies have gone out of business because of loss of accreditation. Some OSHA surveys in health care facilities have resulted in fines of $100,000 or more.

Role of the Patient Care Technician During a Survey

The patient care technician has many important responsibilities in providing direct patient care. View the survey as a positive experience, an opportunity for you to demonstrate work well done. Surveyors will observe your care and may ask you questions. You would feel terrible if your actions resulted in facility punishment, loss of approval, or fines. The best way to prevent this from happening is to take your responsibilities very seriously, follow all facility policies, and always perform procedures the way you were taught. It is easier to develop and use good habits daily than it is to correct deficient practices at the time of a survey. When you know surveyors are in your facility, smile and say hello to them (Figure 18-1) if you pass them in the hallway. Surveyors are guests in your facility and should be treated as such. If a surveyor asks you a particular patient's name,

citation: *a written notice that informs the health care agency of alleged violations of OSHA rules and the time frame within which the condition(s) must be corrected*

deficiency: *a written notice of inadequate care or a substandard practice*

exit conference: *a meeting between surveyors and facility administration upon completion of a survey to discuss the surveyors' findings and the nature of deficiencies*

plan of correction: *a written plan submitted by the health care agency in response to survey findings of deficiency; the plan lists what corrections will be made, by whom, who will monitor the correction, and what will be done to prevent similar deficiencies in the future*

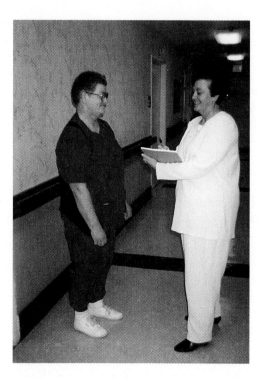

Figure 18-1 Welcome surveyors as you would other guests in the facility.

inform the supervisor. Asking for the name indicates that surveyors are watching some aspect of the patient's care.

SURVEYS FOR FACILITIES HOLDING A LONG-TERM CARE LICENSE

Many different types of agencies are licensed as long-term care facilities. Agencies that may be licensed for long-term care are freestanding nursing homes and rehabilitation centers, skilled units and swing bed units in hospitals, subacute centers, and skilled nursing facilities. Long-term care facilities receive a regular licensure (and certification, if applicable) visit every 9 to 15 months. Surveyors may also visit the facility periodically to evaluate the care that Medicaid recipients receive. This survey is commonly called *inspection of care*. Surveyors return after an annual survey to see if corrections have been made. They also visit facilities in response to complaint calls from residents and families. Long-term care facilities are required to post the state complaint line number (Figure 18-2) in a visible location so residents and family members can call if they are dissatisfied with care.

Because of the many different types of surveys in long-term care, most facilities have two or more surveys a year. Surveyors come to the long-term care facility unannounced and spend several days to a week. The length of time spent in the facility is determined by facility size and the nature of deficiencies noted during the first few days of the visit. If the facility is very large or if the deficiencies are severe, the surveyors will remain in the facility for a longer period of time. When surveyors remain in the facility longer than originally anticipated, this is known as an **extended survey**. During an extended survey, surveyors will examine deficient areas in great detail to determine if a danger to patients exists.

When surveyors arrive at the facility, they usually conduct an **entrance conference** with facility administration. They inform management of the reason for the survey and the nature of any complaints received. If the survey is in response to a complaint, they do not identify the person who registered the complaint. One surveyor may conduct the entrance conference while others go directly to the nursing units to make rounds and observe care. Splitting into

■ **extended survey:** *a survey that lasts longer than originally anticipated so surveyors can examine patient care and facility practices in greater detail*

■ **entrance conference:** *a meeting between surveyors and facility administration to discuss the purpose of a survey; conducted at the beginning of a survey*

NURSING HOME

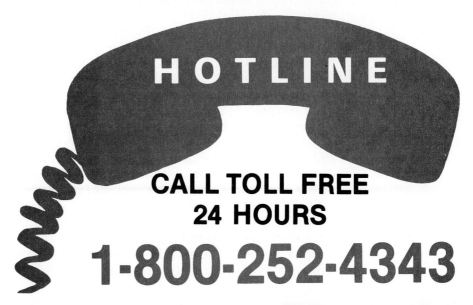

HOTLINE

CALL TOLL FREE
24 HOURS

1-800-252-4343

If you have a complaint concerning this long-term care facility, you may discuss it with the administrator or a person designated by the administrator to discuss complaints. If this does not resolve your complaint, you have the right to contact the Illinois Department of Public Health's Nursing Home Hotline, 1-800-252-4343, or you may write

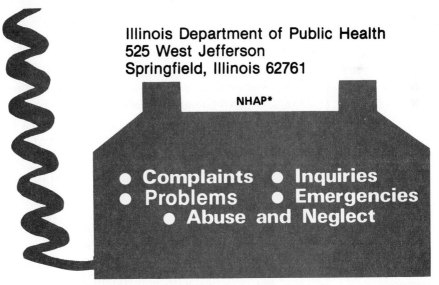

**Illinois Department of Public Health
525 West Jefferson
Springfield, Illinois 62761**

NHAP*

- **Complaints** - **Inquiries**
- **Problems** - **Emergencies**
  - **Abuse and Neglect**

Illinois law requires that all suspected incidents of abuse or neglect shall be reported to the Department of Public Health immediately. (Ill. Rev. Stat. 1983, Ch. 111½, par. 4164).

This information is posted under the authority of Ill. Rev. Stat. 1983, ch. 111½, par. 4153-209(2).

* The Illinois inter-agency Nursing Home Advocacy Program.

Figure 18-2 A sample state complaint line poster

groups like this prevents staff from correcting problems before surveyors arrive on the units to begin the survey. Surveyors want to see the care as it really is on a normal day. There may be very little preparation time from the moment surveyors arrive until they make rounds on the resident care units. This is another reason why you should be survey-ready every day.

During the initial round of the facility, surveyors will make observations of residents and facility conditions. They write down information, then go back and examine certain residents and conditions in greater detail. The first round has a major impact on the survey process. If conditions are not acceptable or problems are suspected, surveyors will immediately go into the extended survey mode.

During the long-term care facility survey, you will be observed while you are providing direct resident care. Surveyors will monitor infection control practices, communication skills, and general facility cleanliness. Your documentation on the medical record will be reviewed. Surveyors also examine incident reports and evaluate how well the staff protects resident rights. Resident quality of life is reviewed to ensure that the staff is meeting both physical and psychological needs. Surveyors will question staff, residents, and families. The OBRA legislation requires long-term care facilities to maintain a homelike environment and accommodate resident needs as much as possible. Surveyors will check to ensure that facilities comply with these requirements. A great emphasis of the survey is an evaluation of how well staff members respect resident rights.

The OBRA survey process is designed to ensure that each resident receives a comprehensive assessment. Care is planned based on this assessment. Risk factors for changes in condition should be identified, anticipated in advance, and avoided whenever possible. Remember that the OBRA legislation requires long-term care facilities to maintain or improve resident conditions unless medical

General Guidelines for Surviving a Long-Term Care Facility Survey

- Know your residents well.
- Know what care is stated on the care plan and deliver it.
- Know facility policies and procedures well and practice them daily.
- Practice good handwashing, standard precautions, medical asepsis, and infection control techniques. Infection control is one of the greatest areas of deficiency in long-term care surveys.
- Use gloves when necessary. Dispose of them according to facility policy, and avoid contaminating environmental surfaces with your gloves.
- Meet the needs of dependent and incontinent residents promptly. Unmet needs are another common area of deficiencies.
- Always try to anticipate problems, such as resident falls, and take measures to prevent them.
- Keep your work area neat and clean at all times.
- Cooperate with your facility **quality assurance** department in pre-survey reviews and audits.
- Communicate with all residents during care, even if the resident has a cognitive impairment. Always explain procedures before you do them.
- Respect all resident rights.
- Give residents as much control over daily routines as possible.
- Know your facility emergency codes, policies, and procedures.
- You can never fully prepare for a survey, so make in-service education a part of your life. The more you learn, the better prepared you are.

■ *quality assurance:* *internal review made by facility staff to identify problems and find solutions for improvement*

complications make this impossible. If residents have suffered declines, this is an indication of problems in the facility. Surveyors will review assessments, care plans, and preventive practices to ensure that residents' conditions have not declined. Surveyors will also evaluate use of restraints, prevention, development, and treatment of pressure sores, resident hygiene and grooming, and correct use of catheters. Staff preparation, training, and in-service records are reviewed.

Another major emphasis of the survey is meal service and food preparation. The entire survey team will observe food preparation and delivery in different areas of the building. Serving food at the proper temperature and providing adequate mealtime assistance are important. Surveyors will monitor pre- and post-meal grooming and hygiene, sanitary food service practices, infection control, and how facility staff care for residents who are incontinent during meals. Surveyors will observe staff feeding residents and will evaluate feeding technique for safety, infection control, and how well staff interacts with the resident during the meal.

The Patient Care Technician's Role During a Long-Term Care Survey

Having surveyors watch you can be very unnerving. Do not call in sick without reason if you know surveyors are in the facility. Trying to replace staff during a survey is stressful for everyone. Facility administration, coworkers, and residents are depending on you, and having a full staff is important. If care providers call in sick, care suffers if replacement workers are not available. Short staffing increases everyone's stress and may cause a negative outcome on the survey. Surveyors will ask you questions about the care you give. They are checking to see if you are following facility policies and procedures. Be proud of your knowledge of the residents, facility policies, and procedures. When a surveyor questions you, remain calm and try to work out why he or she is asking a particular question. Always be honest, but do not volunteer information unrelated to the question. Surveyors generally review resident care plans in advance, so they know if the care you provide is in keeping with the care plan. You must be familiar with the goals and approaches listed on each resident's plan of care.

■■■ JOINT COMMISSION SURVEYS

■ *Joint Commission for Accreditation of Health Care Organizations (JCAHO):* an organization that inspects and accredits health care agencies that meet high quality standards

The **Joint Commission for Accreditation of Healthcare Organizations** (JCAHO) is an agency that inspects and accredits hospitals, nursing homes, home care providers, medical suppliers, ambulance services, and many other health care agencies. JCAHO has very high standards. The Joint Commission evaluates all health care services provided by the organization and makes one accreditation decision and survey report. A health care agency must be prepared to provide evidence of its compliance with each standard. To gain accreditation, a health care facility must demonstrate overall compliance, not necessarily compliance with each individual standard. Participation in the accreditation process is voluntary. The federal government recognizes JCAHO hospital and home health agency accreditation as equivalent to meeting its conditions of participation for Medicare payment. Like other survey agencies, JCAHO inspects all departments of the health care facility. The discussion here applies to all settings in which patient care is delivered.

The JCAHO survey process does not place as much emphasis on observation of the patient care technician as other types of surveys. However, the surveyors will check to see that the overall care delivered is in keeping with established professional standards and infection control guidelines. Maintenance of a safe environment, incident reports, and use of physical and chemical restraints are evaluated to ensure that patient management is in keeping with accepted standards of practice. Emphasis is placed on use of restraint alternatives whenever possible. If patients are in restraints, continuing need for the restraint must be frequently evaluated. Surveyors may question you about emergency fire and disaster codes used in your facility, and about your basic job preparation.

Patient Needs

JCAHO surveyors will determine whether patients receive care that is supervised by a registered nurse and based on a documented assessment of the patient's needs. The assessment must consider the whole person, not just the physical illness. The patient must receive care according to established patient care standards, and may be involved in assessment and care planning if he chooses. The registered nurse must collaborate with other members of the interdisciplinary team to make decisions regarding the patient's care. Teaching the patient about how to live with and manage his medical condition is an important part of the process. Many different care providers are involved in different aspects of the important responsibility of patient teaching. Some teaching is planned by the registered nurse and delivered by the patient care technician.

JCAHO requirements state that care providers should be assigned to care for patients based on identified patient needs and caregiver qualifications, training, and experience. Caregiver qualifications and training are reviewed. Surveyors review the patient's medical record for evidence of assessment, care planning, and quality of services provided. Surveyors also review age-related competencies for patients on each unit.

Facilities are required to develop and maintain policies and procedures based on standards of patient care and nursing practice. Care providers must be familiar with and follow these policies and procedures. The plan for providing patient care must include an internal quality review or evaluation mechanism to identify problems and support improvement. Care provided should be continuously reevaluated by the agency and adjusted to meet patient needs. Surveyors will review facility policies and procedures and determine whether staff is following them. This part of the survey is outcome-oriented and evaluates whether the patient has a positive outcome as a result of the internal quality review process. Emphasis is placed on making sure that health care agency employees followed facility policies and procedures in care of patients.

Staff Requirements

JCAHO standards state that all care providers must be competent in their responsibilities. The health care facility is required to periodically evaluate staff competence and maintain a record of these checks. Staff members must participate in ongoing educational programs, in which their attendance is recorded. Surveyors will check these records to ensure that this requirement is met, and may ask staff members how their competency was evaluated. They may also ask you how you would operate a piece of equipment or perform a procedure.

Accreditation

During the JCAHO survey, the survey team evaluates the level of the health care organization's compliance with the commission's standards. The agency's strengths and weaknesses are identified. Surveyors provide education and consultation throughout the survey. Upon survey completion, a report is issued to the agency. This report details areas in which the agency's performance must improve and includes recommendations for future compliance. If significant issues are identified, accreditation will be awarded upon agreement with the agency to correct the problems promptly. If severe deficiencies are identified, JCAHO will follow up with the agency to assess progress in making corrections.

■■■■ HELPFUL INFORMATION

Many different types of health care agencies employ patient care technicians. It is difficult to provide general rules for doing things correctly in a book that is used in a variety of health care settings. Each health care agency is highly specialized, with specific policies and procedures. Different regulatory agencies survey each type of health care agency. Reviewing your facility-specific policy and procedure manual will provide you with valuable information. Good infection control practices are an emphasis in all health care facility surveys. Infection control and medical asepsis must be practiced regularly to be successful in this area of the survey. Surveyors review patterns of nosocomial infections and other facility practices over the past year to see if there are patterns to nosocomial infections in the facility, which could indicate cross-contamination and inadequate medical asepsis by health care workers. There are many variables. Each care provider should take infection control practices very seriously.

Information You Should Know About Your Health Care Facility

The following is a list of information that can be found in your facility policies, procedures, and orientation information. To deliver patient care in keeping with the standards of the regulatory agencies, follow all policies and learn the answers to these questions for your facility.

- What is the facility's system for patient identification?
- How can you tell the difference between a regular call signal and an emergency signal? How quickly should call signals be answered? Who is responsible for answering signals for patients who are not part of your assignment?
- If you discover a patient in an emergency situation, what is the policy for getting help?
- If you discover a fire, what should you do? How would you prevent smoke from escaping from a room containing a fire? What happens when the fire alarm sounds? Where are the fire extinguishers and emergency exits on your unit? What should you do if you are not on your unit when the fire alarm sounds?
- Where are facility disaster plans located?
- What are your facility fire, disaster, and emergency codes?
- Where are patient care plans located?
- Where are the designated smoking areas, if any, for patients and visitors?
- What are the standard measurements for drinking glasses and other containers in the facility? Where is intake and output recorded? What should you do if the intake or output on your shift appears inadequate?
- How and where do you document what a patient has eaten? What should you do if a patient refuses all or part of a meal?
- In what situations should you complete an incident report?
- What is the proper chain of command in your department?
- What is the facility policy for using restraints? What are the size and application rules for the type of restraints your agency uses?
- What should you do if you suspect that a patient has been abused?
- What are facility policies for separation of clean and soiled items in the patient's room? In other areas of the facility?
- What are the care provider's responsibilities for cleaning utensils, personal care items, and patient care equipment? Where are soiled items cleaned? After cleaning, where are clean items stored?
- What should you do if you find linen that is torn or in poor condition?
- Where is personal protective equipment located? How is it discarded after use?
- Where is biohazardous waste discarded?
- What are facility policies for handling contaminated trash and linen?
- Where are the material safety data sheets located?
- Where is the designated eyewash/body wash station?
- What should you do if you discover broken electrical or mechanical equipment?

PROVIDING CARE THAT COMPLIES WITH ACCEPTED STANDARDS OF PRACTICE

Surveyors may or may not evaluate the care you give. Care involves making observations of the patient's specific condition, the environment, and other factors that influence the patient's well-being. To be successful, you must look at the entire picture. Following these general guidelines will assist you to provide good patient care every day and to ensure that surveyors are satisfied as well.

General Guidelines for Patient Care and Compliance with Accepted Practice Standards

- Follow all facility policies and procedures for patient care.
- Know the care plan for the patients to whom you are assigned including the major diagnosis, approaches to problems, and expected outcomes.
- Perform procedures in the way you were taught. Do not perform procedures for which you have not been trained.
- Practice safety in everything you do.
- All patients should have the call signal within reach at all times. Answer call signals promptly.
- Be polite and treat all patients with dignity and respect.
- Always close the door to the room when providing care. Pull the privacy curtain (Figure 18-3) and close the window curtain. This should be done in the care of all patients, whether alert or confused.
- Cover patients completely in bed, chair, or hallways so they are not exposed.
- Always knock on the door before entering a room (Figure 18-4). If you do not get a response, crack the door and announce your presence.
- If the patient's door is open, knock on the door frame or other surface and wait for permission to enter the room.
- Communicate with patients during care and explain procedures before you perform them.

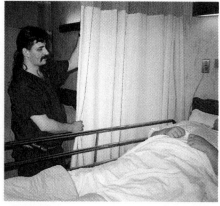

Figure 18-3 Close the door and pull the privacy curtain and window curtain before beginning care.

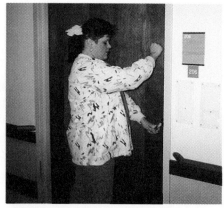

Figure 18-4 Knock on the door and wait for a response before entering a room.

continues

General Guidelines for Patient Care and Compliance with Accepted Practice Standards, *continued*

- Know your responsibility for patients using permanent equipment, such as oxygen, tube feeding, or IV pumps. The flow rate of the pump should match the ordered rate on the care plan. If it does not, notify the supervisor. If an alarm sounds on a piece of medical equipment, notify the supervisor immediately.
- Comb the patient's hair and tend to grooming needs early in the day so the patient is presentable in appearance for visitors. Assist with grooming needs throughout the day, if necessary.
- Check the patient's fingernails to be sure they are clean and neatly trimmed.
- Use handrolls or other props in the hands of dependent patients to prevent contractures. Remove the handrolls and clean the palm of the hand daily, or according to facility policy.
- Shave male patients daily. Follow your facility policy for removing facial hair on female patients.
- Give patients oral care three times a day, or according to facility policy.
- Check patients frequently to be sure they are clean and dry. Give incontinent care as necessary.
- All patients should be clean and odor-free.
- Make sure the patient's appearance is presentable at all times. Remove spilled food from clothing, and change the clothing or gown if necessary. Make sure the patient is clean after meals. If food is spilled on bed linen or the floor, replace the linen or remove the food from the floor. For patients who are up and dressed during the day, clothing should be clean, in good repair, color-coordinated, and appropriate for age and season.
- Patients should have nonslip footwear on their feet during transfers. Feet should be covered when patients are up in a chair so that bare feet are not resting on the floor.
- Pay attention to patient positioning in bed and chair. Preventive mattresses, heel and elbow protectors, and other devices are used if the patient is at risk of skin breakdown. Padding should be used for positioning patients if bony areas will rub against each other or against a firm surface.
- Footboards should be in place for bedfast patients.
- The feet should be supported when patients are up in a chair.
- Patients in wheelchairs should be positioned so their hips are at the rear of the seat. They should be seated upright and not lean to the side. If you are responsible for patients who move about the facility in a wheelchair, find them and check on them periodically to be sure their needs are met.
- If the patient has edema of the hands or feet, the edematous area should be elevated. Report the edema to the supervisor.
- Avoid the use of restraints whenever possible. If restraints are used, apply them only according to the manufacturer's directions.

continues

General Guidelines for Patient Care and Compliance with Accepted Practice Standards, *continued*

- Follow facility safety precautions and post signs if oxygen is in use.
- Clean and soiled equipment should be separated by one room's width in the hallway.
- Items in the refrigerator should be covered, labeled, and dated. The refrigerator should have a thermometer. The temperature should be below 45 degrees, or according to facility policy. Food and beverages should not be stored in the same refrigerator with medications or laboratory specimens.
- Follow your facility policy for storage of chemicals and other potentially toxic items.
- Apply the principles of standard precautions consistently in the care of all patients.
- Wash your hands before and after caring for each patient, and before and after using gloves.
- Avoid environmental contamination with soiled gloves. Remove one glove or use a paper towel under your hand if environmental contact is necessary.
- Discard gloves and other personal protective equipment according to your facility policy.
- Hold both clean and soiled linen away from your uniform.
- Avoid placing soiled linen on the floor.
- Keep clean linen carts covered when not in use.
- Avoid stacking linen in patient rooms; bring only needed linen to the room.
- Avoid overfilling linen hampers and barrels. The lid should fit tightly.
- Be sure each patient has fresh water. The water pitcher must always be covered with a lid. If the lid is missing, replace the pitcher.
- Store bedpans and urinals properly. Follow facility policies for covering them during transport.
- Monitor the position of catheter tubing and bags. The tubing should be secured to the leg and not obstructed or bent. The bag must be below the level of the bladder, but should never touch the floor.
- Personal care items, such as combs, toothbrushes, and hygienic supplies, should be covered if necessary, and stored or labeled so they are used by only one patient.
- Follow facility policies for routine cleaning tasks and dating and labeling clean items.
- Disinfect bathtubs, shower chairs, and pieces of permanent equipment before and after each use.
- Clean and soiled items should be separated in the bedside stand.
- Cover food and beverages when you carry them in the hallway.
- When you are passing ice, keep the ice scoop covered when not in use. Follow your facility policy for preventing contamination of the ice chest or dispenser.

continues

General Guidelines for Patient Care and Compliance with Accepted Practice Standards, *continued*

- Pass trays immediately when they arrive on the unit to maintain food temperature. Cut meat, butter bread, open cartons, put condiments on food, and assist patients with meals as necessary.
- Pass all clean trays before returning soiled trays to the food cart.
- Monitor patient position when eating. Patients should be upright. They should be as close to the table as possible. Tables should not be so high that the patients have to reach up for the food. The patient's feet should be supported on a foot stool or other device if they do not reach the floor.
- Prompt or assist patients who are not eating.
- Offer substitutes if the patient does not eat the meat or vegetable, or follow your facility policy for replacing uneaten food.
- When feeding patients, sit at eye level and maintain a conversation, even if the patient is confused.
- Alternate liquids with solids when feeding.
- Monitor restraints for correct application. Release all restraints every 2 hours for at least 10 minutes.
- Change incontinent patients promptly. Provide perineal care after each incontinent episode.
- Always notify the supervisor of a change in the patient's condition, even if it seems insignificant.
- Document your care completely and accurately. Do not leave blank spaces in flow sheets. Read flow sheets before signing your initials to them. Surveyors review what you have documented. Inadequate documentation can adversely affect the survey. Your documentation is a permanent, legal record of the care provided, and you may have to defend it in court.

KEY POINTS IN CHAPTER

- *Health care facilities must meet quality standards to operate.*
- *Licensure is a process in which the facility is inspected for a state license to operate.*
- *Certification is necessary if health care facilities accept Medicare and Medicaid money as reimbursement for patient care.*
- *Accreditation is a voluntary process in which health care facilities are inspected to ensure that they meet high quality standards of patient care.*
- *OSHA inspects health care facilities to monitor infection control and safety practices that affect employees.*
- *Many agencies survey health care facilities, so the facility must be survey-ready every day.*
- *Most health care facility surveys are unannounced.*
- *Long-term care facility surveyors usually observe the PCT giving direct patient care.*

KEY POINTS IN CHAPTER

- *Infection control practices are a very important part of all health care facility surveys.*
- *The Joint Commission for Accreditation of Healthcare Organizations conducts outcome-oriented surveys.*
- *The patient care technician is responsible for learning and following the policies and procedures of the health care facility.*
- *Following facility policies and doing things the way you were taught will prevent problems during surveys.*
- *The patient care technician is responsible for providing care that complies with accepted standards of practice for health care providers.*

REVIEW QUIZ

Multiple Choice Questions

1. Licensure, certification, and accreditation surveys are done to:
   a. ensure that health care facilities deliver quality care.
   b. maintain compliance with HCFA standards.
   c. check for compliance with OSHA standards.
   d. all of the above.

2. OSHA is:
   a. a governmental agency responsible for patient safety.
   b. a federal agency that studies infections and makes recommendations.
   c. an agency responsible for developing and enforcing job safety standards.
   d. all of the above.

3. Long-term care surveyors evaluate:
   a. quality of care.   c. resident rights.
   b. quality of life.   d. all of the above.

4. Most health care facility surveys are:
   a. announced 24 hours before the survey.
   b. anticipated by the facility administration.
   c. unannounced.
   d. conducted in private.

5. To prepare for a health care facility survey, you should:
   a. provide care in the manner in which you were taught.
   b. follow all facility policies and procedures.
   c. be survey-ready every day.
   d. all of the above.

6. When you pass surveyors in the hallway, you should:
   a. ignore them.
   b. smile and say hello.
   c. ask them what their findings are.
   d. find out the purpose of their visit.

7. The Joint Commission for Accreditation of Health Care Organizations survey is:
   a. outcome-oriented.   c. diagnosis-based.
   b. conducted monthly.   d. all of the above.

8. JCAHO surveyors will check to be sure that:
   a. care providers are clean and well groomed.
   b. sterile technique is used routinely in patient care.
   c. care providers know and follow facility policies and procedures.
   d. all of the above.

9. JCAHO surveys will monitor:
   a. patient teaching.   c. care planning.
   b. infection control.   d. all of the above.

10. When providing care according to accepted standards of practice, you should:
    a. practice safety.
    b. answer emergency call signals for only your assigned patients.
    c. knock on the door before entering the room of alert patients only.
    d. all of the above.

Employment Opportunities

After reading this chapter, you will be able to:

Spell and define key terms.

List six types of health care facilities in which the patient care technician may work.

List four things you can do to improve your success in finding a job.

Demonstrate how to prepare a resume.

List the seven components of a resume.

List nine sources of job leads.

Describe things you should do to ensure a successful interview.

List at least eight things you should do after you begin work to demonstrate that you are a responsible employee.

FINDING A POSITION

Many career opportunities are available for a qualified patient care technician. You must choose the setting in which you feel most comfortable working. Hospitals, nursing facilities, subacute centers, HMOs, doctors' offices, clinics, and other health care facilities hire people with your training and skills.

Finding a job is a full-time job. You must wake up early and set a time to begin looking for work. It may be helpful to list activities to do to look for a job. Apply for jobs early in the day. This makes a good impression and gives you enough time to fill out applications, take tests, or have interviews. Applying at several businesses in the same area will help you organize your time and save time and travel.

Be prepared when looking for a job. Take pens and pencils, paper, a map, reference information, and your resume with you. You will also need a photo identification, such as a driver's license, and your social security card. If you have completed the CNA program, bring a copy of your certificate and state certification. Follow up on all job leads right away. If you hear of a job opening late in the day, call and schedule an appointment for the next day. Network with your friends and relatives. Tell everyone you know you are looking for a job. Ask them to tell you about positions they are aware of.

Determining Your Job Skills and Experience

Before looking for a position, make a listing of your background, experience, and job skills. This includes previous employers, even if you were not employed in the health care field. List names, addresses, and phone numbers of former employers and people you will list as references. Make sure to get permission from these individuals before listing them as references. Also list work experience you have gained as a homemaker, volunteer, and student, or through hobbies and other personal activities. You will use your list to develop a resume, fill out job applications, and provide information for job interviews.

■ *interview: a formal meeting in which the employer assesses the qualifications of an applicant and provides information about the job opening*

■ *networking: communicating with people you know who have similar careers, goals, and interests*

■ *resume: a summary of your professional or work experience and qualifications*

Table 19-1

Activity or Interest	Skill, Knowledge, and Talent Required
Homemaking skills	Manage budgets Manage many priorities at one time Knowledge of human growth and development Child care Cooking Cleaning Laundry
Playing softball	Ability to function as a team player Use basic math to keep track of scores Physical coordination, strength, and agility Ability to direct and teach others
Teaching Sunday school	Ability to teach and direct others Leadership skills Good reading and writing ability Dependability Ability to honor a commitment Desire to serve others
Babysitting	Knowledge of human growth and development Food preparation, cooking Cleaning Dependability Knowledge of household management Basic first aid Child care

Interest and Aptitudes. No one is going to see your list but you, so write everything down that you can think of. List hobbies, clubs, sports participation, school activities, volunteer work, and other interests. Then list your personal qualities and special abilities. This list may appear to have nothing to do with job experience, but it will give you an idea of your abilities. Table 19-1 gives some examples of how to turn this list into useful job information.

After you have listed your interests and activities, list your full- and part-time work experience. List all work that you have done, including self-employment and summer jobs. Next, think about the skills it took to do these jobs. Write them down. Table 19-2 shows how to develop this list of work experience and skills.

Education. List all schools you have attended. Begin with your high school. Add any college, military training, vocational education, and on-the-job training. List your degrees, certificates, awards, and honors. List the date you completed your PCT program, the address and phone number of the agency where you took your course, the instructor's name, and a list of skills you are proficient in.

Physical Condition. Ask yourself if you have any physical problems that could interfere with the type of work you want to do. For example, if you have a back problem, you may not want to work in a care setting that requires frequent, heavy lifting. Some care settings require more strenuous physical effort than others.

Table 19-2

Work Duties	Skills and Talents
Picked fruits and vegetables on a farm	Inspect fruits and vegetables for damage Endurance Ability to bend, stoop, squat, and lift Ability to work with hands Ability to work in extreme temperatures Use garden tools and small equipment Ability to plant vegetables and fruits
Worked as a waitress in a restaurant	Ability to manage many priorities at one time Pleasant personality Ability to keep customers satisfied Desire to serve others Basic math skills to calculate restaurant bills Operate cash register and make change Knowledge of sanitary food service and preparation Ability to bend, lift, and carry heavy trays Endurance—ability to stand on feet for long periods of time Ability to follow directions
Cashier in a convenience store	Trustworthy Honesty Dependability Basic math skills to count money and make change Stocking shelves Maintaining inventory Ability to deal with the public Ability to work with difficult customers Ability to operate cash register and other electrical equipment Physical endurance—ability to stand for long periods of time Ability to bend and lift heavy boxes

Personal Circumstances. Ask yourself what limits you have in the location or hours of work you will accept. How far are you willing to travel? Do you have a car, or are you depending on public transportation? If you will be using public transportation, what hours is it available? Do you need a babysitter for your children while you are at work? What time is the babysitter available? Are there any other circumstances in your life that would affect your attendance and dependability at a job?

Career Goals. What kind of work do you want to be doing in 10 years? What type of job will help you reach this goal?

Matching Your Background and Experience to a Job. Look at the skills, talents, and abilities you listed. Find out what types of health care jobs match these abilities. This textbook provides an overview of the responsibilities of the patient care technician in many different health care settings. You can also find information in the public library. The U.S. Department of Labor publishes books that describe work duties, skills and abilities required, how to enter an occupation, where jobs are located, earnings, work conditions, and future opportunities. Your state employment commission office also has valuable information and free publications about many different jobs and careers. Match your skills, talents, abilities, needs, and interests to the jobs listed. This will give you an idea of the type of job that will best meet your needs.

▬▬ PREPARING A RESUME

The next step to finding a job is to prepare a resume. Use the list you developed of your talents, abilities, interests, and jobs to help you prepare your resume. A resume should be typed or prepared on a computer (Figure 19-1). Many computer programs are available to assist you. There are also professional services that will prepare your resume for a nominal fee. Your resume and cover letter should be printed on good quality paper. Avoid listing personal information such as race, age, sex, height, weight, national origin, marital or family status, and religion. Your completed resume should be as concise as possible; one or two pages is best. After you have completed your resume, proofread it for errors and make corrections. Then make one copy of the resume and inspect the photocopy for stray marks. If the photocopy is clear, print additional copies to distribute to potential employers.

The Seven Components of a Resume

Your resume should be clearly and concisely written. The resume represents you, so you want it to appear as professional as possible. (See the sample resume format in the Appendix.) There are seven components to the resume:

■ **cover letter:** *a letter of introduction sent to a prospective employer with your resume*

■ The cover letter is a business letter of introduction. It should be written in business letter format and be no more than one page long. A cover letter is sent each time you send a resume, stating the position you are applying for. Emphasize why your qualifications meet the requirements of the position. In the cover letter, state that you have enclosed your resume and request to schedule an interview.

■ **personal data:** *the section of your resume that lists your name, address, telephone number, and professional license or certification number*

■ The first section of your resume consists of personal data. This includes your name, address, telephone number, and professional license or certification number.

■ **job objective:** *the section of your resume that lists the type of position you are seeking and states how your ability and skills qualify you for this position*

■ The next section is for the job objective. This part of your resume lists the type of position you are seeking and states how your ability and skills qualify you for this position.

■ Next, list your educational background. Begin with high school and list all education after high school. Include trade or vocational school, college, and continuing education classes. List when and where you went to school and degrees or certificates you earned.

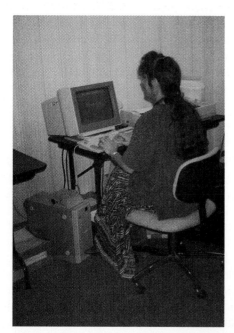

Figure 19-1 Your resume should be written on a computer or typewriter.

■ extracurricular activities: clubs, hobbies, volunteer work, and special interests

■ reverse chronological order: the order in which your previous jobs are listed on your resume, beginning with most recent job first

■ references: individuals who know you and who will recommend you to the prospective employer for the job you are seeking

■ Extracurricular activities may be listed with your educational background, or may be listed separately.

■ After you have completed the information listed here, list your employment. Begin with your most recent employer first. List all employers in reverse chronological order, even if the job was not in the health care field. Add another page if necessary.

■ After you have listed your previous employers, list at least three references. These should be people who know you well, but not relatives. List two work-related references and one personal reference. Before listing people as references, call them and get permission to use their names.

SEARCHING FOR A JOB

There are many places to get leads for your job search. Begin with your state job service or employment commission. Many employers list job openings with this agency. There is no cost for employment commission services. Use all of the resources available in your community.

Sources of Job Leads

Leads and referrals for jobs come from many different places. Investigate all of the sources listed and others you know of in your community. Here are some potential sources of job leads.

■ Private employers. Look in the Yellow Pages for health care employers in your area. Contact the employer directly to inquire about employment opportunities. Talk to the person who would supervise you, even if there are no openings now.

■ Federal, state, and local government personnel offices list a wide range of government employment opportunities for clinics, hospitals, and other government health care facilities in your area.

■ Public libraries may post job announcements.

■ Newspaper ads list many career opportunities. Although the want ads are in the paper every day, the Sunday edition usually lists the most employment ads.

■ Private and temporary employment agencies may have temporary, permanent, or "fill-in" positions available. Sometimes temporary work through an agency leads to full-time employment.

■ Community colleges and trade schools may list employment opportunities on their bulletin boards, or may have job placement offices.

■ Community organizations, such as clubs, associations, and women's and minority centers, may list available jobs in their newsletters or bulletin boards.

■ Community newsletters may list job openings.

■ Network with your friends, relatives, and classmates to learn of potential job openings.

Completing Job Applications

Call potential employers early in the day. This sends a message that you are up and ready for work. Identify yourself and inquire about available positions. Do not ask about money. Many employers will ask you to come to the workplace and complete an application.

■ *application:* the form on which employment information is written and a request for employment is made

When you fill out an application, bring your resume or list with you. Having this information will save time and make a good impression on the employer. Read the directions on the application carefully. Fill it out completely in ink. Be neat—a sloppy application sends a negative message. Avoid leaving blank spaces. Fill out all information. If something on the application does not apply, put "N/A" (not applicable) in the space rather than leaving it blank. If a question asks for a narrative answer, plan ahead. Briefly and concisely give the answer, using no more words than necessary to fill the space.

The Job Interview

After you have investigated job leads and completed applications, an employer may contact you to schedule an interview. You will be given a date and time to meet with the prospective employer. The interview is very important. Most hiring decisions are made on the first interview. How you present yourself in the interview is as important as your training, experience, and ability to do the job.

Preparing for the Interview. Before the interview, learn as much as you can about the health care agency, the job, and how your previous experience and training qualify you for the position. Write down the things you will need to complete an application. Have a friend ask you interview questions (Table 19-3). Bring a copy of your resume. You will also need to bring your social security card and driver's license, or another picture identification, with you.

Dress correctly for the interview. Your appearance is very important and helps you make a positive first impression. The first impression you make is visual. Be neat, clean, and well groomed. Do not overdress, but avoid looking too casual.

The Interview. Go to the interview alone. Arrange for babysitters and transportation ahead of time. Arrive a few minutes early so you have time before the

Table 19-3 Sample Interview Questions

Question:	Tell me about yourself.
Answer:	Briefly outline your strengths. Concentrate on your training and professional achievements. Avoid discussing marriage, family, and your personal life.
Question:	Describe your qualifications for this job.
Answer:	Describe your most recent training and experience. List your strongest skills and talents relating to job performance.
Question:	Why do you want this job?
Answer:	Know something about the employer and say something positive about the company. Avoid using money as the reason you want the position.
Question:	Tell me about your last job.
Answer:	Describe your duties and responsibilities. Discuss skills that relate to the position for which you are applying.
Question:	Why did you leave your last job?
Answer:	Be honest, but avoid making negative comments about your previous employer.
Question:	Tell me about your goals and ambitions.
Answer:	State that you look forward to learning new things, and accepting challenges and responsibilities. State your career goals.
Question:	What are your strengths?
Answer:	Describe strong personal qualities such as honesty, dependability, and caring about other people.
Question:	What are your weaknesses?
Answer:	Mention weaknesses or problems, but state how you have learned and grown from them.

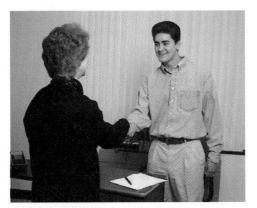

Figure 19-2 A firm handshake makes a good impression.

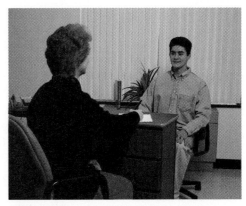

Figure 19-3 This PCT's body language makes a good impression on the interviewer.

interview to fill out an application and other required information. When you are introduced to the interviewer, shake hands (Figure 19-2). Practice shaking hands with your friends so that you have a steady, firm handshake. This sends a message that you have a healthy self esteem. A weak, limp handshake may send a negative message. Make good eye contact with the interviewer. Your eyes should send a message such as, "I like you." Be aware of your posture and the message you are sending through your body language (Figure 19-3). Stand until you are invited to sit. Try to find common ground with the interviewer. This will make you both more comfortable. Pictures, books, plants, and other items in the interviewer's office make good conversation starters. Express your interest in the job or company, using the information you gathered when you prepared for the interview. Let the interviewer direct the conversation. Answer questions clearly and concisely. Show how your experience and training will make you a valuable employee. Speak positively of former employers. Making negative comments about a previous employer is not a good practice.

Listen carefully to the interview questions and be sure you understand them before answering. If you do not understand, ask for clarification. Your answers to questions should reflect your positive features. Avoid discussing negative traits unless you are specifically asked to do so. Be honest with the interviewer. It is easier to defend the truth than to be caught in a lie. Avoid discussing your personal life or financial problems.

Discussing Salary and Benefits. Salary and benefits can be a sensitive issue. Asking questions about them early in the process gives the employer the impression that you are not interested in working at the health care agency, but are, instead, shopping for the highest salary available. This sends a negative message. Save discussions about salary and benefits for late in the interview. Let the employer lead into them. If the interviewer has not discussed salary and benefits by the end of the interview, it is appropriate to ask.

Closing the Interview. If the interviewer does not offer you a position or say when a decision will be made, ask when you may call to find out about it. If the interviewer asks you to call at a certain time, or to return for another interview, note the date, time, and place. If the job is offered to you, make sure you understand the terms and conditions before accepting it. Do not accept a position if you cannot fulfill the responsibilities. For example, if the employer offers you a position on the 10 P.M. to 6 A.M. shift, but you do not have a babysitter during these hours. Arrange for a babysitter before accepting the position. Thank the employer for the interview and reaffirm your interest in the job. Close the interview with a firm handshake.

After the Interview. Use the interview as a learning experience. Make a list of specific ways you can improve your next interview. Have a friend ask you interview questions again. Practice your answers until you are comfortable. Write the interviewer a short personal note thanking him or her for the interview.

In some states, employers are required by law to conduct a criminal history check on each applicant. This background check will show if the applicant has ever been arrested. In these states, if an individual has been convicted of certain felony crimes, he or she cannot work in a health care facility.

Many employers require applicants to pass a physical examination, and undergo drug testing before hire. An initial tuberculin test may also be performed before an individual is allowed to work in a health care facility.

KEEPING A JOB

After you have accepted a position, remember that honesty and dependability are very important qualities of the patient care technician. Arrive for work on time, in proper uniform, and be prepared to work. Follow your facility policies and procedures. Maintain a positive attitude and be willing to learn new things. Avoid bringing your personal problems to work. Be willing to help others and do extra tasks without being asked. Good attendance is very important. Be at work when you are scheduled and avoid calling off unless you are ill. If you will be unable to work your next scheduled shift, notify your facility as far in advance as possible so they can find a replacement.

Review the desirable qualities of the PCT in Chapter 1. It may have been several months since you studied these. List each point on a piece of paper and review it daily after you begin employment. The list will remind you of things you should do to become a valuable employee.

Continue to Learn and Grow

Learn all that you can about your role and responsibilities. Ask appropriate questions of your supervisor, staff development director, and others. Read nursing and medical journals and literature. Medical books are also available from the public library. Attend continuing education classes at your facility and in your community. If you have passed the Certified Nursing Assistant examination, you must attend at least 12 hours of continuing education classes a year to maintain your certification. Your state may have additional continuing education requirements.

RESIGN PROPERLY

If resignation from your position becomes necessary, always leave on a positive note. Your work record follows you, so you must give proper notice of resignation. Each agency has policies on length of resignation notice. It is generally two weeks, or the length of one pay period. Write a formal letter of resignation to your supervisor listing the reasons for resignation. Even if you are unhappy or dissatisfied, the tone of the letter should be positive. State what your last date of employment will be. (Make sure that you work through that day and avoid calling off work during the notice period.) Thank your supervisor for the opportunity to learn and grow at the health care facility.

KEY POINTS IN CHAPTER

- *Many health care agencies employ patient care technicians.*
- *Finding a job is a full-time job.*
- *The best time to look for a job is early in the day.*
- *It is helpful to list your skills, activities, background, and experience before preparing your resume.*
- *Your resume should appear as professional as possible and accurately reflect your education, experience, skills, and interests.*

KEY POINTS IN CHAPTER

- *Information such as race, age, sex, height, weight, national origin, marital and family status, and religion should not be listed on your resume.*

- *The state employment commission, private employers, government personnel offices, public libraries, newspaper ads, employment agencies, colleges and trade schools, clubs, newsletters, friends, and relatives are all sources of potential job leads.*

- *Present a professional appearance when you arrive for a job interview.*

- *Honesty, dependability, and a positive attitude are important characteristics of the patient care technician.*

- *Classes are just the beginning of your education; you will continue to learn and grow throughout your health care career.*

- *If resignation is necessary, always give proper notice to the employer.*

REVIEW QUIZ

Multiple Choice Questions

1. When searching for a job, you should bring:
   a. pen.
   b. resume.
   c. reference information.
   d. all of the above.

2. Before seeking a job, you must consider:
   a. what limits you have on hours and location of the employer.
   b. the employer's starting salary.
   c. the employer's benefit plan.
   d. all of the above.

3. Sources of job information include the:
   a. public library.
   b. state employment commission.
   c. Department of Labor.
   d. all of the above.

4. Your resume should be:
   a. neatly written in pencil.
   b. typed or computerized.
   c. written with carbon copies.
   d. typed in red ink.

5. When mailing your resume to a potential employer, you should include a:
   a. self-addressed, stamped envelope.
   b. copy of the want ad in which the job was advertised.
   c. cover letter.
   d. personal note stating why you need a job.

6. The following information should be included in the personal data section of your resume:
   a. name.
   b. religion.
   c. age.
   d. all of the above.

7. Which of the following is true about a job interview?
   a. Dress very casually.
   b. First impressions are important.
   c. Body language is not important.
   d. All of the above.

8. When you are invited into the interviewer's office:
   a. stand until you are invited to sit.
   b. shake hands with the interviewer.
   c. make good eye contact with the interviewer.
   d. all of the above.

9. It is acceptable to ask about salary:
   a. on the telephone before making application with an employer.
   b. at the beginning of the interview.
   c. at the end of the interview.
   d. when the employer calls you to schedule an interview.

10. When it becomes necessary to resign from your position:
    a. give proper notice of resignation.
    b. call the employer and state that you are not coming back.
    c. do not return to work.
    d. tell a coworker to inform your employer of your resignation.

APPENDIX

Measurement Equivalents

Common U.S. Measurement	Metric Equivalent (approximate)	Common U.S. Measurement	Metric Equivalent (approximate)
1 teaspoon	5 cc	1 quart	1,000 cc (or 1 liter)
1 ounce	30 cc	½ gallon	2,000 cc
½ pint	250 cc	1 gallon	4,000 cc
1 pint	500 cc		

Vital Signs

Temperature	Normal	Report Changes Above	Report Changes Below
Axillary temperature	97.6°F	99°F	96°F
Oral temperature	98.6°F	100°F	97°F
Rectal temperature	99.6°F	101°F	98°F
Pulse	76	100	60
Respiration	16	12	20
Blood pressure	120/80	140/90	100/60

Important Observations of Diabetic Patients

Inadequate food intake	Excessive activity
Eating food not allowed on diet	Complaints of dizziness, shakiness, racing heart
Refusal of supplements or snacks	Signs or symptoms of diabetic coma or insulin shock

Signs and Symptoms of Diabetic Coma and Insulin Shock

Diabetic Coma (blood sugar too high)	Insulin Shock (blood sugar too low)
Nausea, vomiting	Complaints of hunger, weakness, dizziness, shakiness
Weakness	Skin cold, moist, clammy, pale
Headache	Rapid, shallow respirations
Full, bounding pulse	Nervousness and excitement
Fruity smell to breath	Rapid pulse
Hot, dry, flushed skin	Unconsciousness
Labored respirations	No sugar in the urine
Drowsiness	Low blood sugar by finger stick
Mental confusion	
Unconsciousness	
Sugar in the urine	
High blood sugar by finger stick	

Observation and Reporting Summary

System or Problem	Observation to Report
Signs/symptoms of infection	Elevated temperature Sweating Chills Skin hot or cold to touch Skin flushed, red, gray, or blue Inflammation of skin as evidenced by redness, edema, heat, or pain
Cardiovascular system	Abnormal pulse below 60 or above 100 Blood pressure below 100/60 or above 140/90 Unable to palpate pulse or hear blood pressure Chest pain Shortness of breath Headache, dizziness, weakness, vomiting Cold, blue, or gray appearance Cold, blue, painful feet or hands

continues

Observation and Reporting Summary, *continued*

System or Problem	Observation to Report
Respiratory system	Respiratory rate below 12 or above 20 Irregular respirations Noisy, labored, respirations Dyspnea Shortness of breath Wheezing Coughing Blue color of lips, nail beds, or mucous membranes
Integumentary system	Rash Redness Irritation Bruises Skin discoloration Swelling Open areas/skin breakdown Drainage Foul odor Complaints such as numbness, burning, tingling, itching Signs of infection Pressure sores Skin growths "Tenting" of skin Sunken, dark appearance around eyes
Gastrointestinal system	Unusual or abnormal appearance of bowel movement Blood, mucus, or other unusual substances in stool Unusual color of bowel movement Complaints of pain, constipation, diarrhea, bleeding Complaints of indigestion or excessive gas Nausea, vomiting Abdominal pain Coffee-ground appearance of emesis or stool
Genitourinary system	Urinary output too low Oral intake too low Fluid intake and output not balanced Abnormal appearance of urine: dark, concentrated, red, cloudy Unusual material in urine: blood, pus, particles Complaints of pain, burning, urgency, frequency, pain in lower back Edema Sudden weight loss or gain Respiratory distress Change in mental status
Mental status problems	Change in level of consciousness, awareness, or alertness Changes in mood or behavior Change in ability to express self or communicate Mental confusion Threats of harm to self or others

STANDARDS OF CARE AND PRACTICE

The patient care technician cares for patients under the supervision of a licensed health care provider. *Patient* includes all individuals who receive care. Your primary responsibility is to promote health and preserve life. The patient care technician acknowledges the worth, uniqueness, and dignity of all persons. You are a caregiver, not an authority figure. You are responsible for assisting the supervisor with assessment and evaluation information, such as obtaining vital signs and making observation of the patient's skin condition. Your findings are documented on the medical record, which is a permanent, legal record of the patient's care. Safety is a primary consideration in everything you do.

The care plan is the foundation for care delivered to the patient. Each problem has a measurable goal, and your interventions are consistent with the goal and established plan of care. Share your knowledge and ideas with other team members to ensure the best care possible. Organize your work to ensure that the care plan is implemented accurately. Your focus is always on the patient. You will monitor the patient's condition and report changes to the supervisor in a timely manner. The patient care technician must be willing to share information, observations, knowledge, and experience with others. Recognize that you are a member of a team in which all team members focus their efforts on the patient's well-being.

The patient care technician should be adequately prepared by virtue of education and experience to fulfill the responsibilities and perform the procedures listed in the job description. The health care profession is constantly changing, and the patient care technician must be willing to change with it. You must attend classes and learn new things. Be willing to change your thinking and practices and you will grow with your profession.

The patient care technician must practice within the limits of preparation for the job. Function within your scope of practice and ask questions if you are uncertain about procedures. Never perform procedures for which you have not been trained. Be enthusiastic about learning new skills and broadening your scope of practice. Conduct yourself in a professional manner at all times. This ensures a safe and comfortable environment for the patient.

The patient care technician must respect authority and accept constructive criticism. Acknowledge your strengths and limitations. Your performance will be continuously evaluated to identify strengths and areas for further development. You are responsible for taking action to achieve professional goals identified during your performance appraisals.

Show respect for your coworkers and treat them in the same way you would like to be treated. Be dependable and enthusiastic about your work. Be willing to help others when needed. Understand that you must be tolerant of others' personalities. Be reliable, honest, and trustworthy in your interactions with others. Be positive, constructive, and professional by offering solutions to problems instead of complaining. Keep your personal and professional life separate and avoid bringing personal problems to work.

Always follow the policies and procedures of your health care facility. Concentrate on doing the best job possible. This involves being at work on time when scheduled, managing your time well, and maintaining your knowledge and competence in your job. Respect your employer and use the chain of command. Respect the employer's property. The care provided must be cost-effective and conserve the facility's resources as much as possible.

Respect the patient and treat all patients as you would like your family members to be treated. Always promote independence, self-esteem, and respect. Encourage patients to make decisions about their care by offering choices whenever possible. Treat all patients fairly, without criticism or judgment. Respect for the patient continues after death in the care provided to the body and support given to the family.

You will deliver care that protects and preserves the patient's autonomy, dignity, and basic human rights. Respect the dignity and privacy of each patient in the care you give. Remember that information about patients and families is confidential and is not divulged to others, except when necessary to provide care.

Respect the patient as a person. Always show consideration and respect for the patient's life experiences. You are responsible for providing culturally and ethnically sensitive care. Respect the patient's feelings, thoughts, culture, and belief system even if you do not agree with them. Demonstrate respect for the patient's personal property and belongings. Provide privacy when families, clergy, and significant others are visiting. Respect patients' and families' decisions. Actively support and observe the Patient's Bill of Rights.

You are responsible for providing compassionate, considerate, conscientious care to all patients, regardless of age, sex, race, religion, physical disability, or national origin. Consider the type of care you would want for yourself and your family and strive to deliver this type of care to the patients you serve.

Demonstrate respect for the patient's family and visitors. Exercise good judgment and maintain a supportive, professional role by being responsive to their needs. Refer family members to the appropriate health care professional to answer questions or resolve problems.

Your personal appearance and behavior represent the health care industry to the general public. Choose your words carefully. Present a positive impression at all times. You are an ambassador to the community and represent the health care professionals that care for its members. Follow recommended personal and professional health practices to maintain your personal health and safety. You must care for and about yourself in order to properly care for others. The patient care technician teaches others by setting a positive example.

You have chosen a respected, valuable profession. Be proud of your occupation and the care you deliver. The importance of your contribution to the interdisciplinary team and the patient's well-being should never be minimized. There are many personal and professional rewards for the patient care technician in your chosen profession.

Sample Resume

NAME
Street Address
City, State, Zip Code
(area code) and telephone number

OBJECTIVE

I am seeking a position in the health care field where I can use my basic care skills to provide nursing care to hospital patients. I have completed a 100-hour training program at ABC Hospital and have experience caring for patients on medical and surgical units.

EDUCATION

Name of Degree   **Year(s)**
INSTITUTION NAME   CITY, STATE

Major:	Describe major field of study here.
Minor:	Describe minor field(s) of study here.
Activities:	Describe related activities and accomplishments here.

EMPLOYMENT

Job Title   **Year(s)**
ORGANIZATION NAME   CITY, STATE
Address and telephone
Supervisor's name
Responsibilities and accomplishments

Job Title   **Year(s)**
ORGANIZATION NAME   CITY, STATE
Address and telephone
Supervisor's name
Responsibilities and accomplishments

SKILLS

- Use bulleted list here to develop a list of skills.
- Study the duties for the job and list skills that you can perform that will be useful to the employer.
- Review your background and experience list. List talents and accomplishments that demonstrate your ability to perform these job skills.
- Use simple, short, active verbs to start each sentence.

REFERENCES

List names and addresses of three persons. Avoid listing relatives. It is best to list two work references and one personal reference.

Sample Cover Letter

Date of Letter

Human Resources Department
XYZ Hospital
234 Main Street
Capitol City, USA, 00000

To Whom It May Concern: [fill in name of person, if known]

Enclosed is my resume in application for the position of Patient Care Technician I, which was advertised in the *Capitol City Register* on September 20, 1997.

I have completed the 100-hour patient care technician training program at ABC Hospital. The program consisted of 60 hours of classroom and 40 hours of clinical experience. I have worked on both medical and surgical units and provided direct patient care to patients of all ages.

I am anxious to schedule an interview with you to discuss employment opportunities at XYZ Hospital. I can be reached at (000)-888-0000. Thank you for your consideration.

Sincerely,

[sign your name here in ink]

Mary Barton

◼◼ ABSENTEEISM

The following was included in a thought-provoking article about absenteeism and how it affects patients, co-workers, and the health care agency. The article was written by Roberto Taloria, CNA, who has been a CNA for almost 50 years. He is the president of the CNA Association of Georgia, and has done much to further nursing assistant practice in his state. Although the article was written for CNAs, the principles apply to all health care workers. Mr. Taloria's article was originally published in the *Journal of Nurse Assistants,* September/October 1996 issue.

ABSENTEEISM—HOW MUCH IS EXCESSIVE?

Before you "call in," ask yourself these questions:

- Do I really feel too sick to work?
- Do I have an appointment to be somewhere else?
- Can I get my appointment changed to my day off?
- How do my co-workers feel about my calling in?
- Am I putting more work on my co-workers?
- Will my residents or patients miss me?
- How many days have I called in this year?
- Do I have a right to take time off my job whenever I feel like it?
- Does my employer have the right to fire me for always calling in?
- Did I sign an agreement to come to work every day?
- How do I feel when my co-workers call in?
- Who really gets hurt when I am absent?
- Would I put up with this if I were the boss?
- Will all of the days I am absent be on my record?
- Will this hurt me when applying for another job or promotion?

GLOSSARY

abandonment: leaving or walking off the premises before another worker has been assigned to care for your patients.

abbreviation: a shortened form of a word.

abdominal distention: enlargement of the abdomen due to excess gas, fecal matter, or urinary retention.

abduction: moving an extremity *away from* the body.

abrasion: a scrape or injury that rubs off the surface of the skin.

abuse: the willful infliction of injury, unreasonable confinement, intimidation, or punishment that results in physical harm, pain, or mental anguish.

acceptance: the final stage in the grieving process, in which the patient is calmly waiting for death.

accident: an unexpected, undesirable event.

accreditation: a process that health care facilities participate in voluntarily to ensure that high standards of care are maintained.

active assistive range of motion: exercises that are started or completed by the patient with some assistance from the care provider.

active range of motion: moving all joints through their normal movements independently.

activities of daily living (ADLs): personal care activities that people do each day to meet their human needs.

acute illness: illness that develops suddenly and lasts for a short time.

adaptive devices: pieces of equipment used to help a patient perform a task independently.

adduction: moving an extremity *toward* the body.

admission: procedure for checking a patient into the health care agency and getting him or her settled.

advance directive: a document that designates the patient's wishes for a time when the patient is unable to speak for himself or herself.

afternoon care: routine care given after lunch.

AIDS (acquired immune deficiency syndrome): a progressive fatal disease caused by the HIV virus and spread by contact with blood or moist body fluids.

airborne method of transmission: when very small germs suspended in dust and moisture in the air are inhaled by a susceptible host.

airborne precautions: practices that health care workers use to protect themselves from airborne pathogens.

alignment: placement; anatomical position.

Alzheimer's disease: an incurable disease that causes loss of mental abilities and judgment.

AM care: routine care given to prepare the patient for breakfast.

ambulation: the act of walking or moving from one place to another.

aneroid gauge: a gauge that operates with a spring-loaded dial.

anger: the second step in the grieving process, in which the patient is angry because of a terminal diagnosis.

antecedent: an event that causes or triggers a behavior.

antecubital space: the space in front of the elbow.

antibiotics: medications used to eliminate pathogens from the body.

anti-embolism stockings: elastic hosiery used on some patients to relieve edema and prevent blood clots.

antiseptic: chemical agent designed to cleanse the skin

anus: the outlet of the colon to the outside of the body.

apathy: indifference; lack of feeling or emotion.

apical pulse: the pulse taken at the apex of the heart.

apnea: absence of respirations.

appliance: a plastic collection device used to contain the excretions from an ostomy.

application: the form on which employment information is written and a request for employment is made.

aseptic technique: practices used that are free of all microbes.

aspiration: inhalation of food, fluid, or other objects into the lungs.

assess: gather information and facts to identify the patient's problems and needs.

atrophy: weakness and muscle wasting from lack of use.

attending behavior: means and techniques used to improve the transfer of verbal communication.

attitude: the outer reflection of your feelings.

aura: a sensation of smell, taste, or bright light that precedes the onset of a seizure.

aural (tympanic) temperature: the temperature taken at the tympanic membrane inside the ear.

axilla: the area under the arm; the armpit.

axillary temperature: the temperature taken in the armpit or groin.

bacteria: one-celled microorganisms that can cause disease.

bargaining: the third stage in the grieving process, in which the patient attempts to buy more time.

barrier: something that interferes with communication.

barrier equipment. *See* personal protective equipment.

bath blanket: a soft cotton or flannel blanket used to protect patient privacy and provide warmth during procedures in which the body is exposed.

bed bath: the bathing procedure used for a patient who is unable to get out of bed.

bedpan: a device used for elimination in bed.

bed rest: a medically prescribed treatment in which the patient cannot get out of bed.

bedside stand: the nightstand used to store personal possessions and grooming and hygiene items.

bedsore. *See* pressure sore.

belt restraint: a safety device that encircles the patient's waist and/or hips and serves as a reminder to prevent rising.

biohazardous waste: disposable items that are contaminated with blood or body fluids.

bladder: a hollow muscle that stores urine until it is eliminated from the body.

bland diet. *See* soft diet.

bloodborne pathogens: microbe-caused diseases that are spread through contact with blood or body fluid.

blood pressure: the force of blood on the walls of the arteries.

body mechanics: correct use of the body to lift or move heavy objects or patients.

bony prominences: places where the bones are close to the surface of the skin.

bowel movement. *See* feces.

brachial artery: the artery in the antecubital space, in front of the elbow.

bradycardia: slow pulse rate, usually under 60 beats per minute.

bruises: injuries to the skin caused by hitting or striking; the area turns black and blue in color.

burnout: complete physical, mental, or emotional fatigue or exhaustion.

calorie: a unit of energy-producing potential equal to the amount of heat that is contained in food and released upon use by the body.

calorie-controlled diet: a diet that restricts the total number of calories served to the patient; usually served to overweight patients.

carbohydrates: foods that produce heat and energy in the body.

cardiac arrest: a condition that occurs when the heartbeat and respirations cease.

care plan: a plan developed by the interdisciplinary health care team that describes the goals and approaches that all team members should use when caring for the patient.

carrier: a person who can give a disease to others; the person may not know of or show symptoms of the infection.

catastrophic reactions: uncontrolled emotional outbursts in response to feeling completely overwhelmed or fearful; may include crying, sudden mood changes, anger, and combative behavior.

catheter: a hollow tube used to drain secretions from the body.

Celsius (centigrade) scale: a scale for measuring temperature in which the boiling point is 100.

Centers for Disease Control and Prevention (CDC): a federal agency that studies diseases and makes recommendations on protective measures.

centigrade scale. *See* Celsius scale.

certification: an inspection process for facilities that accept state or federal funds as payment for health care.

chain of command: the line of authority in each department.

chain of infection: description of the factors necessary for an infection to spread.

chart: the notebook or binder containing the patient's medical record.

chemical restraint: a medication or drug used to alter behavior only for staff convenience and not required to treat a patient's medical symptoms.

chemicals: substances that may be harmful if they touch the skin or mucous membranes, and are usually dangerous if swallowed.

chemotherapy: a cancer treatment that uses specific chemical agents or drugs to destroy cancer cells.

Cheyne-Stokes respirations: periods of dyspnea alternating with periods of apnea.

chronic illness: an illness or disease that lasts for a long time.

citation: a written notice that informs the health care agency of alleged violations of OSHA rules and the time frame within which the condition(s) must be corrected.

clean-catch (midstream) specimen: a urine sample collected from the middle of the urinary stream.

cleansing enema: introduction of fluid into the lower bowel to remove solid waste.

clear liquid diet: a diet high in water and carbohydrates, with little nutritive value.

clergy: a minister of the gospel, a pastor, priest, or rabbi or other religious worker.

client: the person being cared for in his or her own home.

closed drainage system: a drainage bag and tubing connected to a catheter that is not opened.

coccyx: the bone at the base of the spine.

code blue: an emergency designation to alert staff and summon help when a cardiac arrest occurs.

cognitive impairment: a decline in intellectual functioning.

colostomy: a surgical procedure in which the colon is attached to the outside of the body and waste is eliminated into a plastic bag attached to the skin.

combative: hitting or fighting the care provider.

combative behavior: physically aggressive behavior such as hitting, kicking, scratching, or biting.

commercially prepared enema: an enema solution pre-packaged in a small dispenser.

compassion: kindness and mercy.

compensation: using strength and overachieving in one area to overcome a weakness in another area of life.

complete bath: washing the entire body of a patient.

condom (external) catheter: a catheter applied to the outside of the penis in incontinent males.

confidential: personal, not known to other people.

consent: permission to perform care, treatments, and procedures.

consequences: the outcome of a behavior.

consistent: same; approaches to care that are the same with all care providers.

constipation: difficult passage of hard, dry stool from the lower bowel.

continuity of care: all staff working on the same goals and providing the same approaches to the patient 24 hours a day.

contractures: permanent shortening and deformity of muscles from lack of use.

contraindicated: not indicated, inappropriate.

coping mechanisms: responses to stress and loss that people use to protect feelings of self-esteem.

cover letter: a letter of introduction sent to a prospective employer with your resume.

cubic centimeter: a metric unit of measure used in health care facilities; 30 cc equals one ounce. One cubic centimeter is the same as one milliliter.

cues: brief verbal hints to tell the patient what you want him or her to do.

culture: the pattern or life-style of an individual or group.

dangling: sitting on the side of the bed with the legs over the edge of the mattress.

decline: worsening or deterioration in the resident's physical or mental condition.

decubiti: more than one pressure sore or decubitus ulcer.

decubitus ulcer. *See* pressure sore.

defamation of character: making false or damaging statements about another person verbally.

defecation: elimination of solid waste from the lower bowel.

deficiency: a written notice of inadequate care or a substandard practice.

deformity: disfigurement of the body.

dehydration: a serious condition resulting from inadequate water in the body.

delirium: an acute confusional state indicative of a treatable illness.

delusions: false beliefs.

delusions of persecution: thinking that others are trying to cause personal harm.

dementia: a set of symptoms affecting the patient's thinking, judgment, memory, and ability to reason.

denial: refusal to accept something as the truth; also, the first stage in the grieving process, in which the patient denies the terminal diagnosis.

dentures: artificial teeth.

dependable: trustworthy; able to be relied on.

dependent: unable to care for one's self.

depression: feelings of despair and discouragement; also, the fourth stage in the grieving process, in which the patient is trying to deal with the loss of everything he or she has.

developmental disability: a severe physical and/or mental impairment that is apparent before the age of 22 and is likely to continue indefinitely.

diabetes: a chronic disease caused by a disorder of carbohydrate metabolism.

diabetic diet: a diet calculated by the dietitian to meet the needs of a patient with diabetes mellitus; the diet limits free sugar and some other foods.

diagnosis: the term describing the patient's disease or condition; determination of what is wrong with the patient.

dialysis: a process of removing waste products from the blood in patients with kidney disease.

diarrhea: passage of loose, watery, liquid stools.

diastolic blood pressure: the last sound heard when taking the blood pressure; taken during the relaxation phase of the heartbeat.

dignity: honor or esteem.

dilate: to become larger.

direct contact: the spread of infection by touching.

disability: inability to function normally because of a physical or mental problem.

discharge: procedure for helping a patient to leave the health care agency.

discharge planner: a social worker who is responsible for helping the patient make the transition between the health care facility and the community.

disinfection: a cleaning process that destroys most microorganisms; a chemical is usually used to disinfect reusable items.

disorientation: lack of awareness of person, place, or time.

distal: situated farthest away from the center of the patient's body.

do-not-resuscitate (DNR) order: a physician order indicating that no CPR or life-sustaining measures will be performed.

drainage bag: a bag connected to a catheter to collect urine.

draw sheet: a small sheet placed horizontally across the center of the hospital bed.

droplet method of transmission: when germs are spread by secretions produced when laughing, talking, singing, sneezing, or coughing; these germs are large and usually do not spread more than three feet in the air.

durable power of attorney for health care: a document that designates another individual to make medical decisions on behalf of the patient.

dyspnea: difficulty breathing; labored respirations.

edema: swelling.

emesis basin: a kidney-shaped basin used for oral care procedures.

empathetic: being able to understand how someone else feels.

empathy: understanding how someone else feels.

EMS: Emergency Medical Services; usually an ambulance or fire department.

enabler: a device that empowers patients and allows them to function independently.

enema: introduction of fluid into the lower bowel.

entrance conference: a meeting between surveyors and facility administration to discuss the purpose of a survey; conducted at the beginning of a survey.

environmental services department: the housekeeping department; the department responsible for cleanliness and sanitation in most health care agencies. May also include maintenance.

evaluation: the determination of how the patient's plan of care is working.

eversion: turning a joint outward.

excretions: human waste products eliminated from the body.

exhalation (expiration): breathing air out of the lungs.

exit conference: a meeting between surveyors and facility administration upon completion of a survey to discuss the surveyors' findings and the nature of deficiencies.

expiration. *See* exhalation.

exposure control plan: a written program that the employer is required to have; describes what to do if an employee contacts blood or body fluids.

extended survey: a survey that lasts longer than originally anticipated so surveyors can examine patient care and facility practices in greater detail.

extension: straightening a joint.

external catheter. *See* condom catheter.

extracurricular activities: clubs, hobbies, volunteer work, and special interests.

extremity restraint: a safety device that encircles the arm or leg and prevents movement.

factual: known to be true.

Fahrenheit scale: a scale commonly used for measuring temperature.

false imprisonment: holding or restraining a patient against his or her will.

fats: food products, such as butter and oil, that are used for heat and energy production in the body.

fecal impaction: a large, hard, dry mass of stool that the patient is unable to pass.

fecal material. *See* feces.

feces (fecal material, stool, bowel movement): solid waste eliminated from the digestive system.

feedback: confirmation that a message was received as intended by the sender.

flammable: combustible; catches fire or burns readily.

flank: the area of the back immediately above the waist where the kidneys are located.

flatus: gas expelled from the digestive tract.

flexion: bending at a joint.

fluid restriction: limiting the total amount of fluid the patient can have in a 24-hour period.

food pyramid: a U.S. Department of Agriculture diagram that provides a guide to a well-balanced diet.

footboard: a piece of wood or plastic placed at the end of the hospital bed for positioning the patient's feet.

foot cradle: a metal or plastic frame suspended over the foot of the hospital bed to keep the weight of the linen off the patient's feet.

force: energy, strength, or power.

force fluids: an order to encourage the patient to drink as much liquid as possible.

foreskin: the loose tissue at the tip of the penis.

Fowler's position: a position that places the patient in a semi-sitting position in bed.

fractures: broken bones.

friction: rubbing, usually of the skin against bed linen.

full liquid diet: a diet, used for patients with digestive disorders, that includes clear and milk-based liquids.

functional incontinence: inability to control the passage of urine due to physical inability to get to the toilet.

gait belt (transfer belt): a heavy canvas belt used to assist the patient with ambulation.

gastrostomy: a surgical procedure in which a feeding tube is placed directly into the patient's stomach, with the end extending through the abdominal skin.

gatch handles: handles at the foot of a bed that raise and lower the head, knee, and height of the bed.

generalized: spread throughout the entire body.

generalized application: applied to the patient's entire body.

genital area: the area of the body where the external reproductive organs are located.

geriatrics: care of the elderly.

Good Samaritan laws: laws that protect health care workers who provide emergency care to injured persons outside the place of employment.

graduate: a measuring device with markings on the side.

grieving process: five steps that people go through when they anticipate or suffer a loss.

habit training: a type of bladder management program used for mentally confused patients who urinate at the same time every day.

hallucinating: seeing, hearing, or feeling something that is not real.

handrolls: props that are placed in the hands to prevent contractures.

head lice: human parasites that feed off blood; cannot be contracted from contact with pets or other animals.

Health Care Financing Administration (HCFA): a governmental agency that sets policy and administers payment of Medicare and Medicaid money to health care facilities.

health care proxy: an individual who has been legally designated to make medical decisions on behalf of the patient.

health maintenance organizations (HMOs): groups of health care providers and hospitals paid by insurance companies to care for patients for a monthly fee.

hemorrhage: excessive bleeding.

hepatitis B: an infection of the liver caused by a virus; can cause liver cancer and death.

hepatitis C: an infection of the liver caused by a virus; can be spread through contact with blood or body fluids.

high-efficiency particulate air (HEPA) filter mask: respirator used to protect employees working in rooms of patients who have diseases spread by air.

HIV disease: disease caused by the human immunodeficiency virus, which may progress to AIDS; spread by direct or indirect contact with blood and body fluids.

hospice: an organization that cares for dying patients.

hospice care: physical, psychological, and spiritual care provided to patients who have a limited life expectancy and their families.

hospitals: institutions that care for people with acute illnesses.

host (reservoir): the place where a disease-causing germ can grow.

HS care: routine care given at bedtime to prepare the patient for sleep.

humidifier: a device that adds moisture to the oxygen supply before the oxygen is delivered to the patient.

hygiene: personal cleanliness.

hyperalimentation (total parenteral nutrition (TPN)): a method of feeding a patient total nutrition intravenously, allowing the gastrointestinal system to rest.

hypertension: high blood pressure, usually 140/90 or above.

hypotension: low blood pressure, usually 100/60 or below.

identification band: a plastic bracelet, usually worn on the wrist or ankle, that contains the patient's name and other identifying information.

immobility: being motionless; the inability to move.

immobilize: to support an area in a way that prevents movement.

immune system: part of the circulatory system that recognizes invading germs and works to eliminate them from the body.

implementation: the process of carrying out a plan.

inactivity: being still, quiet, sedentary, or immobile.

incident: an occurrence or event that interrupts normal procedures or causes a crisis.

incident report: a special form that is completed for each accident or unusual occurrence in a health care facility; describes what happened and contains other important information.

incision: a cut in the skin made with a knife.

incontinence management program: a routine in which the patient is taken to the toilet at regular intervals.

incontinent: unable to control the bladder, bowel, or both.

independent: self-reliant, able to care for self.

indirect contact: touching objects, equipment, or dishes contaminated with harmful microorganisms.

indwelling catheter: a hollow tube inserted into the bladder to remove urine; remains in the body for a period of time.

infection: a state of sickness or disease caused by pathogens in the body.

infection control. *See* medical asepsis.

infusion site: the site where the intravenous needle is inserted into the body.

inhalation: breathing air into the lungs.

intake and output (I & O): an estimated measurement of all the liquid the patient takes in and all the fluid he or she loses in a 24-hour period.

interdisciplinary team: a group of caregivers who work together for the good of the patient, resident, or client.

intermittent: alternating or cyclic.

interview: a formal meeting in which the employer assesses the qualifications of an applicant and provides information about the job opening.

intravenous feeding (IV): administering sterile liquid and nutrients into a vein with a needle.

inversion: turning a joint inward.

involuntary seclusion: isolation of a patient as a form of punishment.

isolation: measures used when a patient has an infectious disease to prevent the spread of pathogens to others.

IV standard: a metal pole used to hang an IV bag, bottle, or pump above the infusion site.

jaundice: a yellow color of the skin caused by hepatitis and other liver diseases.

job objective: the section of your resume that lists the type of position you are seeking and states how your ability and skills qualify you for this position.

Joint Commission for Accreditation of Health Care Organizations (JCAHO): an organization that inspects and accredits health care agencies that meet high quality standards.

Kegel exercises: exercises used to make the muscles around the bladder stronger.

Kelly: a special clamp used to close tubes quickly.

kidneys: the organs that filter waste and remove it from the bloodstream.

labia majora: two large, hair-covered structures on the external female genitalia.

labia minora: two small, liplike structures inside the labia majora on the external female genitalia.

laboratory requisition: a document with identifying patient information that specifies the type of lab test to be performed on a specimen.

lateral position: lying on the left or right side.

leg drainage bag: a bag attached to a catheter to collect urine that is secured to the leg with an elastic or Velcro® strap.

lethargy: abnormal drowsiness or sleepiness.

level of consciousness: the degree of awareness or alertness, which ranges from fully awake and alert to confusion and unconsciousness.

libel: making false statements about another person in writing.

lice: parasites that feed on animals and humans.

license: a state permit allowing the health care facility to operate.

licensed vocational nurse (LVN): same as a licensed practical nurse.

licensed practical nurse (LPN): a nurse who has completed one to two years of nursing school and passed a state licensing examination.

living will: a document that specifies the patient's wishes in the event that the patient is in a terminal condition.

localized: confined to a specific area of the body.

localized application: applied to a specific area of a patient's body.

lockout: placing a locking tag on a broken piece of equipment so it cannot be used.

long-term care facilities: health care institutions that care for residents with chronic diseases and personal care needs.

low-cholesterol diet: a diet that is low in fat and cholesterol for patients with heart, blood vessel, liver, and/or gallbladder disease.

low-fat diet: a diet that is low in fat for patients with heart, blood vessel, liver, and/or gallbladder disease.

malpractice: negligence that results in harm to the patient.

Maslow's hierarchy of needs: a chart based on a widely accepted theory of physical and psychological needs of all human beings.

Material Safety Data Sheets (MSDS): information sheets on chemicals used in the workplace that list the health hazards, safe uses, and emergency procedures for chemical exposure.

mechanically altered diet: a diet that is changed in texture to meet the needs of patients with chewing, swallowing, or digestive problems.

mechanical soft diet: a diet that is finely ground or chopped for patients with chewing or swallowing problems.

Medicaid: a program funded by the state and federal governments that pays for health care for individuals with a low income.

medical asepsis (infection control): practices used in health care facilities to prevent the spread of infection.

medical record: written documentation of the patient's true condition and a record of progress and care.

Medicare: a program administered by the federal government that helps the elderly and disabled pay for care in the hospital, long-term care facility, and home health care settings.

mentally retarded: a person with lower than average intellectual development ranging from mild to severe.

message: the information the sender wants to communicate.

methicillin-resistant *staphylococcus aureus* (MRSA): a common pathogen in health care facilities that causes illness or infection; resists treatment with most antibiotics.

microorganism (microbe): living germ that cannot be seen with the eye.

micturition. *See* urination.

midstream specimen. *See* clean-catch specimen.

milliliter: a metric unit of measure used in health care facilities; 30 mL equals one ounce. One milliliter is the same as one cubic centimeter.

minerals: inorganic compounds in food used to build body tissues.

mite: a tiny parasite that cannot be seen with the eye.

miter: tuck a sheet in by forming a 45-degree angle perpendicular to the mattress.

mixed incontinence: a combination of urge and stress incontinence.

mobility: the ability to move about.

morning care: routine care that is given after breakfast.

mucous membranes: tissues of the body that secrete mucus; these areas open to the outside of the body.

myths: common beliefs that are not true.

N95 respirator: a mask with very small pores that may be worn when caring for patients in airborne precautions.

nasogastric tube: a tube inserted into the nose and threaded through the esophagus into the stomach; can be used for feeding or medical procedures.

negative-pressure environment: a description of the ventilation system used in an airborne precautions room; the room air is drawn upward into the ventilation system and is either specially filtered or exhausted directly to the outside of the building.

neglect: failing to provide services to patients to prevent physical harm or mental anguish.

negligence: failing to provide services to a patient in the same manner as a reasonably prudent person would do.

networking: communicating with people you know who have similar careers, goals, and interests.

nits: the eggs left by lice; if untreated, the eggs will hatch into more lice.

nonintact skin: skin that is broken, chapped, or cracked.

normal flora: microorganisms that are healthful and necessary for the body to function correctly; they are not harmful in the area in which they reside, but can cause infection if spread to other parts of the body.

nosocomial infection: an infection acquired by a patient while in a health care facility.

NPO: nothing by mouth.

nursing process: the four-step process of assessment, planning, implementation, and evaluation of the patient and care provided to meet the patient's needs.

nutrients: chemical substances in food that are necessary for life.

objective observations: factual observations that you make by seeing, hearing, feeling, touching, and smelling.

OBRA (Omnibus Budget Reconciliation Act): legislation that made sweeping reforms of the long-term care industry and describes requirements for nursing assistant training.

obstructed airway: food or a foreign body blocking the trachea or windpipe, making it impossible to breathe.

Occupational Safety and Health Administration (OSHA): a government agency responsible for developing and enforcing job safety and health standards to protect employees.

occupied bed: a bed with a patient in it.

oral temperature: the temperature taken by placing the thermometer in the mouth.

orthotic (orthosis): a device that restores or improves function and prevents deformity.

osteoporosis: a decrease in bone mass that leads to fractures with minimal trauma.

ostomy: a surgically created opening into the body.

overbed table: a narrow table on wheels used to hold the patient's water, meal trays, and clean items.

overflow incontinence: the escape of urine that occurs when the bladder is very full and can hold no more urine.

paralyzed: absence of movement and sensation due to an illness or injury.

paraphrasing: a method of restating the message communicated to you in clear, simple terms.

parasites: tiny animals that survive by feeding off humans or other animals.

partial bath: washing the face, hands, underarms, back, and genital area.

passive range of motion: joint exercises performed on the patient by the care provider.

pathogen: a microorganism that causes disease.

patients: persons who are cared for in a hospital.

Patient's Bill of Rights: a list of the rights of patients in hospitals, published by the American Hospital Association.

penis: the external male organ used for sex and elimination.

perineal care (peri-care): washing the genital and anal areas of the body.

perineum: the area between the anus and vagina in the female; the area between the anus and scrotum in the male.

peripherally inserted central catheter (PICC): an intravenous line inserted in the arm and threaded through the venous system to the superior vena cava; used for long-term intravenous therapy and TPN.

peristalsis: muscular contractions of the digestive tract that move food and waste products through the intestines.

perseveration: repetitious behavior, movements, or actions.

personal data: the section of your resume that lists your name, address, telephone number, and professional license or certification number.

personal protective equipment (PPE): equipment worn to protect the health care worker and the patient from contact with disease-causing pathogens; also called barrier equipment.

personal space: a comfortable distance in which to communicate with others.

PFR95 respirator: a mask with very small pores that may be worn when caring for patients in airborne precautions.

physical restraint: physical, manual, or mechanical device attached or adjacent to the patient's body that the patient cannot remove easily; prevents access to the body.

planning: deciding what to do with information gathered in an assessment.

plan of correction: a written plan submitted by the health care agency in response to survey findings of deficiency; lists what corrections will be made, by whom, who will monitor the correction, and what will be done to prevent similar deficiencies in the future.

popliteal artery: the artery behind the knee in which the pulse can be felt.

portal of entry: the place where a pathogen enters the body.

postmortem care: physical care of the body after death.

postoperative care: care given to patients after surgical procedures.

postural support: a device that maintains good body alignment and posture.

preferred provider organization (PPO): listed physicians and health care agencies that contract with insurance companies to provide health care to insurance company subscribers.

prefix: the word element at the beginning of a word.

pressure sore: an ulcer that forms on the skin over a bony prominence as the result of pressure.

pressure ulcer. *See* pressure sore.

priorities: things that are very important that must be taken care of first.

privacy: separation from others; alone; personal.

probe: the attachment on an electronic thermometer that senses temperature.

probe cover: the plastic, disposable cover used on the thermometer probe when taking a patient's temperature.

professional: a skilled practitioner who is capable, competent, and efficient.

prognosis: a prediction of the course or outcome of a disease.

projection: placing the blame for an illness or situation on someone or something else.

prompted voiding: a bladder management program used for patients who know that the bladder is full, but do not communicate the need to use the toilet.

pronation: moving a joint to face downward.

prone position: lying on the abdomen with the head turned to one side.

prostate: a gland surrounding the urethra in the male patient.

prosthesis: an artificial body part.

prosthetic: a device that takes the place of a body part.

protective isolation. *See* reverse isolation.

protein: a nutrient in food that builds and repairs tissues.

pulse: the expansion and contraction of an artery, which can be felt on the outside surface of the body.

pulse points: locations on the body where the pulse can be felt.

pulse pressure: the difference between the systolic and diastolic blood pressure.

pulse rate: the number of pulse beats per minute.

pureed diet: a diet blenderized to a smooth consistency.

quality assurance: internal review made by facility staff to identify problems and find solutions for improvement.

RACE System: the steps to be followed in case of fire.

radial pulse: the pulse felt on the thumb side of the wrist.

range of motion: normal joint movements.

rationalization: providing an acceptable but untrue reason for the illness or behavior.

receiver: the person for whom a message is intended.

rectal temperature: the temperature taken by inserting the thermometer into the anus.

references: individuals who know you and who will recommend you to the prospective employer for the job you are seeking.

reflexes: unconscious or involuntary movements.

reflex incontinence: a loss of urine that occurs without awareness in patients who are paralyzed or have other neurologic problems.

registered nurse (RN): a nurse who has completed two to four years of nursing school and has passed a state licensing examination.

regular diet: a normal diet based on the six food groups in the food pyramid.

rehabilitation: program(s) designed by a therapist to help patients regain lost skills or teach new skills.

reimburse: to repay an institution for the cost of services provided.

reservoir. *See* host.

residents: persons who are cared for in a long-term care facility.

Resident's Bill of Rights: a legal document listing the rights of residents in long-term care facilities.

resolved: through, over, completed.

respiration: the act of breathing in and out.

responsible behavior: behavior that is dependable and trustworthy.

restoration: basic nursing care measures designed to maintain or improve a patient's function and assist the patient to return to self-care.

restorative care: nursing care designed to assist the patient to attain and maintain the highest level of function possible.

restorative environment: an environment that has been modified so the patient can function as independently as possible.

restraint: a device attached or adjacent to the patient's body that the patient cannot remove easily; prevents access to the body.

resume: a summary of your professional or work experience and qualifications.

retention enema: introduction of fluid into the lower bowel to soften, lubricate, and remove solid waste.

reverse chronological order: the order in which your previous jobs are listed on your resume, beginning with most recent job first.

reverse isolation (protective isolation): used in some health care facilities to protect patients with weakened immune systems from contacting pathogens in the environment.

rhythm: a recurring action or movement.

rigor mortis: a condition that occurs two to four hours after death in which the muscles and limbs become stiff.

risk factors: conditions that have the potential to cause the patient, resident, or client's health to worsen; conditions that indicate a problem may develop.

root: the element that gives meaning to a medical word.

rotation: moving a joint in, out, and around.

scabies: a skin condition caused by a mite; causes a rash and severe itching and is highly contagious.

scheduled toileting: a bladder management program used for patients who cannot use the bathroom without physical help; the patient is taken to the bathroom on a fixed schedule developed by the nurse.

secretions: drainage, discharge, or seeping from the body.

seizure: a convulsion or condition characterized by severe shaking and jerking of the body.

self-actualization: the realization of one's full potential.

self-esteem: how a person feels about himself or herself.

semiprone position: a modified prone position in which the body is supported on pillows to relieve pressure from most of the bony prominences.

semisupine (tilt) position: a modified side lying position in which the body is supported on pillows to relieve pressure from most of the bony prominences.

sender: the person who originates communication.

sensory losses: difficulty seeing, hearing, smelling, or touching.

sepsis: systemic poisoning of the body caused by bacteria; a serious infection.

sexual abuse: forcing a patient to perform a sexual act.

shearing: skin damage caused by stretching of a patient's skin between the bone inside and the sheet outside.

shock: the result of blood loss that causes inadequate blood flow to the vital organs.

shroud: a cloth, paper, or plastic covering used to wrap the body after death.

shunt: a passage between two blood vessels, commonly under the forearm skin in patients who are receiving hemodialysis.

sign: observations about the patient that can be observed by others.

Sims' position: a side-lying position in which the patient is placed on the left side with the right leg flexed and bent; used for rectal examinations and treatments.

slander: making false statements about another person.

sodium-restricted diet: a diet prepared with no or limited sodium.

soft (bland) diet: a diet containing foods that are low in residue, with limited or no seasoning.

source: a pathogen that causes disease.

sphygmomanometer: instrument used to measure blood pressure.

splints: devices used to maintain position of an extremity or joint.

standard precautions: measures that health care workers use to prevent the spread of infection to themselves and others.

standards of care: common health care practices based on current information about health care and facility policies.

stereotyping: fixed images or beliefs that categorize an individual or group.

sterile: free from all microbes.

sterilization: processes used to kill all microorganisms.

stethoscope: instrument used to listen to sounds inside the body.

stoma: the opening of an ostomy to the outside of the body.

stool. *See* feces.

strains: injuries to muscles from stretching or overuse.

stress: physical or emotional strain and tension.

stress incontinence: inability to control the passage of urine due to muscular weakness.

strict I & O: an accurate measurement of all the liquid the patient takes in and loses in a 24-hour period.

stump sock: a stocking that is placed over an amputated extremity before the prosthesis is applied.

subacute: a level of care in which the patient has complex care needs but is not critically ill.

subjective observations: observations based on what you think or what the patient tells you; may or may not be factual.

suffix: the word element at the end of a word.

sundowning: increased restlessness and confusion in the late afternoon, evening, and night.

supination: moving a joint to face upward.

supine position: lying on the back; face up.

supplemental feedings: nourishments given to the patient in addition to meals to meet special nutritional needs.

suprapubic catheter: a hollow tube surgically inserted into the bladder through the abdomen.

survey: a review and evaluation of a health care facility to ensure that the agency is maintaining acceptable standards.

surveyor: a representative of a private or governmental agency who reviews health care facility policies, procedures, and practices for quality of care.

susceptibility: the ability of the body to resist disease.

symptom: something the patient reports about his or her condition.

syncope: fainting.

systolic blood pressure: the first sound heard when taking the blood pressure; taken during the contraction phase of the heartbeat.

tachycardia: rapid pulse rate, usually over 100 beats per minute.

tactful: considerate, polite, and thoughtful.

tagout: placing a tag on a piece of broken equipment that warns not to use the equipment until it is repaired.

task analysis: analyzing the steps of a procedure and determining which steps the patient can complete independently.

temperature: measurement of heat within the body.

tepid: lukewarm.

terminal illness: an illness for which there is no cure.

therapeutic diet: a special or modified diet prepared to treat a patient's individual nutritional needs.

thermometer: instrument used to measure temperature.

tilt position. *See* semisupine position.

tornado watch: a state of alert suggesting that conditions are right for a tornado to develop.

tornado warning: a state of alert that occurs when a tornado is in the area.

total parenteral nutrition (TPN). *See* hyperalimentation.

transfer: moving the patient from one place, unit, or facility to another.

transfer belt. *See* gait belt.

transmission: the way in which a germ is spread.

transport bag: a sealed plastic bag labeled with a biohazard emblem, used to contain laboratory specimens during transport.

tremor: involuntary shaking.

tuberculosis (TB): a contagious disease spread by airborne contact; commonly affects the lungs, but can cause illness in other parts of the body.

tympanic temperature. *See* aural temperature.

tympanic thermometer: instrument used to measure temperature inside the ear.

unit: the patient's personal space, which may include a bed, chair, overbed table, nightstand, dresser, wastebasket, and closet.

universal choking sign: one or both hands on the throat.

ureters: two hollow tubes leading from the kidneys to the bladder.

urethra: the hollow tube leading from the bladder to the outside of the body.

urge incontinence: inability to control the passage of urine when the need to urinate is very strong and sudden, preventing the patient from getting to the toilet on time.

urinal: a container used for urinary elimination by the male patient.

urinary meatus: the external opening to the urethra where urine leaves the body.

urinary retention: inability to empty the bladder completely.

urination (voiding, micturition): the act of passing liquid waste to the outside of the body.

vancomycin-resistant *enterococcus* **(VRE)**: a drug-resistant pathogen seen in health care facilities that commonly causes infections.

vector: an insect, rodent, or small animal that spreads disease.

vehicle: food, water, or other items in or on which pathogens can live and multiply.

ventilator: a device used to assist or control breathing.

vest restraint: a safety device applied to the patient's upper body to limit movement and prevent rising.

viruses: tiny pathogens that cause disease; antibiotics will not eliminate them.

vital signs: temperature, pulse, respiration, and blood pressure.

vitamins: organic substances in food that are necessary for normal body function.

voiding. *See* urination.

INDEX

Note: Page numbers ending with "f" refer to a figure on the cited page.